Radiology of Non-Spinal Pain

Mubin I. Syed
Azim Shaikh

Radiology of Non-Spinal Pain Procedures

A Guide for the Interventionalist

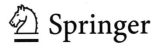

Springer

Mubin I. Syed, MD, FSIR, FACR
Dayton Interventional Radiology
3075 Governors Place Blvd.
Suite 120, Dayton, OH 45409
USA
mubinsyed@aol.com

Azim Shaikh, MD, MBA
3049 Westminster Drive
Unit 208, Beavercreek, OH 45431
USA
azimmail@yahoo.com

ISBN 978-3-642-00480-3   e-ISBN 978-3-642-00481-0
DOI 10.1007/978-3-642-00481-0
Springer Heidelberg Dordrecht London New York

Library of Congress Control Number: 2010933083

Cover design: eStudio Calamar, Figueres/Berlin

Printed on acid-free paper

Springer is part of Springer Science+Business Media (www.springer.com)

Acknowledgements

We appreciate the special assistance of Talal Akhter, Judy Crable, and Robin Osborn, DO. We also would like to acknowledge our families for their patience and support. A special thanks to Dr. Mubin Syed's wife, Afshan Syed and father, Ibrahim Syed.

Contents

Introduction to Radiology

Understanding radiology has always been integral to any interventional procedure. With advances in technology and its applications the breadth and depth of imaging has dramatically increased over the past few years. Therefore, it behooves the interventionalist to have a basic awareness of the various imaging modalities including their strengths and weaknesses, as well as the underlying radiological anatomy, especially in cross section. This knowledge can be helpful in understanding the imaging of the indications for a given procedure, choosing a guidance modality, and for evaluation of the patient who has had a possible complication.

1.1 Plain Film Radiographs and Fluoroscopy

This is the most common and usually the initial type of imaging performed. It is helpful to have more than one view of a particular object. These are generated by X-rays directly creating an image based on the various densities of the underlying structures that the X-rays have passed through. There are five basic densities:

- Air – black on radiography
- Fat – black on radiography
- Bone – white on radiography
- Metal – bright white on radiography
- Soft tissues and water – spectrum of gray on radiography

Contrast can be used for angiography, arthrography, genitourinary, and for alimentary tract imaging. Fluoroscopy is continuous or real-time imaging using X-ray radiography. Its strengths include that it is fast, readily available, is able to perform complex angulations, and that the imaging is in real time. Weaknesses include limited tissue contrast, inability to directly visualize targeted soft-tissue structures, radiation exposure and potential allergic reactions when iodinated contrast is used.

1.2 Computed Tomography

Computed tomography (CT) is widely available in almost all hospitals. It is rapidly performed, has a large field of view, and is not operator dependent. It uses X-rays detectors to generate values called a Hounsfield unit corresponding to shades of gray, black or white. This is then used to create a cross-sectional image through a computer algorithm. Iodinated contrast can be utilized to detect enhancement and thereby improving the diagnostic sensitivity of CT. Two- (2D) and three-dimensional (3D) reconstruction is now available on many modern spiral CT scanners. Its strengths include the following: fast, less motion-sensitive compared to MRI; readily available; cross-sectional capability with better soft-tissue contrast than plain films or fluoroscopy; allows one to visualize vessels and sometimes nerves, enhancing the safety of some image guided procedures; it is helpful in situations with anatomic variation (i.e., pathology) or obese patients for guidance.

However, it has the following weaknesses: it is more expensive than plain films or ultrasound; the radiation dose is higher than plain films; there is a potential for allergic reactions if using iodinated contrast; it is slower than fluoroscopy when used for image guidance; multiple needle insertions and repositionings may be required resulting in longer procedure times; complex angulation is not available for image guidance.

M.I. Syed and A. Shaikh, *Radiology of Non-Spinal Pain Procedures*,
DOI: 10.1007/978-3-642-00481-0_1, © Springer-Verlag Berlin Heidelberg 2011

1.3 Magnetic Resonance Imaging

Magnetic resonance imaging (MRI) is widely available in most hospitals and in many outpatient imaging centers. It has excellent soft-tissue contrast, multiplanar imaging, but is more expensive and has long scan times (issues with patient claustrophobia and motion artifact). Images are formed by exposing the patient to a strong magnetic field while radio waves are transmitted into the patient. The hydrogen protons absorb the energy of the radio waves and resonate to varying degrees. Once the radio wave energy is discontinued the hydrogen protons relax. The radio waves that are generated by this relaxation or decay are detected by a receiver coil. The number and location of the protons can thus be detected by assigning digital values to this information. A cross-sectional image is thus created.

T1-weighted images are obtained receiving the information early during the proton relaxation process when fat gives a white signal, water a dark signal. Anatomic resolution is better than T2-weighted imaging.

T2-weighted images are obtained late during the proton relaxation process when water and fat give a bright signal. This gives better contrast than T1-weighted images and is excellent for identifying pathology.

Proton density or spin density weighted images are intermediate between T1 and T2 weighted images. It is useful in musculoskeletal imaging due to its ability to distinguish between marrow, hyaline cartilage, fibrocartilage (present within menisci) and yet still identify fluid.

Gadolinium contrast demonstrates enhancement on T1-weighted images to identify pathology. The contrast is of much lower volume and has a better safety profile than the iodinated contrast used in CT.

Fat saturation or suppression is routinely used in T2-weighted or proton density-weighted images as well as T1-weighted images post gadolinium enhancement to remove fat signal. This is done to improve the sensitivity of the study to underlying pathology. Both fat and pathology are bright after enhancement or on T2-weighted or proton density-weighted imaging. Therefore, the bright fat signal is subtracted out to better reveal the underlying pathology. Short tau inversion recovery (STIR) is another commonly used technique to remove fat signal.

Magnetic resonance angiography (MRA) may be useful for imaging vessels.

MRI's strengths include: highest soft-tissue contrast of any imaging modality; multiplanar imaging is readily available; no ionizing radiation is used; infinite obliquities are available for guidance if MR guidance is available. Its weaknesses include: more expensive than CT; long imaging times; less available for guidance; limited to use in patients with ferromagnetic cerebral aneurysm clipping, implanted electrical devices (pacemakers, ICDs, spinal cord stimulators), metal foreign bodies in and around the eyes, and recent coronary stenting.

1.4 Ultrasound

Ultrasound is widely available in almost all hospitals. It is relatively inexpensive compared to CT or MRI. In addition, real time imaging is possible. It uses high frequency sound waves transmitted into a patient by a transducer, which are then reflected back and detected intermittently by the same transducer. The information is converted into digital data and processed by a computer to generate a cross-sectional ultrasound image.

Sound waves can be deflected, reflected, or absorbed in a given structure when there is a difference in acoustic impedance (amount of sound energy that can be transmitted) between two adjacent differing structures. Sound waves that are reflected back to the transducer are utilized for image formation where water is anechoic (dark), soft-tissue organs are echoic (gray), margins between adjacent structures are hyperechoic (white) and air is very bright (white), which may not allow use of ultrasound to image. Doppler ultrasound imaging allows one to identify and characterize vascular structures in the field of view.

The major strengths of ultrasound imaging include the following: less expensive than CT or MRI; easily available; no radiation exposure; real-time imaging capability; allows direct visualization of blood vessels and nerves that enhances the safety for guidance; allows complex angulation and multiplanar imaging; portable; expanding role in musculoskeletal application, complimentary to MRI in tendon and nerve evaluations. However, it also has the following weaknesses: operator dependency; requires high technical skill; small field of view; limited in evaluating thorax and bones; limited use in obese patients.

1.5 Nuclear Medicine

Nuclear medicine is widely available in almost all hospitals; however, it has limited applications in the context of pain interventions. It uses an intravenously injected or orally ingested radiopharmaceutical which is then distributed throughout the body based on its uptake (usually metabolically based). Uptake appears as a relative increase or decrease depending on the type of pathology. Nuclear medicine's strength is its sensitivity in evaluating physiology such as inflammatory processes. Its weakness is its lack of anatomic definition and its lack of specificity. Often it must be combined with other modalities to be clinically relevant.

1.6 Book Overview

The purpose of this book is to introduce the interventionalist to the possible applications of radiology both for guidance and diagnoses of indications/contraindications and complications. An introduction to relevant cross-sectional anatomy for each procedure is included, as well as a subsection on anatomic structures to be avoided during a given image-guided procedure.

The chapter is divided into sections of interventions: head and neck, thorax, abdomen, pelvis, and upper and lower extremities.

In the extremity section, however, cross-sectional anatomy was not emphasized since most of the relevant structures are relatively superficial. Clinical presentation was included for a given procedure only if it was usually performed for a clinical pain syndrome and not if the procedure was performed for regional anesthesia.

Contraindications are not specifically listed for every procedure because it is understood that infection and coagulopathy is a contraindication for every procedure and that infection can be imaged radiologically at every location of the site of injection. On the other hand, coagulopathy is not an entity that can be imaged radiologically.

Complications are specifically listed for each procedure only if they are specific to a particular procedure. Complications that can occur for any procedure include: bleeding/hematoma; infection; ischemia/infarction (which can be caused by intravascular injection, vessel thrombosis, embolus, dissection, and spasm); local anesthetic toxicity/allergy; disulfiram reaction (if alcohol is used); nerve damage/neuritis (pain, hypoesthesia, dysesthesia, abnormal sensory or motor function, etc.); reactivation of herpes zoster; tendon rupture if tendon is directly injected; sloughing of skin or mucosa.

** Signifies that the entity may be imaged. It is understood that an entity may represent a clinical syndrome but that its underlying pathology may actually be imaged [cervical radiculopathy** may be imaged via imaging of cervical spondylosis or disc herniation (herniated nucleus pulposus/HNP)]

Disclaimer: This book is not intended to be a procedural manual on how to perform the injection. The book is not intended to entail any type of clinical decision-making process involved in deciding when to perform the injection. In fact, it is often inappropriate to perform the injection but rather preferable to refer the patient for definitive treatment surgically. In addition, conservative measures (rest, anti-inflammatory medications (NSAIDs), physical therapy, ergonomic adjustments, etc.) should be instituted before injections are attempted. Furthermore, it is not a manual on how to perform the diagnostic workup. Many of these diagnoses are made on the basis of patient history and physical examination, and radiology is in fact not necessary. Radiology may only be necessary to confirm the diagnosis if the patient does not respond to initial treatment. Moreover, radiology may not necessarily comprise a first-line diagnostic modality. For instance, EMG or arthroscopy may be better suited as an initial technique in confirming or excluding pathology.

Below we examine the strengths and weaknesses of the various imaging modalities used for diagnosis in the head and neck.

CT (American College of Radiology) is sensitive for benign and malignant paranasal sinus pathology. It is also excellent for lymphadenopathy and evaluating bone invasion from malignancy. It has proven to be superior for the work-up of distant metastasis. CTA should be used for carotid and vertebral dissection, while PET/CT is the most sensitive in the work-up for cancer.

MRI (American College of Radiology) demonstrates superior soft tissue contrast in the head and neck while capable of distinguishing between neoplastic, inflammatory, and obstructive processes in nasal cavity tumors. It is sensitive for trigeminal neuralgia (neurovascular compression for cranial nerve V root entry zone). The migraine phenomenon may be demonstrated in the brain. It is more sensitive for infection than CT, including herpes zoster ophthalmicus. Moreover, it is superior to CT in evaluating the tongue/oral cavity, palate and intracranial extension from the skull base, as well as for detecting malignant perineural and intracranial invasion. MRA can demonstrate carotid and vertebral artery dissection (mimics cluster headache).

Angiography is useful in the evaluation of carotid and vertebral dissection if CTA or MRA is inconclusive. Pseudoaneurysm can be detected as a complication.

PET (American head and Neck Society; Coleman): PET/CT is used for the work-up of suspected malignancy with negative CT or MRI. FDG identifies a primary cancer in 20–40% of patients who present with metastatic disease in the neck with an unknown primary tumor. PET and CT have similar accuracy in the initial staging of nodal disease. PET is more accurate

than CT or MRI in detecting recurrent tumor (study of choice for follow-up). It is sensitive for staging neck cancer, unknown primary, distant metastasis, and response to therapy. However, it is limited by tumor size to less than 3–4 mm. Moreover, it may provide false positive results in inflammation, muscular activity, and healing bone. A thorough understanding of artifacts is required.

Ultrasound is useful in characterizing palpable masses (thyroglossal duct cysts, branchial cysts, cystic hygromas, salivary gland tumors, abscesses, carotid body tumors, vascular tumors, and thyroid masses). It is also capable of characterizing vascularity in real-time and in duplex mode.

2.1 Sphenopalatine Nerve Block

2.1.1 Anatomy

The sphenopalatine ganglion is the largest collection of neurons exterior to the cranium in the head. The ganglion is positioned within the pterygopalatine fossa. It has a complex of nerves attaching to it (Fig. 2.1). The ganglion hangs from V2 via the pterygopalatine nerves. The vidian nerves (composed of greater and lesser petrosal nerves) project posteriorly, which travel through the pterygoid canal. The vidian nerve contains sympathetic fibers from the superior cervical ganglion, which pass through the sphenopalatine ganglion into the lacrimal gland and nasal/palatine mucosa.

The greater and lesser palatine nerves extend inferiorly from the ganglion. The superior posterior lateral nasal and pharyngeal nerves also emanate from the ganglion.

M.I. Syed and A. Shaikh, *Radiology of Non-Spinal Pain Procedures*,
DOI: 10.1007/978-3-642-00481-0_2, © Springer-Verlag Berlin Heidelberg 2011

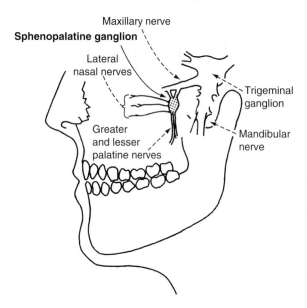

Fig. 2.1 Anatomy of the sphenopalatine ganglion and its immediate connections (Raj et al.)

The parasympathetic innervation arises in the superior salivatory nucleus. It then courses through the facial nerve to constitute the greater petrosal nerve. The greater petrosal nerve combines with the deep petrosal nerve to become the vidian nerve. The vidian nerve terminates in the sphenopalatine ganglion and then post ganglionic fibers supply nasal mucosa and V2 on route to the lacrimal gland.

The pterygopalatine fossa is a small cavity through which many important structures are associated. V2 travels through the foramen rotundum which is located at the upper, medial, and posterior portion of the fossa. The vidian nerve courses through the pterygoid canal at the lower lateral and posterior portion of the fossa. The maxillary artery is contained within the fossa.

The ganglion is separated from the nasal cavity by a thin layer of lateral nasal mucosa at the posterior aspect of the middle turbinate (sphenopalatine foramen). The ganglion communicates to the oral cavity via the greater palatine canal, which contains the greater and lesser palatine nerves. The ganglion communicates to the cranial cavity through the pterygoid canal, foramen rotundum, and foramen lacerum.

The roof of the pterygopalatine fossa is the sphenoid sinus, the outer border is the infratemporal fossa,

the inner border is the palatine bone, and the anterior border is the maxillary sinus.

2.1.1.1 Function

It is a parasympathetic terminal ganglion. Preganglionic parasympathetic fibers from the greater petrosal nerve (of the facial nerve CNVII) via the vidian nerve synapse at the ganglion. Postganglionic sympathetic axons arrive via the vidian nerve from the deep petrosal nerve and pass through the ganglion without synapsing.

The postganglionic parasympathetic axons exit via the greater and lesser palatine nerves, nasopalatine nerve, sphenopalatine nerves, and zygomatic nerves.

It provides secretomotor innervation to the mucous glands of the palate, nasal cavity, lacrimal gland, and the mucosa of the nasopharynx posterior to the auditory tube.

2.1.1.2 Injection Site

There are various approaches that are used including: a lateral approach (discussed below only) including suprazygomatic and infrazygomatic arch approach, intranasal topical application to the back of the nasal pharynx along the middle turbinate, and the greater palatine foramen approach.

2.1.2 Cross-Sectional Anatomy: Lateral Approach

2.1.2.1 What Does the Needle Traverse?

The needle traverses the structures within the infratemporal fossa (infrazygomatic masticator space) prior to entering the pterygopalatine fossa as its final destination (applies to the infrazygomatic approach). The path is just superior to the coronoid process of the mandible. Alternatively, a transnasal or transoral approach (using the pterygopalatine canal to enter the sphenopalatine foramen) can be used. The structures traversed within the infratemporal fossa (within the infrazygomatic masticator space) include (Figs. 2.5–2.6):

- Superficial layer of the deep cervical fascia
- Masseter muscle
- Temporalis muscle/tendon
- Lateral pterygoid muscle
- Pterygoid venous plexus (Harnsberger et al. 2006a)
  - Located both medial and lateral to the lateral pterygoid [http://www.emory.edu/ANATOMY/ Anatomy Manual/fossae.html]
- Retromaxillary fat pad (Buccal space)
- Internal maxillary artery (Harnsberger et al. 2006b)
  - Travels anteromedially within the masticator space lateral to the pterygoid muscle to end up within the pterygopalatine fossa
- Pterygopalatine fossa (Harnsberger et al. 2006c)
  - Communicates with the masticator space via the pterygomaxillary fissure between the maxilla and lateral pterygoid plate

2.1.2.2 Which Structures the Needle Should Avoid

Pterygoid venous plexus: This is a prominent venous plexus medial and lateral to the surface of the lateral pterygoid muscle. It may be difficult to avoid; however, it is a venous structure and therefore under low pressure for potential hematoma formation.

Maxillary artery: The artery travels from its origin within the parotid gland through the masticator space anteromedially on the lateral aspect of the lateral pterygoid (usually) to terminate in the pterygomaxillary fissure as the sphenopalatine artery. It may be difficult to purposefully avoid puncture unless a blunt-tipped needle is used in the infrazygomatic approach.

Inferior orbital fissure: If the needle is advanced too far the orbital structures including the globe can be punctured.

2.1.2.3 Imaging/Radiology

CT and fluoroscopic approaches can be combined (Vallejo et al. 2007) (Figs. 2.2–2.6).

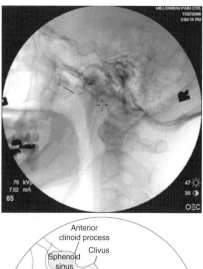

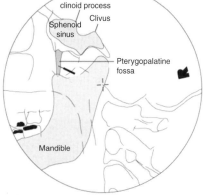

Fig. 2.2 Lateral fluoroscopic view, with the mandibles aligned, the pterygopalatine fossa is seen as an "inverted vase," with the needle inside

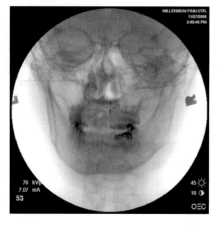

Fig. 2.3 AP fluoroscopic view with the tip of the needle at the lateral wall of the nose

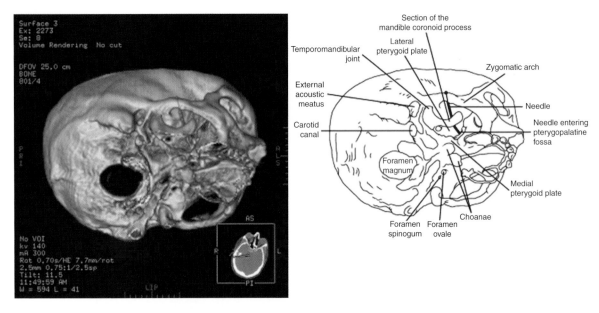

Fig. 2.4 Reconstructed CT image showing the needle inside the pterygopalatine fossa (Vallejo et al. 2007)

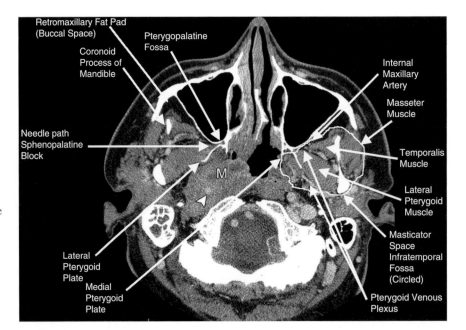

Fig. 2.5 CT at the level of the needle tract for a sphenopalatine block. Needle path is delineated and pertinent anatomic structures are labeled. A mass (*M*) is noted within the right pharyngeal mucosal space encasing the internal carotid artery (*arrowhead*) (Gupta et al. 2007a)

2.1.3 Indications

The following are common indications for intervention in the head and neck:

- Sphenopalatine neuralgia – Sluder's (sphenopalatine) neuralgia is pain of the eyes and nose, with radiation to the ear. The greater superficial petrosal nerve (GSPN) is most likely the pathway along

which this pain radiates to the ear. It is crucial to exclude benign and malignant sinus disease before making the diagnosis of (idiopathic) sphenopalatine neuralgia (Weissman 1997).

- Paranasal sinus infection** – Causing irritation of the sphenopalatine ganglia (SPG) – disputed.
- Intranasal deformities** – deviated septum, septal spurs and prominent turbinates.
- Vasomotor syndrome.

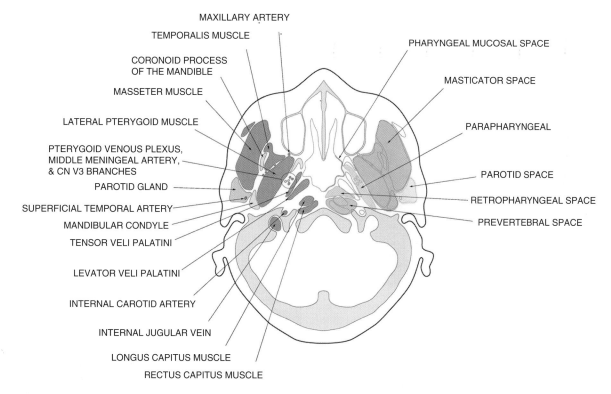

MAXILLARY ARTERY

TEMPORALIS MUSCLE

CORONOID PROCESS
OF THE MANDIBLE

MASSETER MUSCLE

LATERAL PTERYGOID MUSCLE

PTERYGOID VENOUS PLEXUS,
MIDDLE MENINGEAL ARTERY,
& CN V3 BRANCHES

PAROTID GLAND

SUPERFICIAL TEMPORAL ARTERY

MANDIBULAR CONDYLE

TENSOR VELI PALATINI

LEVATOR VELI PALATINI

INTERNAL CAROTID ARTERY

INTERNAL JUGULAR VEIN

LONGUS CAPITUS MUSCLE

RECTUS CAPITUS MUSCLE

PHARYNGEAL MUCOSAL SPACE

MASTICATOR SPACE

PARAPHARYNGEAL

PAROTID SPACE

RETROPHARYNGEAL SPACE

PREVERTEBRAL SPACE

Fig. 2.6 Axial cross-sectional anatomy at the level of the upper maxillary antrum. Anatomic structures are shown on the *left side* of the diagram; spaces are shown on the *right side*. *CN* cranial nerve (Gupta et al. 2007a)

- Trigeminal neuralgia.**
- Head and neck cancer** – cancer of the tongue and floor of the mouth (intranasal approach) (Varghese et al. 2002).
- Lethal midline granuloma** (intranasal approach) (Saade and Paige 1996).
- Migraine** (Fig. 2.7) and cluster headaches – imaging is useful in excluding structural lesions that can mimic cluster headache (i.e., herpes zoster, sinusitis, subarachnoid hemorrhage, trigeminal neuralgia, meningiomas of the cavernous sinus, arteriovenous malformations, pituitary adenomas, nasopharyngeal carcinoma, etc) (Sargeant 2007; Mendizabal 2005).
- Atypical facial pain
- Herpes zoster ophthalmicus** (Fig. 2.8)

2.1.4 Contraindications

Contraindications may include invasion of the pterygopalatine space** (contraindication for percutaneous approach, but not for intranasal approach) (Fig. 2.9) (Varghese and Koshy 2001).

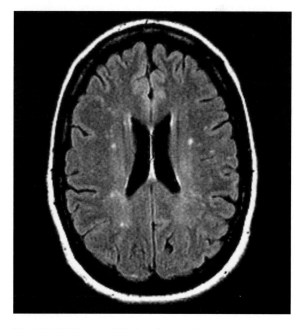

Fig. 2.7 WM increased T2 signal in migraine headache (Fazekas et al. 1992)

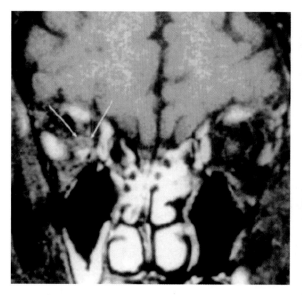

Fig. 2.8 Herpes zoster ophthalmicus in a 68-year-old patient with shingles surrounding the right orbit. Coronal T1-weighted (600/20, two excitations) MR image with gadopentetate dimeglumine and fat suppression shows shaggy, perineural enhancement surrounding right optic nerve (*arrows*). (Reprinted with permission from Tien et al. 1993)

2.1.5 Complications

The six main complications include: (1) Infection**; (2) epistaxis** (this can be imaged angiographically if there is an associated pseudoaneurysm); (3) hematoma – large venous plexus overlying the pterygopalatine fossa or the maxillary artery is punctured** (Figs. 2.10–2.11); (4) hypesthesia, dysesthesia or numbness of the palate, maxilla, or the posterior pharynx; (5) blindness due to needle advancement into the inferior orbital fissure; (6) Parotid gland injury.

2.2 Maxillary and Mandibular Nerve Block

2.2.1 Maxillary Nerve Block
(Fig. 2.12)

2.2.1.1 Anatomy

The maxillary nerve (V2) originates from the trigeminal ganglion, crosses the cavernous sinus, and exits

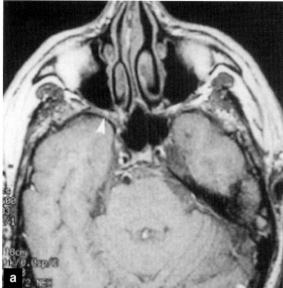
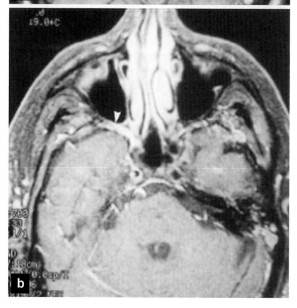

Fig. 2.9 (**a**) Axial T1-weighted (600/33/2) MR image shows subtle but definite loss of the normal fat signal hyperintensity in the right pterygopalatine fossa (*arrowhead*), representing tumor. (**b**) Axial postcontrast, fat-suppressed, T1-weighted (700/33/2) MR image shows excessive, abnormal enhancement in the right pterygopalatine fossa (*arrowhead*), representing tumor (Ginsberg and DeMonte 1998)

the foramen rotundum to leave the cranium. It traverses the pterygopalatine fossa and approaches the orbit through the inferior orbital fissure. It then traverses the infraorbital groove and canal at the floor of the orbit. Finally, it enters the face through the infraorbital foramen where it is known as the infraorbital nerve.

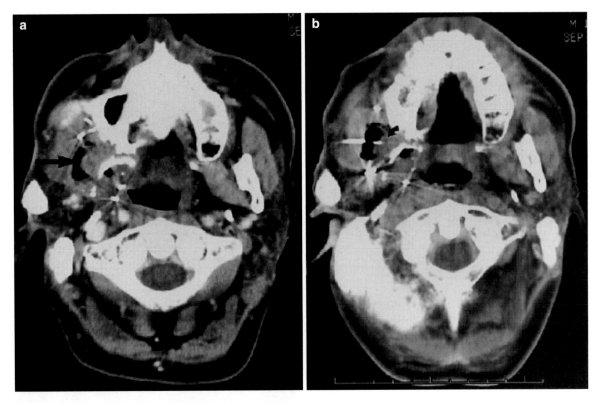

Fig. 2.10 (**a, b**) CT-directed fine-needle biopsy. (**a**) Contrast-enhanced axial CT image shows a focal soft-tissue mass within the masticator space (*arrow*). Gas surrounding the lesion is related to a postsurgical defect that communicates with the oral cavity. (**b**) Axial nonenhanced CT image shows the tip of a 22-gauge Chiba needle within the anterior aspect of the soft-tissue abnormality (*curved arrow*). The region was sampled twice

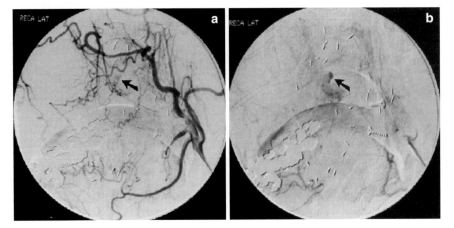

Fig. 2.11 Histologic analysis showed only inflammatory changes. (**a, b**) Pseudoaneurysm of the buccal branch of the distal internal maxillary artery. (**a**) Selective right external carotid arteriogram, lateral projection, shows mild irregularity of the distal internal maxillary artery and focal dilatation of the distal buccal branch (*arrow*). (**b**) Delayed image from same injection shows filling of a 5-mm pseudoaneurysm (*arrow*) (Walker et al. 1996)

2.2.1.2 Function

The maxillary nerve is purely sensory. It supplies sensation to the skin and mucosa between the palpebral fissure and the mouth, including the upper lip, nose, nasal cavity, sinuses, dura mater, temporal and lateral zygomatic region, and maxillary teeth.

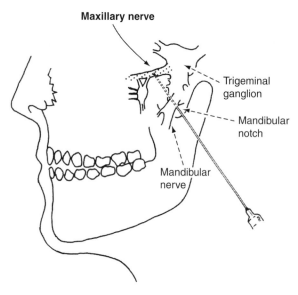

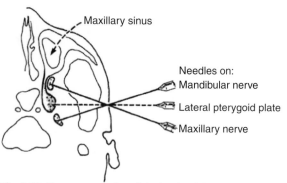

Fig. 2.13 Transverse section of the head and face at the level of the mandibular notch showing needle placement on the mandibular nerve, on the lateral pterygoid plate, and on the maxillary nerve. After the pterygoid plate is touched, the needle is slightly withdrawn and pushed posterior until it slips off the pterygoid plate (Raj et al.)

Fig. 2.12 A patient with the needle on the maxillary nerve entering through the mandibular notch (Waldman 2001a)

2.2.1.3 Injection Site

The classic approach for the maxillary block is a lateral approach anterior to the coronoid process of the mandible through the mandibular notch. This block is usually performed using external anatomical landmarks and by eliciting paresthesia (Fig. 2.12).

2.2.1.4 Cross-Sectional Anatomy

What Does the Needle Traverse? Maxillary Nerve

The needle traverses the structures within the infratemporal fossa (infrazygomatic masticator space) prior to entering the pterygopalatine fossa as its final destination (applies to the infrazygomatic approach). The path is just superior to the coronoid process of the mandible (Figs. 2.13–2.14).

A suprazygomatic approach has also been described with the pterygopalatine fossa as the final destination (Fig. 2.15).

Alternatively, a transnasal or transoral approach is used; however, this is predominately performed by oral surgeons (using either the pterygopalatine canal to enter the sphenopalatine foramen or around the maxillary tuberosity).

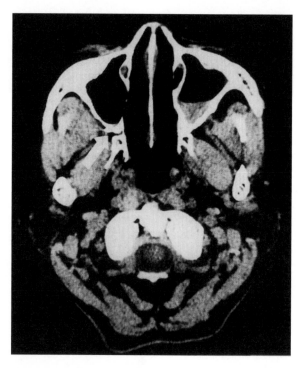

Fig. 2.14 Axial CT of head. An *arrow* indicates the needle tip located at the entrance of the pterygopalatine fossa (Okuda et al. 2000)

The structures traversed within the infratemporal fossa (within the infrazygomatic masticator space) include:

- Superficial layer of the deep cervical fascia
- Masseter muscle

Fig. 2.15 (**a**) Maxillary nerve block by the suprazygomatic route. A skin wheal is raised just above the superior edge of the zygomatic arch. (**b**) The needle is in the pterygopalatine fossa (Okuda et al. 2000)

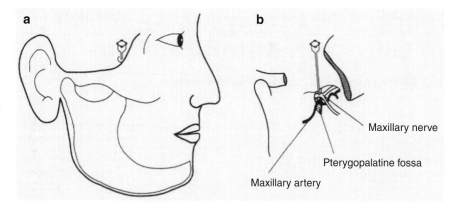

Maxillary nerve

Pterygopalatine fossa

Maxillary artery

- Temporalis muscle/tendon
- Lateral pterygoid muscle
- Pterygoid venous plexus (Harnsberger et al. 2006a)
  - Located both medial and lateral to the lateral pterygoid [http://www.emory.edu/ANATOMY/AnatomyManual/fossae.html]
- Retromaxillary fat pad (Buccal space)
- Internal maxillary artery (Harnsberger et al. 2006b)
  - Travels anteromedially within the masticator space lateral to the pterygoid muscle to end up within the pterygopalatine fossa.
- Pterygopalatine fossa (Harnsberger et al. 2006c)
  - Communicates with the masticator space via the pterygomaxillary fissure between the maxilla and lateral pterygoid plate

Which Structures the Needle Should Avoid

Pterygoid venous plexus: This is a prominent venous plexus medial and lateral to the surface of the lateral pterygoid muscle. It may be difficult to avoid; however, it is a venous structure and therefore under low pressure for potential hematoma formation.

Maxillary artery: The artery travels from its origin within the parotid gland through the masticator space anteromedially on the lateral aspect of the lateral pterygoid (usually) to terminate in the pterygomaxillary fissure as the sphenopalatine artery. It may be difficult to purposefully avoid puncture unless a blunt tipped needle or meticulous aspiration is used in the infrazygomatic approach.

A suprazygomatic approach may avoid the maxillary artery more successfully. This is because the maxillary artery is more ventrally positioned in the pterygopalatine fossa compared to the maxillary nerve. Also, with this approach, there is minimal distance between the point of entry of the needle and the pterygopalatine fossa (see Fig. 2.15).

Emissary veins from the orbit.

CSF space: The needle should not be advanced farther than 1.5 cm medially past the lateral pterygoid plate.

Posterior aspect of the orbit/optic nerve: Avoid by not advancing too cephalad or deeply in the pterygomaxillary fissure to allow entry of injectate into the infraorbital fissure.

Pharynx: if the needle is placed too posterior and air is aspirated (Raj et al.).

Strengths and Weaknesses of Each Image Guidance Modality

- Fluoroscopy
  - Fast
  - Easy
  - Allows complex angulation
  - May be slightly less accurate and reliable than CT

A reliable block can be difficult because fluoroscopy does not always show the relationship of the pterygopalatine fossa and foramen rotundum (Okuda et al. 2000).

- CT with contrast
  - Accurate
  - Safe
  - Vascular structures can be identified initially under contrast administration
  - Cancer may be avoided reliably compared to fluoroscopic guidance with lateral approach

- Reliable/more efficacious
- Anatomic variations better visualized
- Complex angulation more difficult
- Slower than fluoroscopy
- Approaches of CT and fluoroscopy can be combined (Vallejo et al. 2007)

Strengths and Weaknesses of Each Imaging Modality for Diagnosis (Indications/Contraindications and Complications)

(Please see beginning of Head and Neck section, Chapter 2, page 5 for listing of strengths and weakness of various imaging modalities)

2.2.2 Mandibular Nerve Block

2.2.2.1 Anatomy

The mandibular nerve (V_3) (see Fig. 2.16) is composed of sensory and motor roots. It originates from the trigeminal ganglion and exits through the foramen ovale.

2.2.2.2 Function

The mandibular nerve is a combined motor and sensory nerve that innervates:

- Mylohyoid muscle and digastric muscle
- Mucous membrane of the anterior two-thirds of the tongue
- The inside of the cheek (the buccal mucosa)
- Teeth and gums of the mandible
- Skin of the temporal region
- Auricula
- Lower lip and chin
- Muscles of mastication
- The muscles tensor tympani and tensor veli palatini

2.2.2.3 Injection Site

The classic technique involves external landmarks with or without fluoroscopy. The needle is placed through the mandibular notch and is directed posteriorly to the posterior margin of the lateral pterygoid plate (see Figs. 2.16 and 2.17).

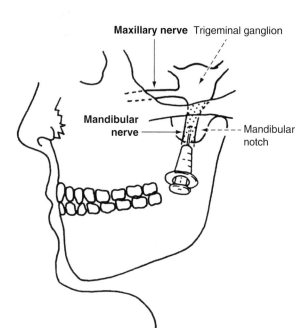

Fig. 2.16 Point of needle entry in the mandibular notch for extraoral mandibular nerve block (Waldman 2001a)

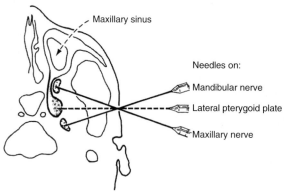

Fig. 2.17 Transverse section of the head and face at the level of the mandibular notch showing needle placement on the mandibular nerve, on the lateral pterygoid plate, and on the maxillary nerve. After the pterygoid plate is touched, the needle is slightly withdrawn and pushed posterior until it slips off the pterygoid plate (Raj et al.)

2.2.2.4 What Does the Needle Traverse? Mandibular Nerve

The needle traverses the same pathway as in the maxillary nerve block until reaching the lateral pterygoid plate. The needle is then directed posteriorly (see Fig. 2.18).

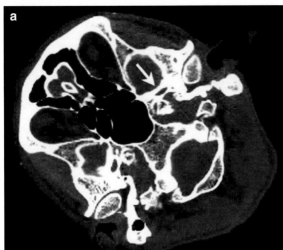

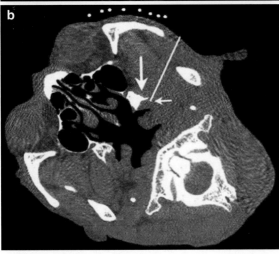

Fig. 2.18 Axial CT sections of the head. (**a**) *Arrow* indicates foramen ovale, which is a landmark to identify the location of nerve exit from the cranium on CT images in this patient. (**b**) The safest and shortest route (*white line*) to the target site (*small arrow*) is determined on the CT image (**b**, caudal section to **a**). The mandibular nerve immediately caudal to the foramen ovale in the posterior margin of lateral pterygoid plate (*large arrow*) is considered to be the target site (Koizuka et al. 2006)

2.2.2.5 Which Structures to Avoid

The same structures should be avoided as in maxillary nerve block, except that there is much less risk of entering the CSF and orbit.

2.2.2.6 Strengths and Weaknesses of Each Image Guidance Modality

Again, the same strengths and weaknesses are seen in image guidance as with the maxillary nerve.

2.2.3 Imaging/Radiology for Both Maxillary and Mandibular Nerve Blocks

Fluoroscopy. The foramen rotundum may be visualized for the maxillary nerve. The foramen ovale may be visualized for the mandibular nerve.

CT. The structure that exits through the foramen rotundum is the maxillary nerve. The structure that exits inferior through the foramen ovale is the mandibular nerve.

MRI. This is the procedure of choice for directly imaging the nerve (see Figs. 2.19–2.20) (Barakos et al. 1991).

2.2.3.1 Indications (Waldman 2001a)

The main indications for imaging/radiology for maxillary and mandibular nerve blocks include: Acute pain emergencies; acute herpes zoster refractory to stellate block** (Fig. 2.22); cancer** (Fig. 2.21); trigeminal neuralgia**; cluster headaches refractory to sphenopalatine (SPG) block; trismus.

2.2.3.2 Contraindications (Waldman 2001a)

A relative contraindication for maxillary or mandibular nerve blocks is altered anatomy due to surgery.

2.2.3.3 Complications

Complications of maxillary and mandibular nerve blocks are the following: Activation of herpes/labialis and herpes zoster**; postprocedure dysesthesias,

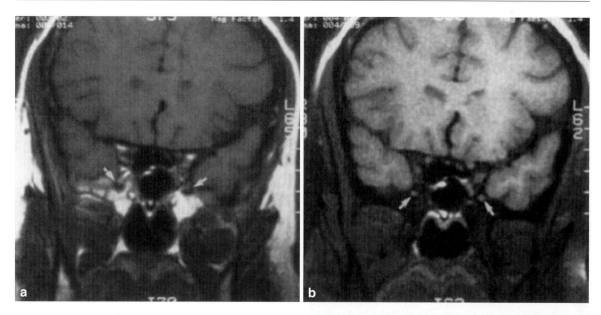

Fig. 2.19 (**a**) Coronal T1-weighted (600/20) image. Chemical shift artifact results in partial obscuration of the maxillary division of the mandibular nerve as it courses through the foramen rotundum (*arrows*). (**b**) After fat suppression, the chemical shift artifact is eliminated, allowing better visualization of the second division of the trigeminal nerve (*arrows*) (Barakos et al. 1991)

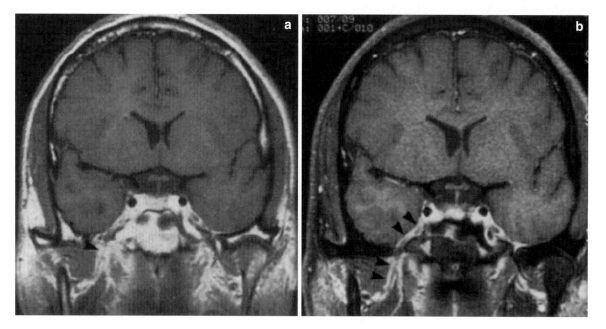

Fig. 2.20 (**a**) Coronal T1-weighted (600/20) image obtained after contrast material administration. The enhancing perineurium of the mandibular division of the trigeminal nerve is difficult to distinguish from surrounding fat (*arrowhead*). (**b**) Coronal fat-suppressed T1-weighted image. Note the uniform suppression of the subcutaneous and diploic space fat. After fat suppression, the perineurium that envelopes the trigeminal nerve (*arrowheads*) is easily defined. Note the enhancement of the perineurium but not the normal nerve itself (Barakos et al. 1991)

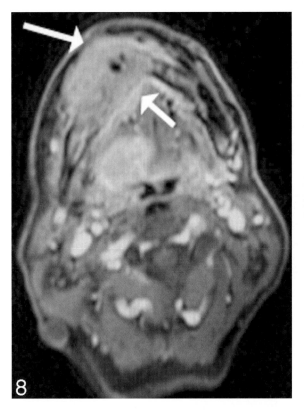

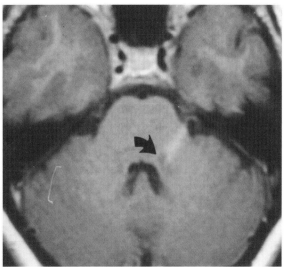

Fig. 2.22 A 33-year-old woman with herpes zoster. Axial contrast-enhanced T1-weighted spin-echo MR image shows enhancement along pontine course of trigeminal nerve and low signal intensity at the site of the main trigeminal sensory nucleus (*arrow*) (Kamel and Toland 2001)

Fig. 2.21 Postgadolinium-enhanced scan through the floor of the mouth demonstrates a contrast-enhancing mass (*arrows*) infiltrating the right side of the mandible and extending into the subcutaneous tissue. There is an associated mass at the right lateral base of the tongue. Note infiltration of the mandible extends across the midline (Yousem et al. 2006). This cancerous mass would result in pain that could be treated with a mandibular block

including anesthesia dolorosa; facial asymmetry; Horner's syndrome; facial ecchymosis and hematoma**; ocular subscleral hematoma**; middle meningeal artery injection (mandibular block).

2.3 Trigeminal Ganglion Block: Trigeminal (Gasserian) Ganglion Block for Trigeminal Neuralgia (Tic Douloureux)

2.3.1 Anatomy

The trigeminal nerve is the largest of the cranial nerves. The preganglionic trigeminal nerve arises (at the root entry zone) from the lateral pons at its superior to mid portion as a large sensory and small motor root. The preganglionic nerve travels forward in the posterior cranial fossa above the superior aspect of the petrous temporal bone. It then merges with trigeminal ganglion at the apex of the petrous temporal bone (Meckel's cave) in the middle cranial fossa. The ganglion is bordered by the cavernous sinus, trochlear nerve, and optic nerve medially, the inferior surface of the temporal lobe superiorly, and the brain stem posteriorly. There are three postganglionic nerve divisions: V1, which exits via the superior ophthalmic fissure into the orbit; V2, which exits via the foramen rotundum and crosses the pterygopalatine fissure and inferior orbital fissure into the orbit; V3, which exits the foramen ovale towards the mandible.

2.3.2 Function

The trigeminal nerve provides sensation for the face and mouth. It supplies the muscles of mastication as well as the tensor tympani, tensor veli palatini, the mylohyoid, and anterior belly of the digastric muscle.

2.3.3 Clinical Presentation

Trigeminal neuralgia presents as episodic excruciating pain of the unilateral face, forehead, jaw, or any isolated facial structure (eye, lip, nose, etc).

2.3.4 Etiology

Etiologies include vascular compression (superior cerebellar artery, aneurysm),** trauma** (root canal), tumor,** arachnoid cyst** in the cerebellopontine angle, multiple sclerosis,** and postherpetic neuralgia.**

2.3.5 Differential Diagnosis

Differential diagnoses include cluster headache, sinusitis,** temporomandibular joint syndrome,** atypical facial pain syndrome, odontogenic pain,** acute glaucoma, and intracranial aneurysm.**

2.3.6 Injection Site

The needle is inserted at the lateral margin of the lips (Fig. 2.23). It is then advanced along the inner aspect of the mandible between the mandible and the oral mucosa. The index finger is positioned inside the mouth to stabilize the needle and prevent it from puncturing the oral mucosa on its way to the foramen ovale. The needle is pushed past the posterior margin of the mandible to the skull base under fluoroscopic guidance. The needle tip is then advanced just inside the foramen ovale. In the lateral view the needle tip should not be advanced past a line between the tips of the anterior and posterior clinoid processes (Figs. 2.24–2.26).

2.3.7 Cross-Sectional Anatomy

2.3.7.1 What Does the Needle Traverse?

- Taking an anterior approach, the needle first penetrates the skin and passes through the fascia. It then enters the buccal space through the inferior portion of the retromaxillary fat pad between the buccinator muscle and the masseter. It may traverse the medial margin of the temporalis muscle. The lateral pterygoid muscle is then traversed to reach the foramen ovale adjacent to the lateral surface of the lateral pterygoid.

A lateral approach to the foramen ovale can also be used similar to the mandibular nerve block (Krol and Arbit 1988).

2.3.7.2 Which Structures the Needle Should Avoid (Kaplan et al. 2007)

It is advisable that the needle avoid the following structures:

- Optic nerve
- Inferior orbital fissure (needle injury to CN III and/or IV)
- Nasociliary nerve or injury to its feeding artery
- Recurrent meningeal artery (feeding vessel for the trochlear nerve)
- Motor branch innervation to masseter muscle
- Abducens nerve (CN VI)
- Greater superficial petrosal nerve
- Geniculate ganglion (if the needle advanced too far within the middle cranial fossa into the petrous bone)
- Carotid artery and cavernous sinus
- Anastomotic veins between cavernous sinus and pterygoid plexus
- Middle meningeal artery

2.3.7.3 Imaging/Radiology

Fluoroscopy: The target is superior and posterior to the foramen ovale. Precise location of the foramen ovale may be difficult in some patients due to osteoporosis or variant anatomy. Moreover, there is a 15% failure rate using this modality.

CT: The trigeminal ganglion is a structure within Meckel's cave, but may not be directly visualized. The foramen ovale can be seen reliably. This method can be combined with CT/fluoroscopy for real-time needle manipulation. 3D volume rendering CT can also be helpful to localize the foramen ovale (Horiguchi et al. 2005).

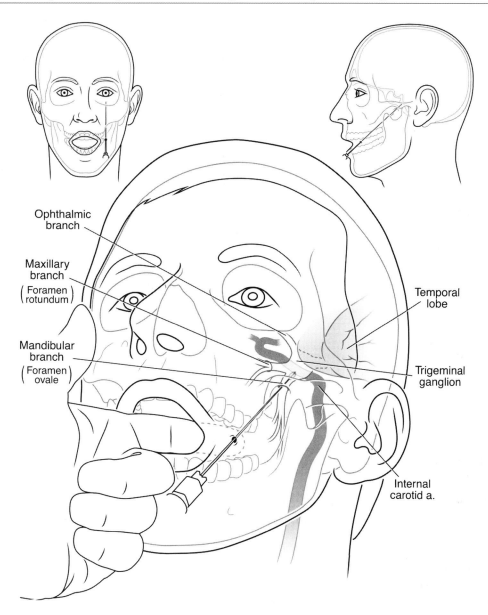

Fig. 2.23 Gasserian ganglion block for trigeminal neuralgia (tic douloureux) (Neal, 2007)

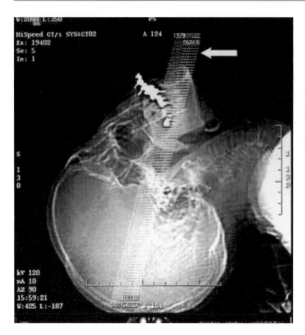

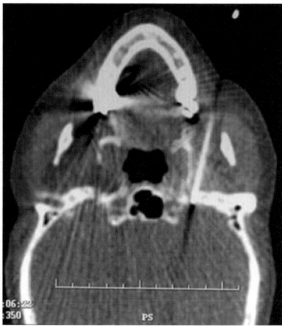

Fig. 2.24 The patient's neck is extended and the angle of the computed tomography (CT) gantry is set vertically to the cranial base on the scout view. The *arrow* points to the *white bar* that indicates the inclination of the CT gantry (Sekimoto et al. 2005)

Fig. 2.26 The needle was advanced following the predesigned route under CT fluoroscopy (Sekimoto et al. 2005)

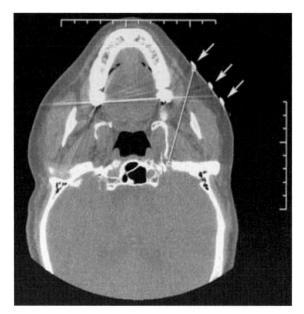

Fig. 2.25 The safest and shortest route to the foramen was designed on the CT image. The *arrows* show the marking devices (Sekimoto et al. 2005)

MRI: This is the procedure of choice for diagnosis of the various indications including trigeminal neuralgia due to arterial compression or AVMs, migraine phenomenon, and cranial nerve invasion. It is the best modality for excluding other diagnosis in cluster headaches. It is also the best modality for the visualization of complications (hematoma) in the middle cranial fossa and masticator space (Figs. 2.27–2.29).

2.3.8 Indications

The following are common indications for trigeminal ganglion block (double asterisks indicate that the pathology can be imaged): Trigeminal neuralgia**; multiple sclerosis **; cancer resulting in direct nerve involvement **; cancer pain in invasive tumors**; cluster headaches; atypical facial pain; and failed sphenopalatine block.

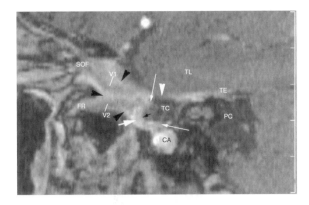

Fig. 2.27 Sagittal enhanced 3D time-of-flight image through the right side of Meckel's cave in a 53-year-old-man. The enhancing ganglion (*thick white arrow*) is shown at the anteroinferior margin of the cave, in continuity with the dural wall (*white arrowhead*). Superior and inferior lips of the ganglion (*thin white arrows*) are well depicted. No sensory rootlets are seen in the trigeminal cistern (*TC*). The ophthalmic nerve (*V1*) and maxillary nerve (*V2*) are hypointense, linear structures surrounded by strongly enhancing venous channels (*black arrowheads*) in the lateral wall and along the inferior border, respectively, of the cavernous sinus. V2 enters the foramen rotundum (*FR*), while V1 passes to the superior orbital fissure (*SOF*). *CA* carotid artery; *PC* prepontine cistern; *TE* cerebellar tentorium; *TL* temporal lobe (Yousry et al. 2005)

2.3.9 Complications

The following are complications of trigeminal ganglion block (double asterisks indicate that the pathology can be imaged) (Kaplan et al. 2007):

- Numbness, hypoesthesia or dysesthesia (trigeminal trophic syndrome) in the entire trigeminal nerve distribution – 29–63% incidence.
- Corneal abnormalities in 3–15% of patients due to nasociliary nerve injury.
- Masticatory weakness (masseter motor innervation injury).
- Reactivation of dormant HSV in 27–94% patients.**
- Hematoma: the pterygopalatine space is highly vascular and significant hematoma of the eye can occur.** Retrobulbar hematoma** can also occur.
- Hemorrhage into temporal fossa (veins into the subtemporal region can be punctured).**
- CSF leak or fistula.**
- Blindness due to optic nerve injury.
- Oculomotor paresis.

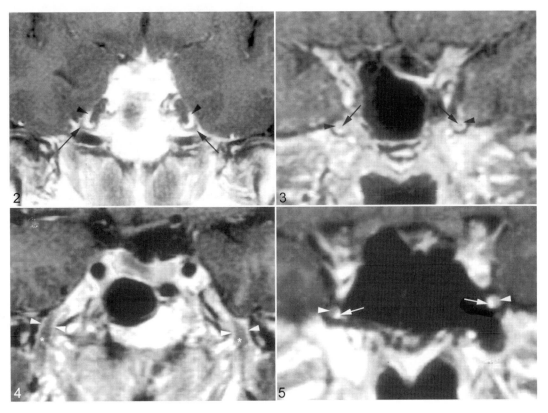

Fig. 2.28 Coronal gadolinium-enhanced T1-weighted image (TR/TE/NEX, 400/15/2) depicts the nonenhancing crescent-shaped trigeminal ganglion (*arrows*) and the prominent perineural venous plexus (*arrowheads*) superior to it. The venous plexus as well as the ganglion are symmetric in appearance (Williams et al. 2003)

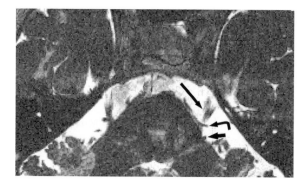

Fig. 2.29 Image obtained in a 55-year-old woman with trigeminal neuralgia, with neurovascular compression caused by both the vein and anterior inferior cerebellar artery. Transverse 3D CISS MR image (12.25/5.9, 70° flip angle) shows that both the vein (*curved arrow*) and the anterior inferior cerebellar artery (*short straight arrow*) have compressed the left trigeminal nerve (*long straight arrow*) at the root entry zone. This finding was confirmed at surgery (Yoshino et al. 2003)

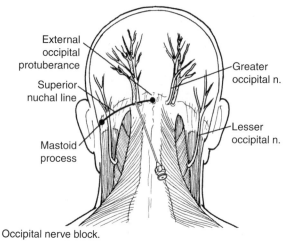

Occipital nerve block.

Fig. 2.30 Occipital nerve block for occipital neuralgia (Weiss 2007)

- Extremely rare injuries to CN 7, 8, and 12.**
- Caroticocavernous fistula.**
- External carotid artery fistula.**
- Meningitis** (Ward et al. 2007; James et al. 1995).

2.4 Occipital Nerve Block: For Occipital Neuralgia

2.4.1 Anatomy

The greater occipital nerve arises from the C2 nerve root and the lesser occipital nerve receives supply from the C2 and C3 nerve roots. The third occipital nerve originates from the medial sensory branch of the posterior division of C3 nerve root. It courses through the splenius and trapezius medial to the greater occipital nerve. Sites of compression of the greater occipital nerve include the atlantoaxial joint, the posterior arches of C1 and C2, and the site of nerve penetration at the trapezius tendon (Figs. 2.30 and 2.31).

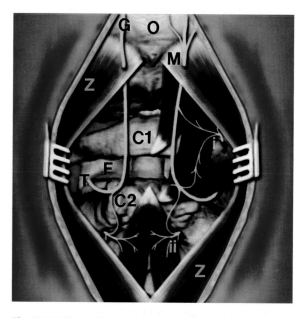

Fig. 2.31 The occipital region and upper cervical vertebrae viewed from behind showing the course of the greater occipital nerve (*G*) with possible sites of compression: *F* due to atlantoaxial joint disease; *M* as it penetrates the tendinous portion of the trapezius muscles (*Z*); *T* as the occipital nerve pierces the posterior atlantoaxial membrane (depicted in *light semitransparent blue*); and between posterior arches of C1 and C2 vertebrae. Note connections between greater occipital nerve (*G*) and C1 (*i*) and C3 (*ii*) nerves. *O* occipital bone (Kapoor et al. 2003)

2.4.2 Function

The lesser and greater occipital nerves provide sensory supply to the upper neck and occipital scalp.

2.4.3 Clinical Presentation

Occipital neuralgia presents as chronic headache pain, which may be aching, burning, and throbbing with intermittent shooting episodes. The headache pain may involve the eyebrows and/or behind the eye. It is usually unilateral. There may be photosensitivity associated with the headaches. There is often associated scalp tenderness. The presentation may be similar to a migraine or a cluster headache.

2.4.4 Etiology

Etiologies include trauma such as whiplash injury** or concussion injury with involvement of the lesser and/or greater occipital nerves. Tumor** of the C2 and/or C3 nerve roots, repetitive use injury, rheumatoid arthritis** or osteoarthritis**of the upper cervical spine, cervical spondylosis,** herniated nucleus pulposus,** C1–C2 facet arthritis,** and ligamentum flavum thickening.** Compression of the greater or lesser occipital nerve or the C2 and C3 nerve roots associated with cervical spine degeneration.** Vascular compression by an anomalous, ectatic vertebral artery** or posterior inferior cerebellar artery.** Arnold–Chiari type I syndrome** (foramen magnum syndrome), gout,** diabetes, arteritis,** or infection.**

2.4.5 Differential Diagnoses

Differential diagnoses include tension headaches, cluster headaches, migraine headaches, and fibromyalgia.

2.4.6 Injection Site

At a theoretical line (level of the superior nuchal margin) between the external occipital protuberance and the mastoid process, the greater occipital nerve is positioned at the inner third. The lesser occipital nerve is positioned between the central and lateral third interface. The subcutaneous tissues at these sites are injected (Figs. 2.30 and 2.32).

2.4.7 Cross-Sectional Anatomy

2.4.7.1 What Does the Needle Traverse?

The needle enters the skin and traverses the trapezius muscle. The superficial layer of the deep cervical fascia that surrounds the trapezius is then traversed. The deep layer of the deep cervical fascia is next penetrated by the needle. The needle then crosses the semispinalis/splenius capitis muscle followed by the rectus capitis muscle. The base of the occipital bone is then reached (Fig. 2.32).

2.4.7.2 Which Structures the Needle Should Avoid

The needle should avoid the following structures:

- Suboccipital venous plexus (complex meshwork of superficial veins between layers of muscle in the suboccipital region)
- Condylar emissary vein (connects the suboccipital venous plexus to the sigmoid sinus via the condylar canal at the occipital condyle)
- Occipital artery (nerve lies just medial to the artery)
- Vertebral artery

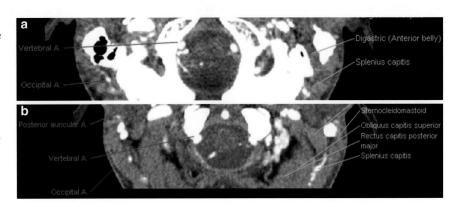

Fig. 2.32 (**a**) Depiction of the occipital artery and posterior scalp musculature at the level of the inferior occipital bone. (**b**) Depiction of the occipital artery and posterior scalp musculature at the level of the occipital condyle [http://www.e-anatomy.org/anatomy/human-body/head-neck-face/skull-face.html] (courtesy of e-Anatomy - Micheau A, Hoa D, www.imaios.com)

2.4.7.3 Imaging/Radiology

Plain film radiographs: Plain films are less sensitive than CT or MRI and are usually not helpful for evaluation of indications for occipital nerve block.

Fluoroscopy is the best technique for guidance. It may not be necessary however, since anatomic landmarks are usually palpable.

Ultrasound: Cadaver study shows that the nerve can be directly visualized and targeted under ultrasound in its proximal portion before its division at the caudal end of the obliquus capitis inferior muscle (Curatolo and Eichenberger 2007). Ultrasound may be of use to localize the occipital artery.

CT: CT is useful for the evaluation of upper cervical spine pathology. It is also useful for guidance of C2–C3 nerve blocks when lesser and greater occipital nerve blocks have failed in the scalp.

MRI: This is the modality of choice for the exclusion of intracranial pathology and to evaluate the cervical spine. It is superior to CT except in subarachnoid hemorrhage and cortical bone invasion/pathology.

2.4.8 Indications

The following are relatively common indications (double asterisks indicate that the pathology can be imaged): Headache (tension, vascular, cervicogenic), occipital neuralgia, cervical arthritis** (Fig. 2.33) and myofascial pain.

Relatively rare indications include: Arnold–Chiari malformation,** (Fig. 2.34) tumor (primary and secondary),** and infection (mastoid and intraspinal)** .

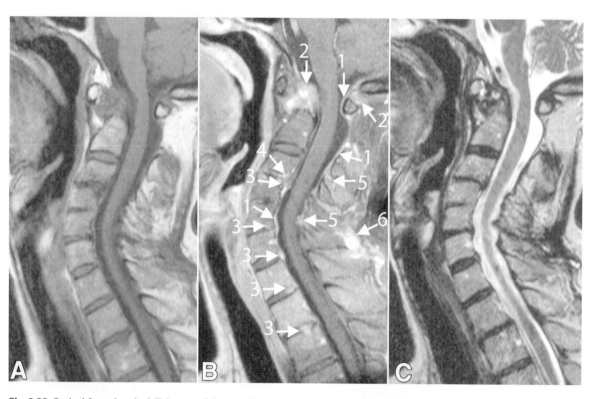

Fig. 2.33 Sagittal fast spin-echo MR images of rheumatoid arthritis with superficial and deep enhancement in a 69-year-old woman (rheumatoid arthritis for 31 years). T1-weighted (500/7) (**a**) and T2-weighted (3,398/150) (**c**) images show stenoses (waisted) at level C1–C2 and levels C3–C4 through C6–C7, presumably caused by pannus and subluxation on level C1–C2 and by discopathy and ligamentum flavum hypertrophy on subaxial levels. (**b**) Gadolinium-enhanced T1-weighted SPIR fat-suppressed image (500/7) shows superficial enhancement lining the cerebrospinal fluid (*arrow 1*) and enhancement involving deeper structures. Deep-enhancing tissue is recognized as bone and presumably pannus on C1–C2 (*arrow 2*), as disk on subaxial anterior levels (*arrow 3*), and as bone on level C3–C4 (*arrow 4*). Ligamentum flavum and interspinal ligaments enhanced posterior (*arrow 5*). Deep enhancement coincides mostly with narrowing of the spinal canal on these levels. Note enhancement of the ligamentum nuchae (*arrow 6*) (Kroft et al. 2004)

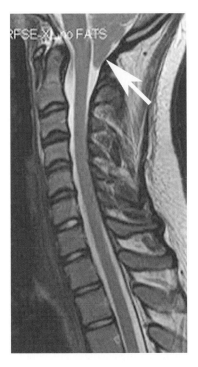

Fig. 2.34 Sagittal T2-weighted MR image in patient with asymptomatic Chiari I malformation. *Arrow* points to herniated cerebellar tonsil extending below the inferior margin of the occipital lobe (Hofkes et al. 2007)

2.4.9 Contraindications

The main specific contraindication is suboccipital craniectomy.** (Figs. 2.35–2.36).

2.4.10 Complications

Uncommon complications include: (1) Intravascular injection of occipital artery; total spinal anesthesia in the sub cranial injection of patients who have had posterior suboccipital cranial surgery.

2.5 Cervical Plexus Blockade

2.5.1 Anatomy

The cervical plexus is formed by the ventral rami of the superior fourth cervical nerves. It lies deep to the sternocleidomastoid. It is lateral to the levator scapulae

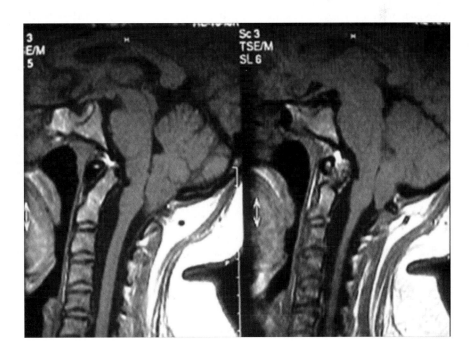

Fig. 2.35 Herniated cerebellar tonsils up to C1

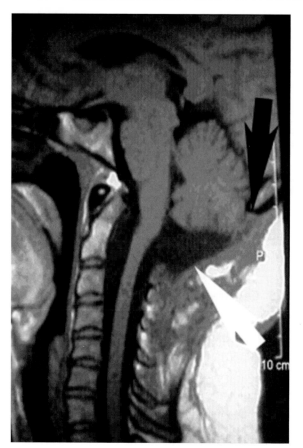

Fig. 2.36 An example of suboccipital craniectomy. Postoperative MRI showing the recently created cisterna magna. Note that the inferior aspect of the occipital bone is now at the level of the mid cerebellum. *White arrow* points to cisterna magna. *Black arrow* points to inferior margin of the occipital bone (Silva et al. 2005)

muscles and middle scalene. This is surrounded by the prevertebral fascia. The plexus has links to cranial nerves 11, 12, and the sympathetic trunk. The cervical plexus becomes superficial at the posterior margin of the sternocleidomastoid along the posterior triangle. There are four cutaneous and one muscular branch. A deep and superficial component to the cervical plexus is present (Fig. 2.37).

2.5.2 Function

The cutaneous branches of the cervical plexus include the lesser occipital nerve, which provides sensory supply to the lateral portion of the occipital scalp; the greater auricular nerve, which provides sensory supply to the auricular region of the ear

(behind the ear); the transverse cervical nerve, which provides sensory supply to the ventral neck; the supraclavicular nerve, which provides sensory supply to the shoulder, upper thorax, and suprascapular region (Fig. 2.37).

The ansa cervicalis provides motor supply to the geniohyoid, thyrohyoid, sternothyroid, sternohyoid, and omohyoid muscles. The phrenic nerve provides motor supply to the diaphragm.

There is a contribution to cranial nerve 11 for the sternocleidomastoid and trapezius muscles.

2.5.3 Injection Site

For the superficial plexus, the site is chosen at the midpoint of the posterior margin of the sternocleidomastoid, one-half the depth of the muscle superiorly and inferiorly along the posterior border (Fig. 2.37).

For the deep cervical plexus, an anterior approach is utilized such that the needle is adjacent to the transverse processes of C2 through C4. The point of injection is chosen along a line between the mastoid process and the C6 transverse process (Chassaignac's tubercle) (Figs. 2.38–2.41).

2.5.4 Cross-Sectional Anatomy: Superficial Cervical Plexus Block

2.5.4.1 What Does the Needle Traverse?

The needle enters the skin and traverses the posterior margin of the platysma. The needle next traverses the superficial layer of the deep cervical fascia at the posterior margin of the sternocleidomastoid to enter the posterior cervical space. The needle is then superficial to the deep layer of the deep cervical fascia surrounding the levator scapulae muscle (Figs. 2.41a and 2.41b).

2.5.4.2 Which Structures the Needle Should Avoid

Care must be taken to avoid cranial nerve 11 (spinal accessory nerve), which runs in the floor of the posterior cervical space. This supplies innervation to the trapezius. The nerve is located within the occipital

Fig. 2.37 Superficial cervical plexus block – anatomy and technique (Brown 1992)

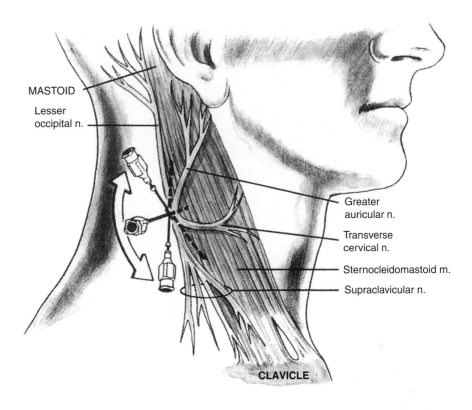

MASTOID

Lesser occipital n.

Greater auricular n.

Transverse cervical n.

Sternocleidomastoid m.

Supraclavicular n.

CLAVICLE

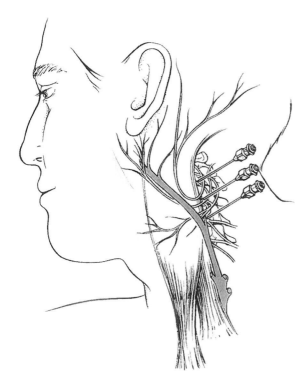

Fig. 2.38 Deep cervical plexus block – anatomic drawing. *Right* to *left*, the needles are noted at the sulci of the transverse processes of C2, C3, and C4 (Carron et. al. 1984)

triangle formed by the sternocleidomastoid antero-medially, the trapezius posterolaterally, and the omohyoid muscle inferiorly. The dorsal scapular nerve should also be avoided. It arises from the brachial plexus (spinal nerve C4 & C5); this supplies motor innervation to the rhomboid and levator scapulae muscles. The internal and external jugular veins should also be avoided (Figs. 2.40–2.41).

2.5.5 Cross-Sectional Anatomy: Deep Cervical Plexus Block Lateral Approach

2.5.5.1 What Does the Needle Traverse?

The needle enters the skin and traverses the sternocleido-mastoid and the superficial layer of the deep cervical fascia, which surrounds the sternocleidomastoid. Next, the middle scalene muscle and/or anterior scalene muscle is crossed until the anterior tubercle of the transverse process is contacted at its lateral most aspect (Figs. 2.38–2.39 and 2.41).

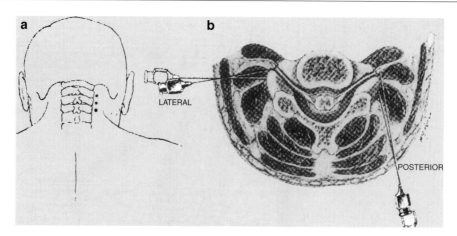

Fig. 2.39 "Deep cervical block" by the original posterior (Kappis) and lateral (Heidenheim) routes. (**a**) With the posterior approach, the needles are inserted 3 cm from the midline and advanced until the articular pillar is contacted, whereupon the needles are withdrawn and reinserted farther laterally until they "walk off" the lateral margin of the transverse processes. At that point the local anesthetic is injected. With the lateral approach, a line is drawn from the mastoid process above to the transverse process of C6 below, indicating the location of the cervical transverse processes. (**b**) Then, using either two or three needles, the lateral margins of the second, third, and fourth cervical transverse process are contacted, whereupon the anesthetic solution is injected (Winnie et al. 1975)

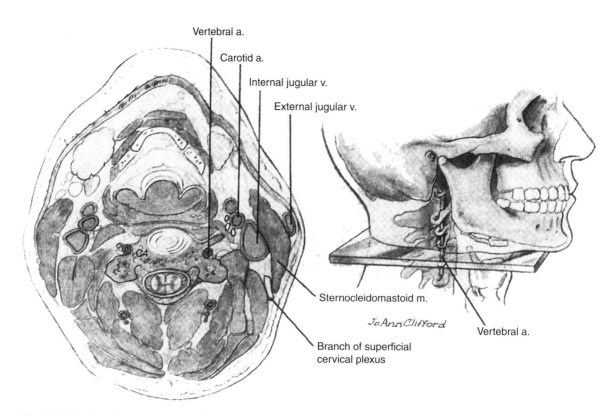

Fig. 2.40 Cervical plexus cross-sectional anatomy: midpoint of sternocleidomastoid muscle (Brown 1992)

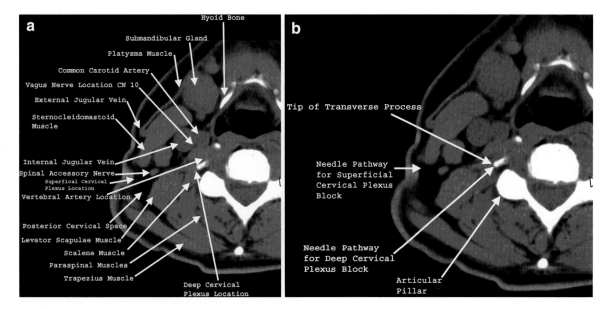

Fig. 2.41 (**a**) CT image of cervical plexus cross-sectional anatomy – midpoint of sternocleidomastoid muscle (at same level as Fig. 2.38). (**b**) CT image depicts needle pathway for cervical plexus blocks

2.5.5.2 Which Structures the Needle Should Avoid?

The vertebral artery should be avoided within the transverse foramen. Care should be taken to limit the volume of anesthetic injected anterior to the transverse processes as this may cause compression of the carotid sheath and anesthesia of cranial nerves 9 and 10. Avoid the intravertebral foramina so as to prevent epidural or subarachnoid injection and even spinal cord injury. The phrenic nerve located ventral to the anterior scalene muscle should also be avoided.

2.5.6 Cross-Sectional Anatomy: Deep Cervical Plexus Block Posterior Approach

This approach is technically more difficult to perform than the lateral approach, but useful when the lateral approach is technically impossible, i.e., neck tumor (Waldman 2001b).

2.5.6.1 What Does the Needle Traverse?

The needle enters the skin and traverses trapezius and the superficial layer of the deep cervical fascia (surrounding the trapezius). The deep layer of the deep cervical fascia is then entered, followed by the posterior paraspinal muscles. Next, the posterior and middle scalene muscles are traversed by the needle until the lateral margin of the transverse process is contacted.

2.5.6.2 Which Structures the Needle Should Avoid

The brachial plexus root lies near the needle path between the anterior and middle scalene muscles.

2.5.7 Imaging/Radiology (Jacobsen et al. 2006)

Ultrasound: This method is useful for characterizing palpable masses (thyroglossal duct cysts, branchial cysts, cystic hygromas, salivary gland tumors, abscesses, carotid body tumors, vascular tumors, and thyroid masses). It is able to characterize vascularity in real-time and in duplex mode.

CT: This represents the first-line imaging technique for masses/lymphadenopathy Superior to MRI in evaluating bony cortex. It is helpful for staging cancer, including capsular penetration and extension beyond the lymph nodes (Fig. 2.42). CTA is recommended for vertebral/carotid artery injury.

MRI: This modality is superior to CT for evaluating intracranial pathology, especially infarcts of the posterior fossa. It is also valuable in assessing the superior extent of nodal involvement of malignancy (intracranial extension). Although is capable of detecting bone marrow invasion, it is not able to detect bone cortex destruction, unlike CT. MRA is useful for vertebral/carotid artery injury.

2.5.8 Indications

The following are common indications (double asterisks indicate that the pathology can be imaged) (Smoker

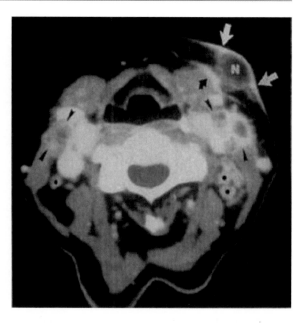

Fig. 2.43 Multispatial tularemia. Enhanced CT scan shows a large suppurative node in external aspect f superficial space (*N*) with thickening and enhancement of overlying skin (*white arrows*) and underlying platysma muscle (*black arrow*). Suppurative adenopathy is also present bilaterally in deep cervical chain nodes of carotid spaces (*arrowheads*), and smaller, reactive-appearing nodes are present in spinal accessory nodes of posterior cervical spaces (*dots*) (Smoker, 1991)

and Harnsberger 1991; Holliday et al. 1995; Parker and Harnsberger 1991):

- Painful infections (tuberculosis) affecting the lymph nodes in the neck (Fig. 2.43)
- Pain after laryngectomy and/or radiation therapy following laryngectomy for cancer
- Surgery involving the inferior or lateral aspect of the neck:
- Dissections of the neck**
- Excisions of masses**
- Tumors**
- Thyroglossal cysts**
- Branchial cysts**
- Operations of the thyroid**
- Parathyroid or lymph nodes**
- Operations on the blood vessels including ligations of the carotid and lingual arteries and carotid endarterectomy**
- Pharyngeal cancer and metastases**
- Occipital and posterior auricular neuralgias associated with acute inflammation or compression of the cervical plexus by tumors** or aneurysms**
- Hiccups

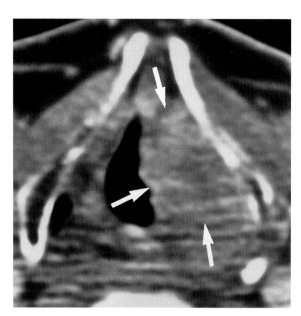

Fig. 2.42 Transverse CT image in a patient with T3 supraglottic carcinoma. Pretreatment image shows a mass (*arrows*) in the region of the left false vocal cord and paraglottic space (Hermans et al. 2000)

2.5.9 Contraindications

The following represent the main unique contraindications: significant respiratory disease due to potential blockage of the phrenic nerve (diaphragm paralysis), especially in bilateral cervical plexus block.

2.5.10 Complications

The range of possible complications is relatively wide, including:

- Intravascular injections of the local anesthetic
- Internal or external jugular vein injections (systemic toxicity, hematoma due to wall tear, air embolism)**
- Vertebral artery injury resulting in convulsions, apnea, total reversible blindness and unconsciousness due to dissection,** thrombosis,** and/or infarction**
- Occlusion of the PICA (Wallenberg syndrome)**
- Compression of the carotid sheath, especially with carotid artery disease**
- Injection into the epidural or subarachnoid spaces – anesthesia of the upper limbs and thorax with bilateral phrenic nerve paralysis
- Spinal cord injury**
- Recurrent laryngeal nerve block** occurs in 2–3% of unilateral cervical plexus block
- Vagus nerve block
- Bilateral hypoglossal nerve block
- Bilateral phrenic nerve block**
- Blockade of the ninth and tenth cranial nerves or a combination of both through the pharyngeal plexus
- Bilateral stellate ganglion blocks
- Occipital headaches

2.6 Stellate Ganglion Block

2.6.1 Anatomy

The stellate ganglion is located ventral to the C7 transverse process. It is ventral to the first rib, medial to the vertebral artery and superior to the subclavian artery, and cupula/apex of the lung (Fig. 2.44).

2.6.2 Function

The stellate ganglion provides sympathetic innervation to the head, neck, upper extremity, and heart. It also receives input from the paravertebral sympathetic trunk. The stellate ganglion is involved in sympathetically mediated pain (i.e., complex regional pain syndrome).

2.6.3 Injection Site

Fluoroscopic: An anterior approach is utilized to the junction between the C6 and/or C7 vertebral body and their respective transverse processes (Fig. 2.45).

CT: An anterolateral approach is utilized with the tip of the needle adjacent to the first rib head (Fig. 2.46).

2.6.4 Cross-Sectional Anatomy: Anterior Approach

2.6.4.1 What Does the Needle Traverse?

After traversing the skin, the needle penetrates the platysma and the infrahyoid strap muscle that is surrounded by the superficial layer of the deep cervical fossa. The middle layer of the deep cervical fascia that surrounds the visceral space is then traversed. The needle may then traverse the thyroid gland and the posterior margin of the middle layer of the deep cervical fascia to enter the retropharyngeal space. The needle is kept medial to the carotid sheath. The deep layer of the deep cervical fascia is then traversed (perivertebral space prevertebral component). The longus coli is then traversed to contact the anterior tubercle of the C6 transverse process (Chassaignac's tubercle) (Fig. 2.47).

2.6.4.2 Which Structures the Needle Should Avoid

It is advisable to avoid the following structures: Carotid artery (carotid artery sheath); vertebral artery (transverse foramen); esophagus (posterior and to the left of trachea); phrenic nerve (anterior to the anterior scalene); recurrent laryngeal nerves (tracheoesophageal groove) (Figs. 2.47 and 2.50).

Fig. 2.44 Axial diagram of stellate ganglion block. The needle is positioned in the vertebral gutter, a shallow depression where the transverse process joins with the vertebral body. Note the position of the vertebral artery within the foramen transversarium, the exiting nerve root, and the carotid artery (Rathmell 2006)

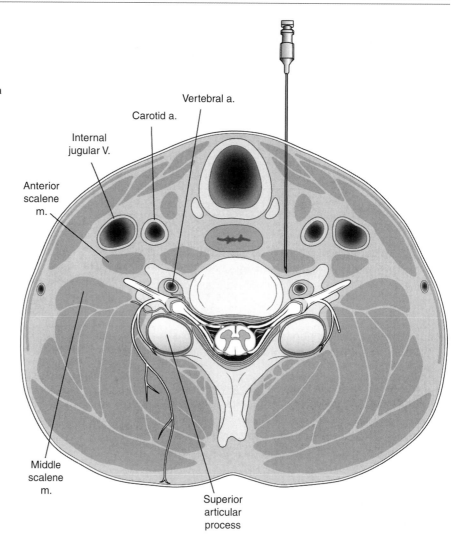

2.6.4.3 Imaging/Radiology

Fluoroscopy: This method allows accurate needle placement at the level of the C6 transverse process, since many individuals lack a bony tranversarium at C7 and thus the needle may enter the vertebral artery at this level (C7).

Arteriography is useful for evaluating upper extremity arterial insufficiency.

CT (Erickson and Hogan 1993)*:* Intravenous contrast allows accurate identification of vascular structures (vertebral artery and carotid sheath). CT also enables identification of the esophagus and allows one to avoid critical nerves such as the phrenic nerve and recurrent laryngeal nerve, and spinal cord/nerve roots. The pneumothorax can also be avoided. It is useful in excluding other sources of upper extremity pain where bony pathology is suspected. Temporal bone CT is useful in excluding other sources of inner ear pathology in the setting of Ménière's disease.

Ultrasound: This imaging modality allows identification of the esophagus in the left-sided approach. It also allows accurate identification of vascular structures (carotid artery, vertebral artery, thyroid arteries) (Fig. 2.49). However, it cannot monitor spread of contrast agent as well as CT or fluoroscopy to prevent intrathecal or recurrent laryngeal nerve involvement.

Nuclear medicine bone scan is useful for evaluating complex regional pain syndrome (reflex sympathetic dystrophy) (Fig. 2.51).

MRI: This method is useful in excluding other sources of upper extremity pain. MRI of the internal auditory canal is useful in excluding other sources of inner ear pathology in the setting of Ménière's disease (Fig. 2.48). The stellate ganglion may be directly imaged.

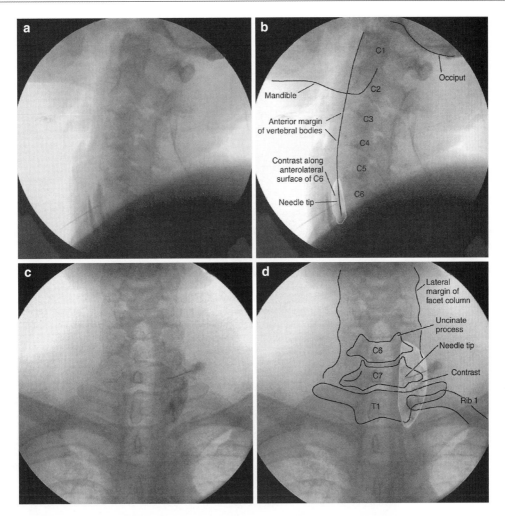

Fig. 2.45 (**a, b**) Lateral radiograph of the cervical spine during stellate ganglion block at C6. (**a**) The needle is seated against the anterior surface of C6. Radiographic contract (1.5 mL of iohexol 180 mg/mL) has been injected and spreads along the anterolateral surface of C6 to reach the adjacent vertebra. A small amount of contrast is seen in a more superficial plane and was placed before the needle was firmly seated against the vertebral body. (**b**) Labeled image. (**c, d**) Posterior–anterior radiograph of the cervical spine during stellate ganglion block at C7. (**c**) The needle is in position at the junction of the C7 transverse process and

the vertebral body, just inferior to the uncinate process of C7. Particular care must be taken when performing stellate ganglion block at the C7 level. The needle tip must remain aligned below the uncinate process or more medial to avoid the vertebral artery, which courses unprotected over the anterior surface of the C7 transverse process in many individuals. Radiographic contrast (1.5 mL of iohexol 180 mg/mL) has been injected, followed by 10 mL of 0.25% bupivacaine, and spreads along the anterolateral surface of C6 to T2. (**d**) Labeled image (Rathmell 2006)

2.6.5 Indications

The following are common indications for stellate ganglion block:

- Sympathetically maintained pain syndromes (reflex sympathetic dystrophy or complex regional pain syndrome) (Schweitzer et al. 1995)
- Vascular disease**
- Raynaud's disease**

- Raynaud's phenomenon**
- Frost bite
- Vasospasm**
- Occlusive vascular disease**
- Embolic vascular disease**
- Scleroderma**
- Chronic pain syndromes involving the upper limb, thoracic structures, and head and neck.
- Phantom limb pain
- Paget's disease**

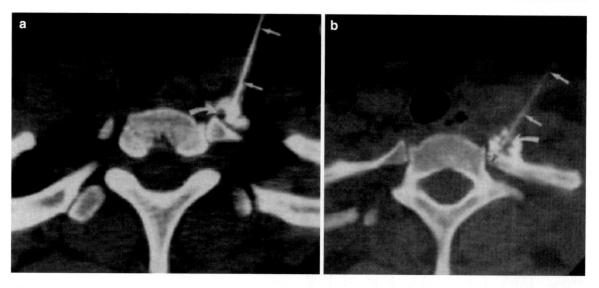

Fig. 2.46 CT-guided stellate ganglion injections in a 32-year-old-woman. (**a**) CT image shows needles (*straight arrows*) and high-attenuation contrast material surrounding the stellate ganglion (*curved arrow*). (**b**) CT image shows the entire course of the needle (*straight solid arrows*), with its tip (*open arrow*) residing on the head of the first rib. Contrast material surrounds the stellate ganglion (*curved arrow*) (Erickson and Hogan 1993)

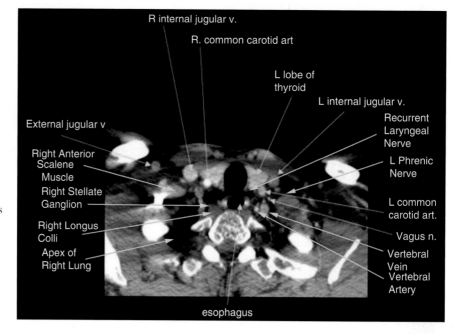

Fig. 2.47 CT showing important anatomic structures at the level of the stellate ganglion block. Similar anatomy is also encountered with brachial plexus block (modified from [http://www.urmc.rochester.edu/smd/Rad/neuroanatomy/neck_anatomy.htm])

- Neoplastic disorders
- Postradiation neuritis**
- Diabetic neuropathy
- Pain from cranial nerve disorders (tic douloureux, Bell's palsy)**

- Postherpetic neuralgia/acute herpes zoster**
- Severe refractory angina** (Chester et al. 2000)
- Hyperhidrosis
- Ménière's syndrome** (Valvassori and Dobben 1984)
- Vascular headaches

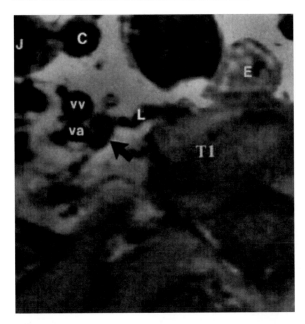

Fig. 2.48 Axial TI-weighted MR image of a 42-year-old woman shows ovoid stellate ganglion (*arrow*) reaching cephalad beyond the first rib. *C* common carotid artery; *J* internal Jugular vein; *vv* vertebral vein; *va* vertebral artery; *L* longus coli; *E* esophagus; *T1* T1 vertebral body (Hogan and Erickson 1992)

2.6.6 Contraindications

Contraindications of stellate ganglion block include myocardial infarction,** bradycardia, glaucoma, contralateral pneumothorax** or compromised function or absence of the contralateral lung.**

2.6.7 Complications (Neal et al. 2007)

The following are uncommon complications of stellate ganglion block:

- Recurrent laryngeal and phrenic nerve block**
- Brachial plexus blockade
- Pneumothorax**
- Generalized seizure
- Total spinal anesthesia
- Severe hypotension
- Transient locked-in syndrome
- Paratracheal hematoma**
- Vertebral artery injection causing dissection/thrombosis or infarction** (Makiuchi et al. 1993) (see Fig. 2.52)

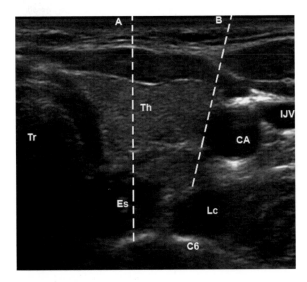

Fig. 2.49 Ultrasound imaging of the left stellate ganglion. *A* the needle path with the anterior paratracheal approach (with fluoroscopic guidance). *B* the needle path with ultrasound guidance. *Tr* trachea; *Es* esophagus; *Th* thyroid; *Lc* longus coli muscle; *CA* carotid artery; *IJV* internal jugular vein. (Reprinted with permission from the Cleveland Clinic Foundation (Narouze et al. 2007))

2.7 Brachial Plexus Block: For Brachial Plexopathy

2.7.1 Anatomy

The brachial plexus is a complex system of nerves, which originates from the C4 through T1 nerve roots. The brachial plexus then travels through the neck between the anterior and middle scalene muscles posterior to the clavicle and cephalad to the first rib next to the subclavian artery, through the axilla into the arm (Figs. 2.53 and 2.54).

2.7.2 Function

The brachial plexus innervates all skin sensation and motor supply to the upper extremity except for the trapezius and the skin adjacent to the axilla (supplied by the intercostobrachialis nerve).

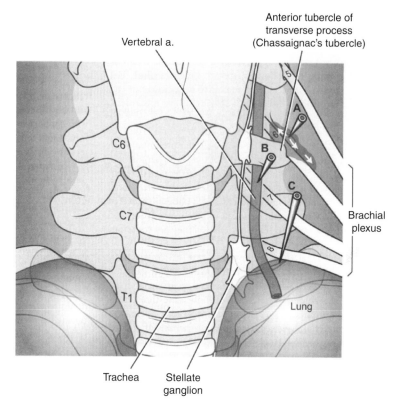

Fig. 2.50 Complications of stellate ganglion block. The stellate ganglion conveys sympathetic fibers to and from the upper extremities and the head and neck. The ganglion is comprised of the fused superior thoracic ganglion and the inferior cervical ganglion and is named for its fusiform shape (in many individuals, the two ganglia remain separate). The stellate ganglia lie over the head of the first rib at the junction of the transverse process and uncinate process of T1. The ganglion is just posteromedial to the cupola of the lung and medial to the vertebral artery, and these are the two most vulnerable structures. Stellate ganglion block is typically carried out at the C6 or C7 level to avoid pneumothorax, and a volume of solution that will spread along the prevertebral fascia inferiorly to the stellate ganglion is employed (usually 10 mL). When radiographic guidance is not used, the operator palpates the anterior tubercle and the transverse process of C6 (Chassaignac's tubercle), and a needle is seated in the location. With radiographic guidance, it is simpler and safer to place a needle over the vertebral body just inferior to the uncinate process of C6 or C7. Incorrect needle placement can lead to: *A* spread of the injectate adjacent to the spinal nerves where they join to form the brachial plexus; *B* damage to the vertebral artery or intra-arterial injection; or *C* pneumothorax. Local anesthetic can also course proximally along the spinal nerves to the epidural space (Rathmell 2006)

2.7.3 Clinical Presentation

Brachial plexopathy presents as pain and decreased sensation in the upper extremity and shoulder as well as weakness.

2.7.4 Etiology

Etiologies include trauma,** stretching injury, tumor,** radiation therapy, birth defects, toxins, drugs, thoracic outlet syndrome,** and acute idiopathic/viral plexitis** as well as autoimmune plexitis.**

2.7.5 Differential Diagnosis

Differential diagnoses include adhesive capsulitis,** amyotrophic lateral sclerosis,** cervical radiculopathy,** herniated nucleus pulposus,** and spondylosis,** polymyalgia rheumatica, rotator cuff disease,** and thoracic outlet syndrome.**

2.7.6 Injection Site

Supraclavicular, infraclavicular, axillary, and interscalene (Fig. 2.53) approaches are used. The axillary approach is described in the upper extremity nerve section.

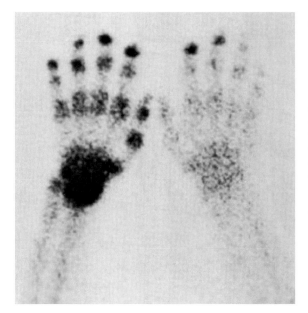

Fig. 2.51 A patient with RSDS shows the typical pattern of increased periarticular activity in the affected hand. Two distal interphalangeal joints on the opposite hand show increased activity at the sites of osteoarthritis (Kozin et al. 1981)

2.7.7 Cross-Sectional Anatomy: Interscalene Approach

2.7.7.1 What Does the Needle Traverse?

The needle enters the skin and traverses the platysma. It then crosses the sternocleidomastoid muscle, which is surrounded by the superficial layer of the deep cervical fascia. The needle then penetrates the deep layer of the deep cervical fascia surrounding the anterior scalene muscle. It then traverses the anterior scalene muscle to the target point between the anterior and middle scalene muscle (Fig. 2.55).

2.7.7.2 Which Structures the Needle Should Avoid

It is advisable that the needle avoid the following structures: phrenic nerve, recurrent laryngeal nerve, pneumothorax (lung apex), and central neuroaxial structures (see Fig. 2.47 for relevant anatomy).

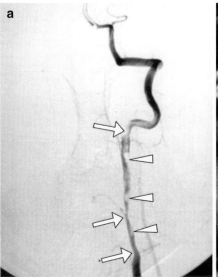

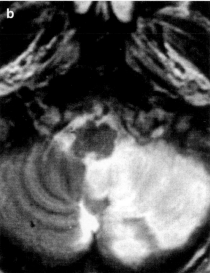

Fig. 2.52 Irregular stenosis with multiple filling defects involving the left VA in a 37-year-old man with dizziness and ataxia (patient 17). (**a**) Anteroposterior left vertebral angiogram shows an irregular long segmental stenosis (*arrows*) and multiple filling defects (*arrowheads*) in left V2, which represent intramural or intraluminal thrombi. The left posterior inferior cerebellar artery was occluded on later angiograms. (**b**) Axial T2-weighted MR image shows regions of high signal intensity, which represent multiple infarcts. The infarcts involve the territory of the left posterior inferior cerebellar artery and middle cerebellar peduncle, an appearance that suggests the embolic nature of the infarction (Shin et al. 2000)

Fig. 2.53 Needle placement for interscalene brachial plexus block. Lateral view of patient lying supine with head to the left. (Waldman 2001c)

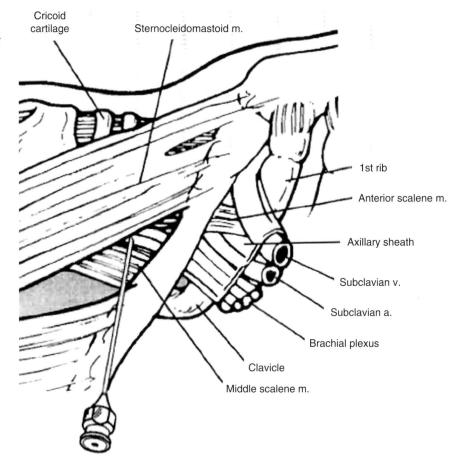

Cricoid cartilage

Sternocleidomastoid m.

1st rib

Anterior scalene m.

Axillary sheath

Subclavian v.

Subclavian a.

Brachial plexus

Clavicle

Middle scalene m.

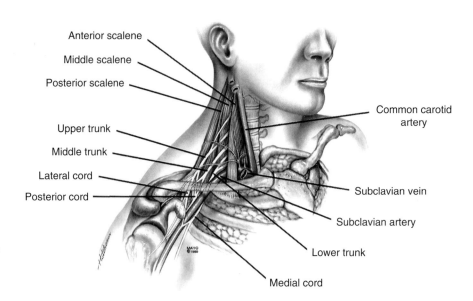

Anterior scalene

Middle scalene

Posterior scalene

Upper trunk

Middle trunk

Lateral cord

Posterior cord

Common carotid artery

Subclavian vein

Subclavian artery

Lower trunk

Medial cord

Fig. 2.54 Normal anatomy of the brachial plexus (Wittenberg and Adkins 2000)

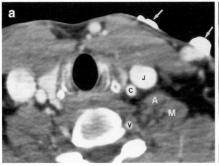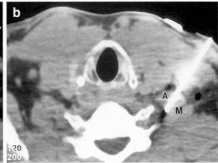

Fig. 2.55 Brachial plexus block to treat a left C7 mononeuropathy. (**a**) Transverse contrast-enhanced CT scan, obtained after the skin over the brachial plexus was marked with barium paste (*arrows*), was acquired to help identify the locations of the common carotid artery (*C*), internal jugular vein (*J*), and vertebral artery (*V*). *A* anterior scalene muscle; *M* middle scalene muscle (Mukherji et al. 2000). (**b**) Transverse CT scan demonstrates the tip of the needle inserted within the plane separating the anterior (*A*) and middle (*M*) scalene muscles (Mukherji et al. 2000)

2.7.8 Imaging/Radiology

Plain film radiographs: Plain films are useful to rule out shoulder impingement syndrome. Chest radiographs are useful to evaluate for sarcoidosis, granulomatous disease, and Pancoast tumor. Cervical ribs may also be excluded.

Image guidance: Although palpable anatomic landmarks may be used for guidance, image guidance may be useful in patients with short thick necks, prior history of surgery or radiation (Mukherji et al. 2000).

Fluoroscopy is the method most commonly used.

CT is safe (avoidance of pneumothorax and neurovascular structures) and can be useful for obese patients and patients with altered anatomy (i.e., neoplastic invasion) (Fig. 2.55). It is capable of imaging thin slices with 2D coronal and sagittal reconstruction. CT myelography may be useful in preganglionic injury evaluation.

Ultrasound can be useful to provide guidance for brachial plexus block. It is helpful with adjunctive color Doppler in altered vascular anatomy/vascular pathology (AVM) and coagulopathy. However, it is limited in neoplastic invasion. It is not able to document spread of contrast solution prior to injection as in CT or fluoroscopy.

MRI excludes cervical radiculopathy within the cervical spine. Furthermore, MRI of the brachial plexus is useful to evaluate for carcinoma or granulomatous disease. It can directly evaluate the brachial plexus for the signal intensity of its nerves, enhancement, and perineural pathology (masses) (Figs. 2.56–2.57). MRI (brachial plexus and cervical spine) is the study of choice in visualizing preganglionic and postganglionic injury to the brachial plexus. MR myelography may be useful in preganglionic evaluation.

2.7.9 Indications

The following are common indications for brachial plexus block: Preoperative analgesia, postsurgical pain, and brachial plexopathy.**

2.7.10 Complications

The five main complications of brachial plexus block are: (1) Intravascular injection of the subclavian artery **; (2) phrenic nerve block**; (3) recurrent laryngeal nerve paralysis** (Fig. 2.58); (4) pneumothorax**; (5) epidural, subdural, and subarachnoid spread of anesthetic**.

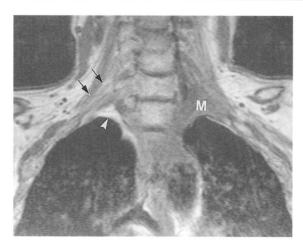

Fig. 2.56 Brachial plexus block for pain relief for recurrent Pancoast tumor. Note the normal appearance of the apical fat (*arrowhead*) and brachial plexus (*arrows*). *M* a mass situated in the apex of the left lung (Mukherji et al. 2000)

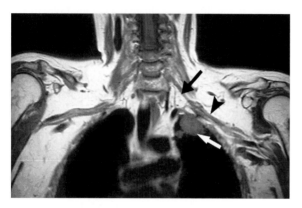

Fig. 2.57 Small left Pancoast's tumor in a 60-year-old woman. Coronal T1-weighted image shows small bilobed mass (*white arrow*) in left lung apex. Note preservation of normal interscalene fat pad (*black arrow*), which on coronal images has triangular appearance. Left brachial plexus (*arrowhead*) is nicely seen "Pancoast's tumor" is a term used to describe a bronchogenic neoplasia that arises in the apical pleuropulmonary groove (the superior sulcus); most are nonsmall cell cancers (squamous cell carcinomas, adenocarcinomas, or large cell carcinomas). They generally progress by direct extension and invasion of the brachial plexus, intercostal nerves, stellate ganglion, neighboring ribs, and vertebrae. Involvement of the brachial plexus and of the adjacent vertebrae is seen in fairly advanced cases. Supraclavicular lymphadenopathy denotes an N3 stage (according to the TNM classification) and also represents an advanced stage of the disease. Perhaps the earliest sign of extrathoracic and brachial plexus involvement is invasion of the interscalene fat pad by the tumor. This fat pad normally lies between the anterior and the middle posterior scalene muscles just cephalad to the lung apex. The trunks of the brachial plexus are found in this fat pad. On coronal T1-weighted MR images, the interscalene fat pads have a triangular appearance and should always be present, bright in signal intensity, and bilaterally symmetric. Obliteration of this normal bright fat signal by a mass arising in a lung apex generally implies invasion of the brachial plexus, and surgical resection may no longer be feasible (Castillo 2005)

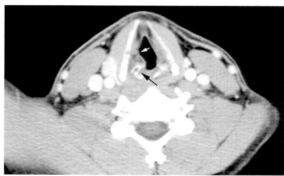

Fig. 2.58 A 45-year-old woman with hoarseness and right recurrent laryngeal nerve paralysis who underwent axial contrast-enhanced CT. The *white arrow* shows dilatation of the right laryngeal ventricle. The *black arrow* shows anterior positioning of the right arytenoid cartilage (Chin et al. 2003)

2.7.11 Contraindications

The contraindications to brachial plexus block are prior neck surgery,** radiation,** phrenic nerve palsy,** recurrent laryngeal nerve palsy on the contralateral side** and advanced COPD.** Altered thoracic anatomy** or clavicle deformity** may be a contraindication for the infraclavicular approach.

References

American College of Radiology. ACR Practice Guideline for the Performance of Computed Tomography (CT) of the Extracranial Head and Neck in Adults and Children. Reston: American College of Radiology. Revised 10/1/06

American College of Radiology. American College of Radiology Practice Guideline for the Performance of Magnetic Resonance Imaging (MRI) of the Head and Neck. Reston: American College of Radiology. Revised 10/1/07

American head and Neck Society. Management of Cancer of the Head and Neck Imaging: GeneralGuidelines. Los Angeles: American head and Neck Society. http://www.headandneck-cancer.org/clinicalresources/docs/imaginggeneral.php

Coleman RE. PET Refining Head and Neck Cancer Management. http://www.medscape.com/viewarticle/439654

Raj PP, Lou L, Erdine S et al. Radiographic Imaging for Regional Anesthesia and Pain Management New York: Churchill Livingstone, c2003. ISBN 0-443-06596-9

Harnsberger R, Macdonald AJ. Diagnostic and Surgical Imaging Anatomy. Brain, Head & Neck, Spine, 1st ed. Salt Lake City: Amirsys, 2006. NLM ID: 101266773, I-380, I-383, I-384

Harnsberger R, Macdonald AJ. Diagnostic and Surgical Imaging Anatomy. Brain, Head & Neck, Spine, 1st ed. Salt Lake City: Amirsys, 2006. NLM ID: 101266773, I-218, I-266

Harnsberger R, Macdonald AJ. Diagnostic and Surgical Imaging Anatomy. Brain, Head & Neck, Spine, 1st ed. Salt Lake City: Amirsys, 2006. NLM ID: 101266773, II-118-123

Vallejo R, Benyamin R, Yousuf N, Kramer J. Computed tomography-enhanced sphenopalatine ganglion blockade. Pain Pract. 2007;7(1):44-6

Gupta S, Henningsen JA, Wallace MJ, Madoff DC, Morello FA Jr, Ahrar K, Murthy R, Hicks ME. Percutaneous biopsy of head and neck lesions with CT guidance: various approaches and relevant anatomic and technical considerations. Radiographics. 2007;27(2):371-90

Weissman JL. A pain in the ear: the radiology of otalgia. AJNR Am J Neuroradiol. 1997;18:1641-51

Varghese BT, Koshy RC, Sebastian P, Joseph E. Combined sphenopalatine ganglion and mandibular nerve, neurolytic block for pain due to advanced head and neck cancer. Palliat Med. 2002;16(5):447-8

Saade E, Paige GB. Patient-administered sphenopalatine ganglion block. Reg Anesth. 1996;21(1):68-70

Sargeant LK. Headache, Cluster. 2007. http://www.emedicine.com/EMERG/topic229.htm

Mendizabal J. Cluster Headache. 2005. http://www.ouch-us.org/chgeneral/choverview.htm

Tien RD, Felsberg GJ, Osumi AK. Herpes virus infections of the CNS: MR findings. Am J Roentgenol. 1993;161:167-76

Varghese BT, Koshy RC. Endoscopic transnasal neurolytic sphenopalatine ganglion block for head and neck cancer pain. J Laryngol Otol. 2001;115(5):385-7

Ginsberg LE, DeMonte F. Imaging of perineural tumor spread from palatal carcinoma. AJNR Am J Neuroradiol. 1998;19:1417-22

Walker AT, Chaloupka JC, Putman CM, Abrahams JJ, Ross DA. Sentinel transoral hemorrhage from a pseudoaneurysm of the internal maxillary artery: a complication of CT-guided biopsy of the masticator space. AJNR Am J Neuroradiol. 1996;17(2):377-81

Waldman SD. Interventional Pain Management, 2nd ed. Philadelphia: Saunders, 2001a. NLM ID: 100959973

Okuda Y, Okuda K, Shinohara M, Kitajima T. Use of computed tomography for maxillary nerve block in the treatment of trigeminal neuralgia. Reg Anesth Pain Med. 2000;25(4):417-9

Koizuka S, Saito S, Kubo K, Tomioka A, Takazawa T, Sakurazawa S, Goto F. Percutaneous radio-frequency mandibular nerve rhizotomy guided by CT fluoroscopy. AJNR Am J Neuroradiol. 2006;27(8):1647-8

Barakos JA, Dillon WP, Chew WM. Orbit, skull base, and pharynx: contrast-enhanced fat suppression MR imaging. Radiology. 1991;179(1):191-8

Yousem DM, Gad K, Tufano RP. Resectability issues with head and neck cancer. AJNR Am J Neuroradiol. 2006;27(10):2024-36

Kamel HA, Toland J. Trigeminal nerve anatomy: illustrated using examples of abnormalities. AJR Am J Roentgenol. 2001;176(1):247-51

Sekimoto K, Koizuka S, Saito S, Goto F. Thermogangliolysis of the Gasserian ganglion under computed tomography fluoroscopy. J Anesth. 2005;19(2):177-9

Krol G, Arbit E. Percutaneous electrocoagulation of the trigeminal nerve using CT guidance. Technical note. J Neurosurg. 1988;68(6):972-3

Kaplan M, Erol FS, Ozveren MF, Topsakal C, Sam B, Tekdemir I. Review of complications due to foramen ovale puncture. J Clin Neurosci. 2007;14(6):563-8. Epub 2006 Dec 13

Horiguchi J, Ishifuro M, Fukuda H, Akiyama Y, Ito K. Multiplanar reformat and volume rendering of a multidetector CT scan for path planning a fluoroscopic procedure on Gasserian ganglion block-a preliminary report. Eur J Radiol. 2005;53(2):189-91

Yousry I, Moriggl B, Schmid UD, Naidich TP, Yousry TA. Trigeminal ganglion and its divisions: detailed anatomic MR imaging with contrast-enhanced 3D constructive interference in the steady state sequences. AJNR Am J Neuroradiol. 2005;26:1128–35

Williams LS, Schmalfuss IM, Sistrom CL, Inoue T, Tanaka R, Seoane ER, Mancuso AA. MR imaging of the trigeminal ganglion, nerve, and the perineural vascular plexus: normal appearance and variants with correlation to cadaver specimens AJNR Am J Neuroradiol. 2003;24:1317–24

Yoshino N, Akimoto H, Yamada I, Nagaoka T, Tetsumura A, Kurabayashi T, Honda E, Nakamura S, Sasaki T. Trigeminal neuralgia: evaluation of neuralgic manifestation and site of neurovascular compression with 3D CISS MR imaging and MR angiography. Radiology. 2003;228(2):539-45. Epub 2003 Jun 11

Ward L, Khan M, Greig M, Dolin SJ. Meningitis after percutaneous radiofrequency trigeminal ganglion lesion. Case report and review of literature. Pain Med. 2007;8(6):535-8

James EA, Kibbler CC, Gillespie SH. Meningitis due to oral streptococci following percutaneous glycerol rhizotomy of the trigeminal ganglion. J Infect. 1995;31(1):55-7

Weiss LD. Easy Injections. Philadelphia: Elsevier, 2007. NLM ID: 101308328, p 112, Figure 6-5

Kapoor V, Rothfus WE, Grahovac SZ, Amin Kassam SZ, Horowitz MB. Refractory occipital neuralgia: preoperative assessment with CT-guided nerve block prior to dorsal cervical rhizotomy. AJNR Am J Neuroradiol. 2003;24(10):2105-10

Curatolo M, Eichenberger U. Ultrasound-guided blocks for the treatment of chronic pain. Tech Reg Anesth Pain Manag. 2007;11:95-102

Kroft LJ, Reijnierse M, Kloppenburg M, Verbist BM, Bloem JL, van Buchem MA. Rheumatoid arthritis: epidural enhancement as an underestimated cause of subaxial cervical spinal stenosis. Radiology. 2004;231(1):57-63. Epub 2004 Feb 27

Hofkes SK, Iskandar BJ, Turski PA, Gentry LR, McCue JB, Haughton VM. Differentiation between symptomatic Chiari I malformation and asymptomatic tonsillar ectopia by using cerebrospinal fluid flow imaging: initial estimate of imaging accuracy. Radiology. 2007;245(2):532-40. Epub 2007 Sep 21

Silva JA, Holanda MM, Pereira CB, Leiros Mdo D, Araújo AF, Bandeira E. Retropulsion and vertigo in the Chiari malformation: case report. Arq Neuropsiquiatr. 2005;63(3B):870-3. Epub 2005 Oct 18. Erratum in: Arq Neuropsiquiatr. 2005;63(4):1120

Brown DLL. Atlas of Regional Anesthesia. Philadelphia: WB Saunders, 1992, pp 165-170

Carron H: Cervical plexus blocks. In Regional Anesthesia: Techniques and Clinical Applications. New York, Grune and Stratton, 1984, pp 10-15.

Winnie AP, Ramamurthy S, Durrani Z, Radonjic R. Intrascalene cervical plexus block: a single-injection technique. Anesth Analg. 1975;54:370-375

Gupta S, Henningsen JA, Wallace MJ, Madoff DC, Morello FA Jr, Ahrar K, Murthy R, Hicks ME. Percutaneous biopsy of head and neck lesions with CT guidance: various approaches and relevant anatomic and technical considerations. Radiographics. 2007;27(2):371-90

Waldman SD. Interventional Pain Management, 2nd ed. Philadelphia: Saunders, 2001b. NLM ID: 100959973, p 356

Jacobsen AS, Urken ML, Teng MS. Head and Neck Diagnostic Procedures from ACS Surgery: Principles and Practice. 2006. http://www.medscape.com/viewarticle/521712_8

Hermans R, Pameijer FA, Mancuso AA, Parsons JT, Mendenhall WM. Laryngeal or hypopharyngeal squamous cell carcinoma: can follow-up CT after definitive radiation therapy be used to detect local failure earlier than clinical examination alone? Radiology. 2000;214:683

Smoker WR, Harnsberger HR. Differential diagnosis of head and neck lesions based on their space of origin. 2. The infrahyoid portion of the neck. AJR Am J Roentgenol. 1991;157(1):155-9

Holliday RA, Swartz JD, Hudgins PA, Dalley RW, Curtin HD, Reede DL, Smoker WR. Head and neck radiology. Radiology. 1995;194(2):613-6

Parker GD, Harnsberger HR. Radiologic evaluation of the normal and diseased posterior cervical space. AJR Am J Roentgenol. 1991;157(1):161-5

Rathmell JP. Atlas of image-guided intervention in regional anesthesia and pain medicine. Philadelphia: Lippincott Williams & Wilkins, 2006

Erickson SJ, Hogan QH. CT-guided injection of the stellate ganglion: description of technique and efficacy of sympathetic blockade. Radiology. 1993;188(3):707-9

Hogan QH, Erickson SJ. MR imaging of the stellate ganglion: normal appearance. AJR Am J Roentgenol. 1992;158(3):655-9. Erratum in: AJR Am J Roentgenol 1992;158(6):1320

Narouze S, Vydyanathan A, Patel N. Ultrasound-guided stellate ganglion block successfully prevented esophageal puncture. Pain Phys. 2007;10(6):747-52

Kozin F, Soin JS, Ryan LM, Carrera GF, Wortmann RL. Bone scintigraphy in the reflex sympathetic dystrophy syndrome. Radiology. 1981;138(2):437-43

Schweitzer ME, Mandel S, Schwartzman RJ, Knobler RL, Tahmoush AJ. Reflex sympathetic dystrophy revisited: MR imaging findings before and after infusion of contrast material. Radiology. 1995;195(1):211-4

Chester M, Hammond C, Leach A. Long-term benefits of stellate ganglion block in severe chronic refractory angina. Pain. 2000;87(1):103-5

Valvassori GE, Dobben GD. Multidirectional and computerized tomography of the vestibular aqueduct in Meniere's disease. Ann Otol Rhinol Laryngol. 1984;93(6 pt 1):547-50

Neal JM, Rathmell JP. Complications in regional anesthesia and pain medicine. Philadelphia, PA: Saunders/Elsevier, 2007

Makiuchi T, Kondo T, Yamakawa K, Shinoura N, Yatsushiro K, Ichi S, Yoshioka M. [Stellate ganglion blocks as the suspected route of infection in a case of cervical epidural abscess]. No Shinkei Geka. 1993;21(9):805-8. Japanese

Shin JH, Suh DC, Choi CG, Leei HK. Vertebral artery dissection: spectrum of imaging findings with emphasis on angiography and correlation with clinical presentation. Radiographics. 2000;20(6):1687-96

Waldman SD. Interventional Pain Management, 2nd ed. Philadelphia: Saunders, 2001c. NLM ID: 100959973, p 383

Wittenberg KH, Adkins MC. MR imaging of nontraumatic brachial plexopathies: frequency and spectrum of findings. Radiographics. 2000;20(4):1023-32

Mukherji SK, Wagle A, Armao DM, Dogra S. Brachial plexus nerve block with CT guidance for regional pain management: initial results. Radiology. 2000;216(3):886-90

Castillo M. Imaging the anatomy of the brachial plexus: review and self-assessment module. Am J Roentgenol. 2005; 185:S196-204

Chin SC, Edelstein S, Chen CY, Som PM. Using CT to localize side and level of vocal cord paralysis. AJR Am J Roentgenol. 2003;180(4):1165-70

Fazekas F, Koch M, Schmidt R, Offenbacher H, Payer F, Freidl W, Lechner H. The prevalence of cerebral damage varies with migraine type: a MRI study. Headache. 1992;32(6):287-91

Diagnostic imaging modalities in the thorax demonstrate both strengths and weaknesses. Radiography may be helpful as an initial diagnostic test to exclude fractures and malignancy. CT, however, is the study of choice to exclude other causes of chest pain. Although not commonly indicated, MRI may be useful for cardiac and vascular (aortic) pathology.

3.1 Thoracic Sympathetic Ganglion Block (Fig. 3.1)

3.1.1 Anatomy

The thoracic sympathetic ganglia are located in the paravertebral region and are usually 12 in number on each side. They form the thoracic sympathetic trunk.

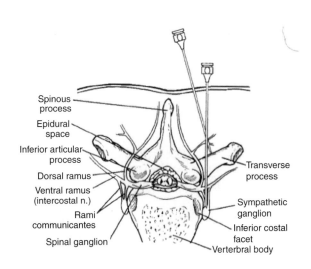

Spinous process
Epidural space
Inferior articular process
Dorsal ramus
Ventral ramus (intercostal n.)
Rami communicantes
Spinal ganglion
Transverse process
Sympathetic ganglion
Inferior costal facet
Verterbral body

Fig. 3.1 Needle placement for thoracic sympathetic ganglion block (Waldman 2001a)

The ganglion communicates with the intercostal spinal nerves via gray and white rami communicantes. The white rami contain preganglionic sympathetic fibers from the spinal cord, which travel into the sympathetic ganglion. The gray rami contain postganglionic sympathetic fibers from the sympathetic ganglion, which connects back to the spinal nerve. Other thoracic postganglionic fibers link with the sympathetic trunk inferiorly or superiorly or may travel to the celiac plexus (via the splanchnic nerves). The first thoracic ganglion fuses with the lower cervical ganglion in most cases to form the stellate ganglion. The thoracic splanchnic nerves (greater, lesser, and least splanchnic nerve) provide sympathetic innervation to the abdominal viscera.

3.1.2 Function

The thoracic sympathetic ganglia provide autonomic sympathetic function "fight or flight" response. They affect the cardiovascular system by increasing the heart rate and blood pressure as well as by constricting the blood vessels. They also enlarge the bronchi within the respiratory system. They decrease gut motility. There are responsible for pupil dilation, piloerection (goose bumps), sweating, etc. They are also responsible for heat, cold, or pain sensation in the afferent nerves. They also carry sympathetically mediated pain in the chest wall for cardiac angina as well as visceral pain.

3.1.3 Injection Site

At the level of the spinous process, a site is chosen 3 cm lateral to this. A posterior paravertebral approach is used to approach the transverse process at this site (Fig. 3.1). Once the transverse process is reached, the needle is redirected superiorly over the transverse process until there is loss-of-resistance or penetration of the superior costotransverse ligament. CT or fluoroscopic guidance may be utilized (Figs. 3.2–3.6).

3.1.4 Cross-Sectional Anatomy

3.1.4.1 What Does the Needle Traverse?

The needles traverses the following muscles: trapezius (midline), rhomboid (deep to trapezius, may be traversed in a more lateral approach), and the erector spinae (deep to trapezius, would be traversed in a more midline approach). It also passes above or inferior to the transverse process and to the anterior aspect of the rib head. The sympathetic ganglion lies in the paravertebral space (extrapleural) (Fig. 3.2).

3.1.4.2 Which Structures the Needle Should Avoid

Descending thoracic aorta: Avoid deviating from the paraspinal space and needle advance anterior to vertebral body; CT guidance is helpful especially in the midthorax below the level of the aortic arch.

Esophagus: Avoid needle advance anterior to and midline of vertebral body.

Thoracic spinal nerve roots: Avoid needle advance into neuroforamen medial to the pedicle. If paresthesia occurs in the distribution of the thoracic paravertebral nerve, the needle should be redirected slightly more cephalad.

Hemiazygous vein: Posterior to thoracic aorta on the left, T9–T12 vertebral body levels.

Accessory hemiazygous vein: Anterior to T4–T8 vertebral bodies on the left side.

Azygous vein: Ascends on the right side anterior to the T5–T12 vertebral bodies.

Intercostal artery, nerve and vein: Avoid needle adjacent to the inferior margin of the rib.

Lung: Avoid needle advance lateral to vertebral body margin (stay close to the vertebral body) (Fig. 3.2).

3.1.5 Imaging/Radiology

Fluoroscopy is the most commonly used technique. However, *CT* (Okuda et al. 2001) allows you to create a paraspinal window to avoid the pleural space (saline can be injected to push the pleura away from the vertebral body). Also, the double needle technique may be helpful to reduce needle insertions and repositionings. Galvanic skin response monitoring may be helpful in improving the accuracy of the block in cases of pleural adhesions (Uchino et al. 2007) (Figs. 3.3 and 3.5–3.6).

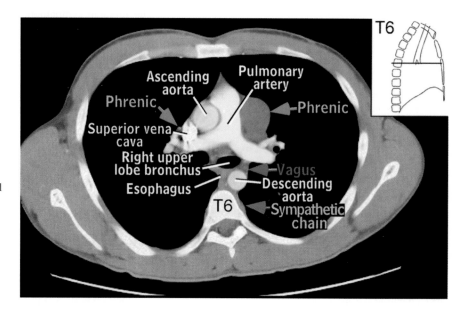

Fig. 3.2 Neurofibromatosis in an asymptomatic 28-year-old man. Serial axial CT scan obtained between the level of T6 and T9 demonstrates neurofibromas involving the phrenic and vagus nerves bilaterally, the sympathetic chain, and a right intercostal nerve (Aquino et al. 2001)

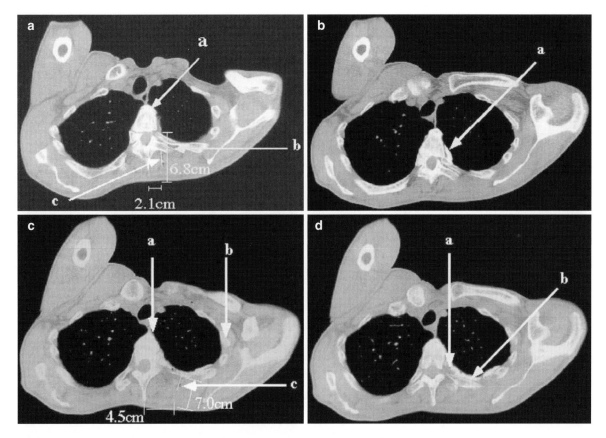

Fig. 3.3 (**a–d**) Procedures for (CT)-guided thoracic sympathetic blockade. (**a**) A needle was inserted until it touched the transverse process. *a* Second thoracic vertebral body; *b* transverse process; *c* nerve block needle. (**b**) Distribution of contrast medium in compartment *a*. (**c**) Advance of needle into compartment. *a* Third thoracic vertebral body; *b* third rib; *c* nerve block needle. (**d**) Distribution of contrast medium in compartment. *a* Distribution of contrast medium; *b* suspected region of adhesion (Uchino et al. 2007)

3.1.6 Indications

The following are common indications for thoracic sympathetic block:

- Sympathetically mediated pain of the upper thorax chest wall, thoracic/upper abdominal viscera evaluation and management.
- With local anesthetics this method can be used as a diagnostic tool when performing differential neural blockade for the evaluation of chest, thoracic and upper abdominal pain. Useful prognosis for degree of pain relief.
- Intractable cardiac and abdominal angina.**
- Post-thoracotomy pain, acute herpes zoster, postherpetic neuralgia, and phantom breast pain after mastectomy (Fig. 3.7).

- Destruction of the thoracic sympathetic chain is indicated for palliation of pain syndromes that have responded to thoracic sympathetic pain blocks.
- Cancer of thoracic area with paraspinal invasion (Fig. 3.4).**

3.1.7 Complications

The four main complications of thoracic sympathetic block are: (1) pneumothorax**; (2) thoracic aorta puncture (hemorrhage)**; (3) azygous, hemiazygous vein puncture**; (4) epidural, subdural or subarachnoid injection and injury to the spinal cord** or exiting nerve roots.**

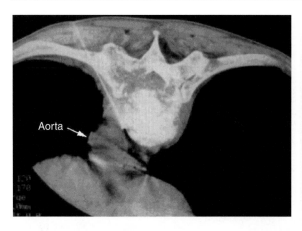

Fig. 3.4 Thoracic sympathetic block in a lung cancer patient with mediastinal and vertebral invasion. With the patient in a prone position, local anesthetic is injection into subcutaneous tissue and muscle and onto the periosteum. CT scan obtained after a few minutes shows the 22-guage needle placed just above the transverse process and the rib. The needle tip is positioned in front of the head of the rib between the vertebral periosteum and the parietal pleura. A solution of local anesthetic and contrast medium is then injected to confirm optimal position of the needle on a CT scan. Finally, 3 mL of ethanol is administered (Gangi et al. 1996)

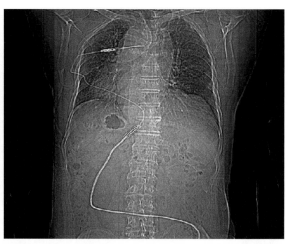

Fig. 3.6 CT coronal scout image showing placement of needle adjacent to the thoracic vertebra (Courtesy of Dr. Mingi Chan-Liao, Jen Ai Hospital)

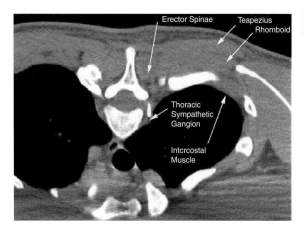

Fig. 3.5 Axial CT anatomy of thoracic sympathetic block. Note needle tip adjacent to thoracic sympathetic ganglion (www. pain-manage.org.tw/ray/ray23.pdf) (Courtesy of Dr. Mingi Chan-Liao, Jen Ai Hospital)

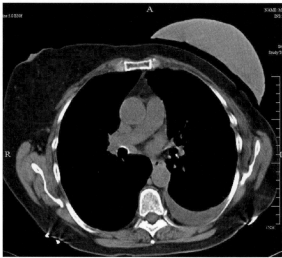

Fig. 3.7 CT of the thorax in a patient status post right mastectomy

3.2 Intercostal Nerve Block: For Intercostal Neuralgia (Figs. 3.8 and 3.9)

3.2.1 Anatomy

The intercostal nerves are formed by the anterior division of the thoracic nerves. Of the 12 nerves, 11 are called intercostal nerves since they lie between ribs (Fig. 3.8). The intercostal nerve communicates just beyond its origin with the sympathetic ganglion via gray and white rami communicantes. The intercostal nerve travels in the intercostal groove at the inferior ribcage adjacent to the artery and vein. The lateral cutaneous nerve arises at the lateral segment of the nerve. The anterior cutaneous nerve arises at the anterior tip of the nerve. The anterior cutaneous nerves may be entrapped as they enter the rectus sheath.

Fig. 3.8 Anatomy of the intercostal nerves. The thoracic nerve roots exit the spinal canal through the intervertebral foramina and divide into anterior and posterior primary rami. The anterior rami course laterally to enter a groove beneath the inferior margin of each rib, where they traverse laterally inferior to the intercostal vein and artery. The posterior cutaneous branch rises in a variable location along the course of the intercostal nerve but always anterior to the posterior axillary line (a line that extends directly inferior from the posterior fold of the axilla). Thus, intercostal nerve block should be carried out medial to the posterior axillary line to ensure the entire sensory distribution of the nerve is blocked. The *inset* shows the orientation of the diagram (Rathmell 2006)

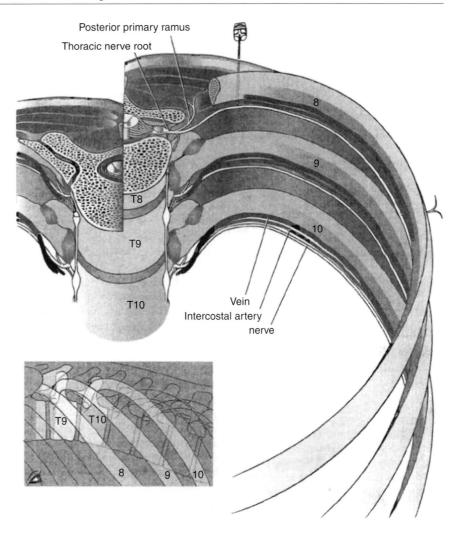

3.2.2 Function

The intercostal nerve supplies sensation to the chest wall including the parietal pleura. It also supplies sensation to the anterior abdominal wall via the anterior cutaneous nerves (T8–L1).

3.2.3 Clinical Presentation

Chest wall pain which worsens with respiration. The pain may follow around the chest or torso in a band-like pattern. Abdominal wall pain may be seen with abdominal cutaneous nerve entrapment syndrome (ACNES) which may otherwise be undiagnosed.

3.2.4 Etiology

(1) Trauma or surgery resulting in intercostal neuroma formation, (2) Herpes zoster, or (3) ACNES.

3.2.5 Injection Site

Fluoroscopy can be used to guide the needle. The images are obtained with roughly 15–20° of C-arm

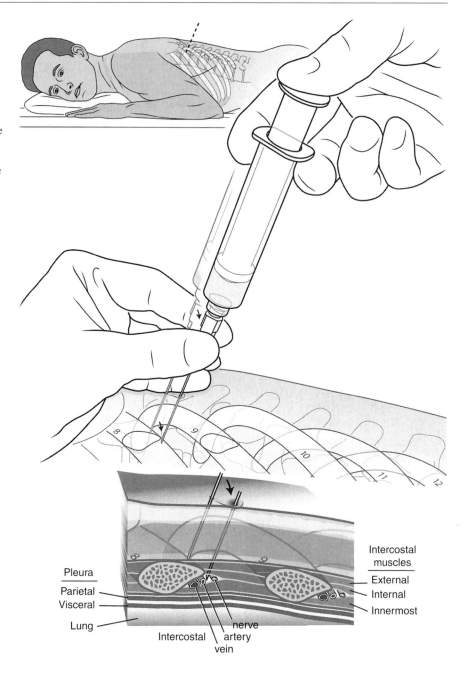

Fig. 3.9 Technique for intercostal nerve block. The needle is advanced with 15–20° of cephalad angulation and is first seated on the inferior margin of the rib. The needle is then walked off the inferior rib margin while maintaining the same cephalad angulation of the needle and advanced 2–3 mm to lie adjacent to the intercostal nerve. The intercostal nerve lies inferior to the intercostal vein and artery, between the internal and innermost intercostal muscles (Rathmell 2006)

caudal angulation centered over the hemithorax. This allows the needle to traverse the inferior margin of the rib in a caudal to cephalad direction. The needle is advanced to the inferior margin of the rib at or medial to the posterior axillary line. The needle is then "walked off" of the inferior rib edge and then advanced 2–3 mm anteriorly past the rib margin. The needle tip should now be adjacent to the intercostal nerves and injection can be performed (Fig. 3.9).

3.2.6 Cross-Sectional Anatomy

3.2.6.1 What Does the Needle Traverse?

It is usual for the needle to traverse the following structures: lumbodorsal fascia, muscle [trapezius, rhomboid, erector spinae (lateral margin)]; rib and just below rib; and intercostal muscle.

3.2.6.2 Which Structures the Needle Should Avoid

It is advisable that the needle avoid the intercostal artery and vein as well as the lung/pleura.

3.2.7 Imaging/Radiology

Fluoroscopy: Intercostal nerve blocks are usually done with palpation only. Fluoroscopy may be helpful in large body habitus patients or variant anatomy (kyphoscoliosis or postoperative) (Fig. 3.10).

CT: The pleural margin is well delineated with this method (Fig. 3.11).

Ultrasound: This technique enables direct real time visualization of the pleural space to avoid pneumothorax.

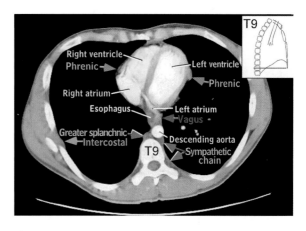

Fig. 3.11 Neurofibromatosis in an asymptomatic 28-year-old man. Serial axial CT scan demonstrates neurofibromas involving the phrenic and vagus nerves bilaterally, the sympathetic chain, and a right intercostal nerve (Aquino et al. 2001)

It may be useful in the midaxillary approach where the risk of pneumothorax is higher (Fig. 3.12).

3.2.8 Indications (Fig. 3.13)

The following are common indications for intercostal nerve block:

* Fractured Ribs,** chest wall contusion,** pleurisy** and flail chest**

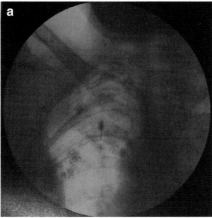

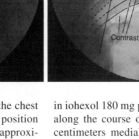

Fig. 3.10 a and **b**: Anterior-Posterior radiograph of the chest during fifth intercostal neurolysis. A. A needle is in position just inferior to the inferior margin of the fourth rib, approximately 5cm from midline. Three milliliters of radiographic contrast containing phenol have been injected (10% phenol in iohexol 180 mg per ml). The neurolytic solution has spread along the course of the intercostal nerve, extending several centimeters medial and lateral from the point of injection. B. Labeled image. Residual contrast is from previous injections

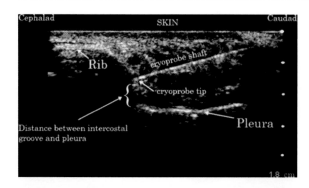

Fig. 3.12 The needle tip is visible and placed at the intercostal groove, within the internal intercostal muscle. In thin patients, the pleura is within 0.5 cm of the intercostal groove, showing how little movements may result in puncture into the pleural space. As cryoablation is initiated, a hyperechoic rim will appear around the probe, signifying the formation of the ice ball (Byas-Smith and Gulati 2006)

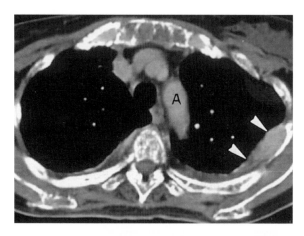

Fig. 3.13 Multiple myeloma in a 59-year-old man. Contrast-enhanced CT scan at the level of the aortic arch (*A*) shows multiple osteolytic lesions involving the sternum, vertebral body, scapulae, and ribs, and a soft-tissue mass (*arrowheads*) that originates from a left rib (Tateishi et al. 2003)

- Pain from median sternotomy,** pericardial window,** fractured sternum** (parasternal blocks)**
- Thoracotomy tubes,** percutaneous biliary drainage,** or liver biopsy**
- Postoperative pain of the chest or abdomen (appendectomy, right lateral intercostals blocks T10, T11, and T12**)
- Chronic pain: in combination or with celiac plexus block may be helpful in distinguishing abdominal wall pain from visceral pain.
- ACNES may be diagnosed and treated with local blocks of the anterior cutaneous nerves as they enter the rectus sheath

- Unilateral paravertebral T12 and L1 nerve block can distinguish nerve entrapment syndrome after inguinal hernia repair**
- Herpes zoster
- Cancer (Fig. 3.13)**

3.2.9 Contraindications

The four principal contraindications to intercostal nerve block are: (1) neurofibromatosis**; (2) Marfan's syndrome**; (3) coarctation of the aorta (Fig. 3.14)**; (4) severe scoliosis (may require image guidance).** Use the smallest needle gauge possible in the setting of respiratory compromise due to flail chest** or multiple rib fractures**.

3.2.10 Complications

Unique complications of intercostal nerve block include:

- Pneumothorax**
- Hypotension (high epidural or total spinal block with central spread of solution)
- Hypotension in ICU patients who are hypovolemic and vasoconstricted (analgesia releases

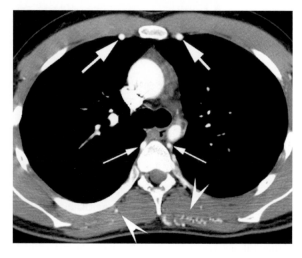

Fig. 3.14 Congenital aortic coarctation. Contrast-enhanced axial CT scan shows enlarged internal mammary arteries (*large arrows*), intercostal arteries (*small arrows*), and descending scapular arteries (*arrowheads*) (Sebastià et al. 2003)

the compensatory vasoconstriction which leads to hypotension)
- Respiratory failure (pain relief of the block unmasks the ventilatory depression of previously administered but ineffective narcotics)

3.3 Suprascapular Nerve Block (Fig. 3.15)

3.3.1 Anatomy

Suprascapular neuropathy results from impingement of the nerve at the suprascapular notch. As the nerve continues distally, it may be impinged at the spinoglenoid notch where it becomes the infraspinatus nerve. The suprascapular nerve is formed from the C4 through C6 nerve roots of the brachial plexus. It continues inferiorly and posteriorly below the coracoclavicular ligament through the scapular notch adjacent to the suprascapular artery and veins. The nerve continues posteriorly past the notch to the dorsal aspect of the scapula deep to the supraspinatus muscle. Here, it divides into the supraspinatus nerve and the infraspinatus nerve. The infraspinatus nerve travels within the spinoglenoid notch into the infraspinatus fossa (Fig. 3.15).

3.3.2 Function

The suprascapular nerve branches proximally into the supraspinatus nerve. This innervates the supraspinatus

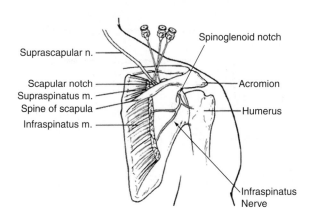

Fig. 3.15 Needle placement for suprascapular nerve block (Waldman 2001b)

Labels in figure:
Spinoglenoid notch
Suprascapular n.
Scapular notch
Supraspinatus m.
Spine of scapula
Infraspinatus m.
Acromion
Humerus
Infraspinatus Nerve

muscle and supplies sensation to the shoulder including the acromioclavicular and glenohumeral joints. The distal branch of the suprascapular nerve is the infraspinatus nerve, which innervates the infraspinatus muscles. It supplies sensation to the shoulder and scapula.

3.3.3 Clinical Presentation

Suprascapular neuropathy presents as nonspecific shoulder pain. It can be analogous to rotator cuff syndrome. In advanced cases, there may be associated atrophy of the supraspinatus and/or infraspinatus muscle.

3.3.4 Etiology

Etiologies include trauma,** scapular fracture,** surgery (rotator cuff surgery**), tumor (soft tissue** or osseous**), ganglion cyst,** or paralabral cyst** (associated with glenoid labrum tears** posteriorly), lipoma,** enlarged spinoglenoid vein**/varicosities,** repetitive overhead upper extremity movement (pitchers, painters, volleyball, weightlifters, and other athletes), congenitally small suprascapular or spinoglenoid notch.**

3.3.5 Differential Diagnosis

Rotator cuff pathology,** glenoid labral tear,** glenohumeral and acromioclavicular joint arthritis**/instability,** subacromial bursitis,** adhesive capsulitis,** bicipital tenosynovitis,** calcific tendonitis,** and cervical radiculopathy (HNP,** spondylosis**).

3.3.6 Injection Site

The scapular spine and acromion is identified and a puncture site is chosen approximately 5 cm medial to the lateral margin of the acromion. The needle is advanced using a posterior approach just above the scapular spine at this site. The needle is then "walked" to the suprascapular notch (Fig. 3.15).

3.3.7 Cross-Sectional Anatomy (Figs. 3.16–3.17)

3.3.7.1 What Does the Needle Traverse?

Using this technique, the needle traverses the supraspinatus muscle, the suprascapular notch, and the coracoclavicular ligament.

3.3.7.2 Which Structures the Needle Should Avoid

The needle should avoid the suprascapular artery and vein as well as the lung.

3.3.8 Imaging/Radiology

Radiography is useful in bone pathology.

Fluoroscopy may be used; however, the procedure is often performed with anatomic landmarks without fluoroscopy.

CT (Schneider-Kolsky et al. 2004; Shanahan et al. 2004) is rarely used for guidance. No improvement was observed in patient outcomes for guidance in randomized single blinded trial comparing it to the use of anatomic landmarks. It is useful for cross-sectional imaging of bone pathology and for the evaluation of fractures and tumors.

Ultrasound is used for guidance (has been described in a case report) (Harmon and Hearty 2007).

MRI is the modality of choice for diagnosis. It allows visualization of suprascapular nerve related muscle denervation (Figs. 3.18–3.19).

Suprascapular nerve entrapment: Paralabral cysts (Fig. 3.21) typically arise adjacent to a torn glenoid labrum. On MRI, they appear as well-defined, uni- or multiloculated, nonenhancing, fluid-filled masses. The cysts may extend into the suprascapular or spinoglenoid notches and compress the suprascapular nerve.

3.3.9 Indications

The following are common indications for suprascapular nerve block:

- Diagnostic tool in the evaluation of shoulder girdle and shoulder pain

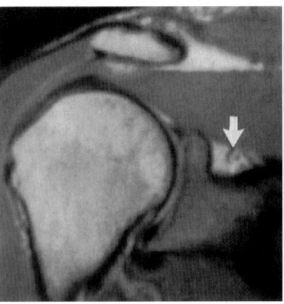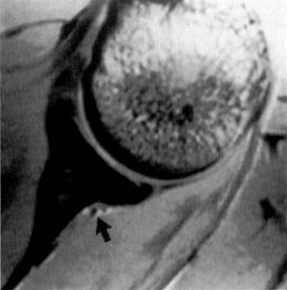

Fig. 3.16 *Left*, normal suprascapular nerve. Oblique coronal proton density-weighted SE MR image (2,000/20) shows suprascapular nerve (*arrow*) within scapular notch. *Right*, normal infraspinatus nerve. Axial gradient-echo MR image (400/20, 25° flip angle) shows infraspinatus nerve (*arrow*) below level of spinoglenoid ligament (Beltran and Rosenberg 1994)

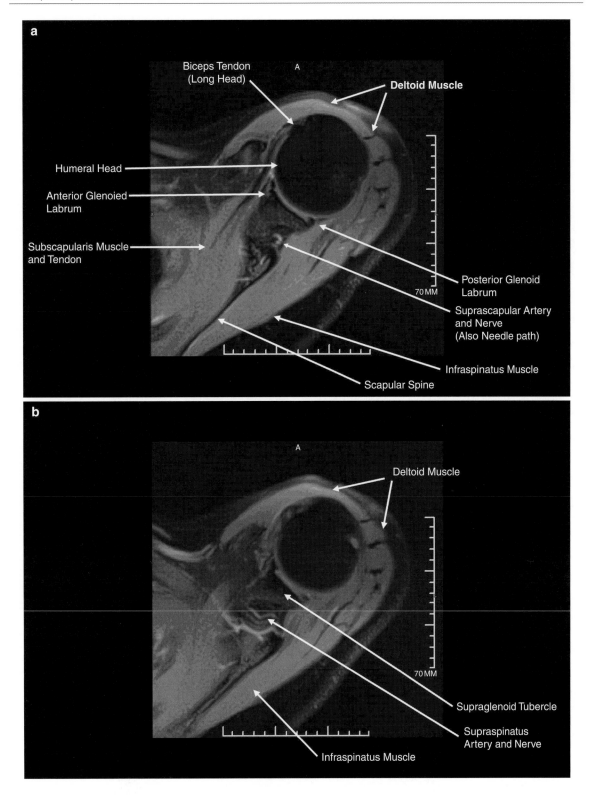

Fig. 3.17 (**a**, **b**) Proton density axial images of the scapula/shoulder depict relevant anatomy at the level of the suprascapular nerve. (Supraspinatus muscle not depicted as it is more cephalad)

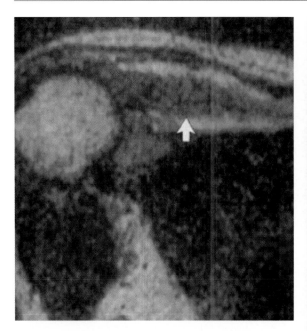

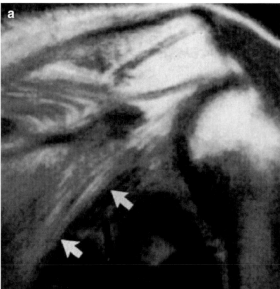

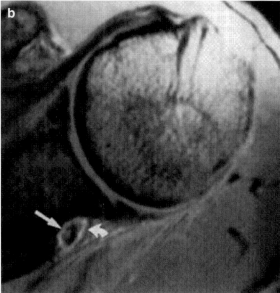

Fig. 3.18 Suprascapular nerve syndrome in a 30-year-old woman with nonspecific shoulder pain referred for MR to rule out rotator cuff tear. Oblique coronal T2-weighted SE MR image shows high signal intensity of supraspinatus muscle (*arrow*) compatible with denervation. Subsequent nerve conduction studies showed denervation. Cause of denervation could not be determined, but was presumed to be related to dynamic entrapment of suprascapular nerve (Beltran and Rosenberg 1994)

- Prognosis indicator of the degree of motor and sensory impairment prior to destruction of the brachial plexus
- Acute pain emergencies
  - Acute herpes zoster
  - Postoperative pain**
  - Cancer pain while waiting for chemotherapy, surgery, and XRT to take effect**
- Decreased motion of the shoulder secondary to RSD** (hand/shoulder variant) or adhesive capsulitis (Fig. 3.20)**
- Suprascapular nerve entrapment**
- Tolerate more aggressive physical therapy after shoulder reconstructive surgery** (adjunct to rehabilitation)
- Cancer pain including that of invasive tumors of the shoulder girdle**

Fig. 3.19 Suprascapular nerve syndrome in a 44-year-old man with shoulder pain. (**a**) Oblique coronal fast SE MR image shows atrophy and hyperintensity of infraspinatus muscle (*arrows*). (**b**) Axial gradient-echo MR image shows marked thickening of infraspinatus nerve (*straight arrow*) at level of spinoglenoid ligament (*curved arrow*). Atrophy was thought to be related to dynamic entrapment of infraspinatus nerve. Suprascapular nerve and its branches were released surgically, and the patient had significant clinical improvement (Beltran and Rosenberg 1994)

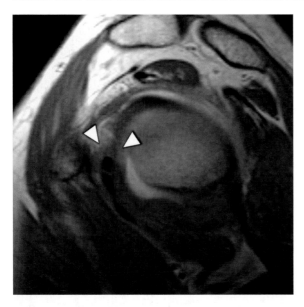

Fig. 3.20 Sagittal oblique T1-weighted (700/12) image shows synovitis-like abnormality (*arrowheads*) with blurred borders and intermediate signal intensity at the superior border of the subscapularis tendon in a 55-year-old patient with frozen shoulder (Mengiardi et al. 2004)

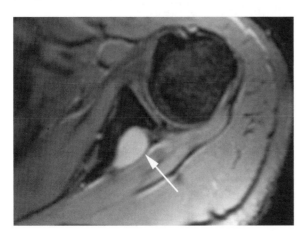

Fig. 3.21 A 20-year-old man with paralabral cyst. T2-weighted axial image reveals mass of fluid signal intensity (*arrow*) in suprascapular notch consistent with paralabral cyst (O'Connor et al. 2004)

3.3.10 Complications

The unique complication of suprascapular nerve block is pneumothorax.**

References

Waldman SD. Interventional Pain Management, Second Edition ISBN 0-7216-8748-2. Philadelphia: WB Saunders, 2001a, p. 400

Aquino SL, Duncan GR, Hayman LA. Nerves of the thorax: atlas of normal and pathologic findings. Radiographics. 2001;21:1275

Uchino H, Sasaki S, Miura H, Hirabayashi G, Nishiyama T, Ohta T, Ishii N, Ito T. Usefulness of galvanic skin reflex monitor in CT-guided thoracic sympathetic blockade for palmar hyperhidrosis. J Anesth. 2007;21(3):403-8. Epub 2007 Aug 1

Gangi A, Dietemann JL, Schultz A, Mortazavi R, Jeung MY, Roy C. Interventional radiologic procedures with CT guidance in cancer pain management. Radiographics. 1996;16(6): 1289-304; discussion 1304-6

Okuda Y, Yamaguchi S, Fujimaki K, Usui Y, Shinohara M, Kitajima T. Application of the double needle technique to CT-guided thoracic sympathetic and splanchnic plexus blocks. J Clin Anesth. 2001;13(5):398-400

Rathmell JP. Atlas of image-guided intervention in regional anesthesia and pain medicine. Philadelphia: Lippincott Williams and Wilkins, 2006

Byas-Smith MG, Gulati A. Ultrasound-guided intercostal nerve cryoablation. Anesth Analg. 2006;103(4):1033-5

Tateishi U, Gladish GW, Kusumoto M, Hasegawa T, Yokoyama R, Tsuchiya R, Moriyama N. Chest wall tumors: radiologic findings and pathologic correlation: part 2. Malignant tumors. Radiographics. 2003;23(6):1491-508

Sebastià C, Quiroga S, Boyé R, Perez-Lafuente M, Castellà E, Alvarez-Castells A. Aortic stenosis: spectrum of diseases depicted at multisection CT. Radiographics. 2003;23 Spec No:S79-91

Waldman SD. Interventional Pain Management, Second Edition ISBN 0-7216-8748-2. Philadelphia: WB Saunders, 2001b, p. 389

Beltran J, Rosenberg ZS. Diagnosis of compressive and entrapment neuropathies of the upper extremity: value of MR imaging. AJR Am J Roentgenol. 1994;163(3):525-31

Schneider-Kolsky ME, Pike J, Connell DA. CT-guided suprascapular nerve blocks: a pilot study. Skeletal Radiol. 2004;33(5):277-82. Epub 2004 Feb 10

Shanahan EM, Smith MD, Wetherall M, Lott CW, Slavotinek J, FitzGerald O, Ahern MJ. Suprascapular nerve block in chronic shoulder pain: are the radiologists better? Ann Rheum Dis. 2004;63(9):1035-40

Harmon D, Hearty C. Ultrasound-guided suprascapular nerve block technique. Pain Physician. 2007;10(6):743-6

Mengiardi B, Pfirrmann CW, Gerber C, Hodler J, Zanetti M. Frozen shoulder: MR arthrographic findings. Radiology. 2004;233(2):486-92. Epub 2004 Sep 9

O'Connor EE, Dixon LB, Peabody T, Stacy GS. MRI of cystic and soft-tissue masses of the shoulder joint. AJR Am J Roentgenol. 2004;183(1):39-47

Abdomen

4

4.1 Celiac Plexus Block and Splanchnic Nerve Block

4.1.1 Anatomy

The celiac plexus or solar plexus is an intricate meshwork of nerves in the abdomen. The celiac plexus lies inferior to the celiac artery at the L1 vertebral level. It may also be located at or above the superior mesenteric artery origin. It lies behind the stomach and omentum. It is also anterior to the crura of the diaphragm. It drapes anterolaterally over the aorta on both sides. The celiac plexus is composed of preganglionic splanchnic nerve endings, sensory fibers from the splenic nerve, preganglionic parasympathetic fibers from the vagus nerve, and postganglionic nerve fibers emanating into the viscera. The celiac plexus block would involve afferent nociceptive nerves fibers from most of the viscera of the abdomen (Figs. 4.1 and 4.2).

The origin of the neural supply of the celiac plexus is from the anterolateral horn of the spinal cord. Preganglionic nerve fibers from T5 to T12 exit the neuroforamen within the ventral rami of the spinal nerves. These preganglionic fibers then diverge to the white rami communicantes, which connect the spinal nerve to the sympathetic ganglion. These preganglionic fibers traverse through the sympathetic trunk, but do not synapse until they reach the celiac ganglia.

The celiac plexus therefore receives its preganglionic nerve supply from the greater, lesser, and least splanchnic nerves. The greater splanchnic nerve arises from the T5 through T10 nerve roots. It travels with the sympathetic trunk traversing the diaphragmatic crus to course into the abdomen where it terminates in the celiac ganglion. The lesser splanchnic nerve courses in a similar path, but originates from T10 to

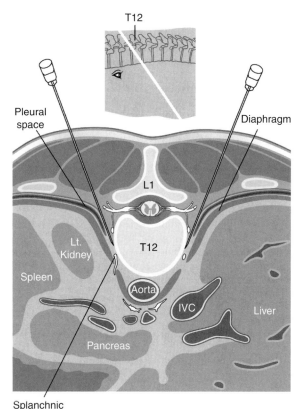

Fig. 4.1 Axial diagram of splanchnic nerve block. Two needles remain posterior to the crura of the diaphragm and are in final position over the anterolateral surface of the T12 vertebral body. The *inset* indicates the approximate plane of the needles (Rathmell 2006)

T11. The least splanchnic nerve originates from T12 and then penetrates the diaphragm to also end up in the celiac ganglion. A pure splanchnic nerve block may be performed for the preganglionic nerves. This may benefit a small group of patients, who are refractory to celiac plexus block.

M.I. Syed and A. Shaikh, *Radiology of Non-Spinal Pain Procedures*,
DOI: 10.1007/978-3-642-00481-0_4, © Springer-Verlag Berlin Heidelberg 2011

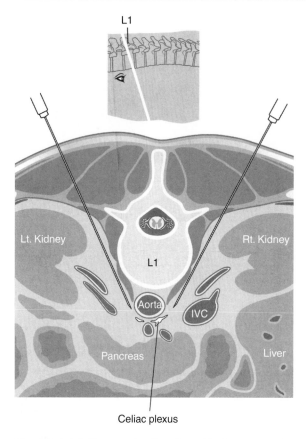

L1

Lt. Kidney

Rt. Kidney

L1

Aorta

IVC

Pancreas

Liver

Celiac plexus

Fig. 4.2 Axial diagram of celiac plexus block. Two needles pass through the crura of the diaphragm adjacent to the L1 vertebral body and are in final position over the anterolateral surface of the aorta. The *inset* indicates the approximate plane of the needles (Rathmell 2006)

The splanchnic nerves occupy a small space. They are bounded by the posterior mediastinum at the anterior aspect, the pleura laterally, the pleural connection to the vertebra posteriorly and the vertebral body medially. The crus of the diaphragm are positioned caudal to most of the course of these nerves, which in fact penetrate the crus.

4.1.2 Function

The celiac plexus and corresponding splanchnic nerves relay pain stimuli from the abdominal viscera including the pancreas, with the exception of the left colon, rectum, and pelvic organs.

4.1.3 Injection Site

A retrocrural approach is usually utilized. A posterolateral approach at the level of T12-L1 may be utilized. An anterior abdominal approach may be used as well as a transaortic and transdiscal posterior approach. Fluoroscopy, CT, or ultrasound guidance may be utilized (Figs. 4.3–4.7).

4.1.4 Cross-Sectional Anatomy Associated with the Needle Tract–Transaortic Approach

The cross-sectional anatomy associated with the needle tract (transaortic approach) is as follows: At the level of L1 the needle first traverses the subcutaneous tissue which has two layers the superficial fatty layer (Camper fascia) and the deep membranous layer (Scarpa fascia). The needle then penetrates the thoracolumbar fascia followed by the erector spinae musculature. Next the psoas muscle is traversed. The retroperitoneal space is then accessed; specifically the posterior pararenal space is traversed. The needle may next traverse the aorta to lie adjacent to the celiac plexus just above the origin of the celiac artery (this allows better spread of the neurolytic agent despite the location of the celiac ganglia just caudal to the origin of the celiac artery). Anterior to the celiac plexus is the superior mesenteric artery and vein. Anterior to this lies the pancreas.

4.1.4.1 Which Structures the Needle Should Avoid?

It is advisable that the needle avoid the artery of Adamkiewicz (major spinal cord feeder originating from the aorta, usually left-sided between level of T9 and L1 along the lateral margin of the vertebral body). In addition, the following structures should equally be avoided: Inferior vena cava; cisterna chyli; lung; kidney; lumbar plexus within the psoas muscle compartment; somatic nerve roots (contrast injection is helpful to make sure the needle tip is within the precrural space to minimize posterior spread in the retrocrural space towards the somatic nerve roots).

Fig. 4.3 Anterior–posterior radiograph of the spine during celiac plexus block. (**a**) A single needle has been inserted from the left oblique approach and is in final position over the anterolateral surface of the aorta. (**b**) Labeled image. The *white arrows* indicate the final needle position for splanchnic nerve block. (**c**) A single needle has been inserted from the left oblique approach and is in final position over the anterolateral surface of the aorta. Radiographic contrast (2 mL of iohexol 180 mg/mL) has been injected followed by 20 mL of 0.25% bupivacaine. The local anesthetic has diluted the contrast and extended the spread. A portion of the contrast spreads along the inferior border of the left hemidiaphragm. (**d**) Labeled image. The approximate position of the aorta is shown (Rathmell 2006)

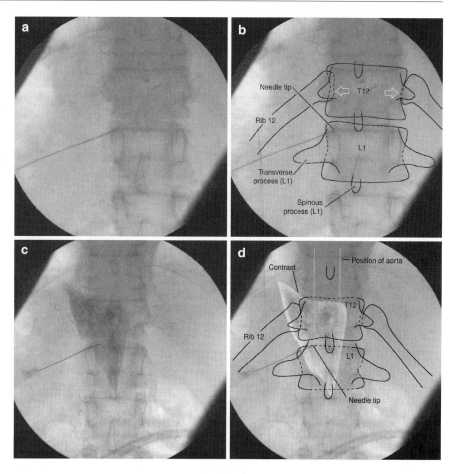

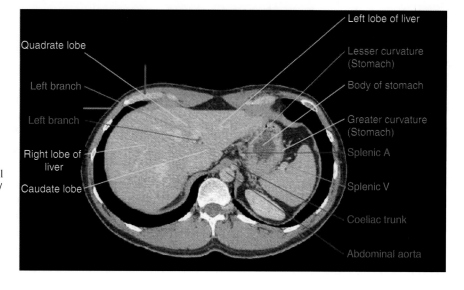

Fig. 4.4 CT anatomy at level of celiac plexus block (http://www.e-anatomy.org/anatomy/human-body/abdomen-pelvis/male-abdomen-ct.html) (courtesy of e-Anatomy - Micheau A, Hoa D,www.imaios.com)

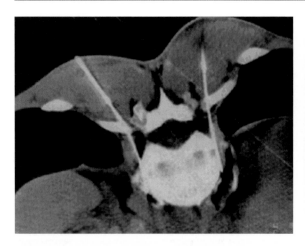

Fig. 4.5 Bilateral splanchnic nerve block with ethanol in a patient with gastric cancer and excruciating epigastric pain. CT scan shows the needle tips positioned just lateral to the anterolateral surfaces of the T11 vertebral body. Complete pain relief was achieved (analgesic score = 4) (Gangi et al. 1996)

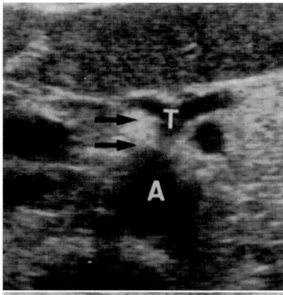

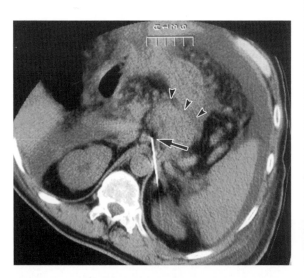

Fig. 4.6 A 62-year-old man with pancreatic adenocarcinoma. CT scan obtained at time of celiac plexus block in patient with carcinoma in body of pancreas (*arrowheads*) shows that the needle tip (*arrow*) is at the level of the celiac axis (Titton et al. 2002)

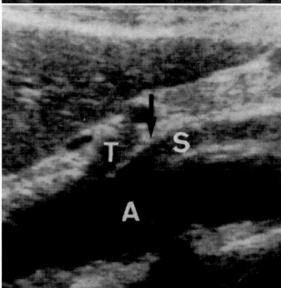

Fig. 4.7 Transverse (*top*) and longitudinal (bottam) sonograms show anatomy of celiac trunk (*T*) and abdominal aorta (*A*). For neurolysis of celiac plexus (*arrows*), the needle is placed anterior to the aorta, between the celiac axis and the superior mesenteric artery (*S*) (Giménez et al. 1993)

4.1.4.2 Cross-Sectional Anatomy Associated with the Needle Tract–Retrocrural Approach

The needle first traverses the subcutaneous tissue which has two layers: the superficial fatty layer (Camper fascia) and the deep membranous layer (Scarpa fascia).

The needle then penetrates the thoracolumbar fascia followed by the erector spinae muscle (sacrospinalis) at its lateral margin overlying the lateral tip of the 12th rib at the level of L2. Next, the needle enters the retrocrural space adjacent to the lateral margin of the vertebral body of L1. The needle is advanced to a point just posterior to the aorta on the left side and the anterolateral aspect of the aorta on the right side.

4.1.4.3 Which Structures the Needle Should Avoid?

It is advisable that the needle avoid the following structures: cisterna chyli (located posterior to the aorta, and anterior to the L1-L2 vertebral bodies), lung, kidney, somatic nerve roots (contrast injection is helpful to make sure the needle tip is within the precrural space to minimize posterior spread in the retrocrural space towards the somatic nerve roots). The aorta and inferior vena cava are generally avoided with the retrocrural approach if possible.

4.1.4.4 Cross-Sectional Anatomy Associated with the Needle Tract–Anterior Approach

The needle first traverses the subcutaneous tissue followed by the fascia. The needle then penetrates the abdominal wall musculature. Next, the peritoneum, left hepatic lobe, stomach, and pancreas plus or minus small bowel are traversed.

4.1.4.5 Which Structures the Needle Should Avoid?

It is advisable that the needle avoid the following structures: Celiac artery, superior mesentery artery, renal arteries, artery of Adamkiewicz, kidney and ureter, superior mesenteric vein, cisterna chyli, and lung.

4.1.5 Imaging/Radiology

4.1.5.1 Imaging Guidance Modalities

Fluoroscopy (Ugur et al. 2007): Failure of the contrast to surround the anterior aorta may occur due to preaortic tumor**, previous pancreatic surgery**, or radiation therapy. In this setting, the chance of success is poor. Selective alcohol neurolysis of the splanchnic nerves may provide better pain relief.

CT: The anterior approach may be the safest technique. The transaortic approach may also be used; however, it should be avoided in the setting of aortic aneurysm**, mural thrombus**, or calcification** (Romanelli et al. 1993; Marra et al. 1999).

Ultrasound: Color Doppler imaging is useful to locate the celiac trunk. However, there is limited visualization due to obscuration of structures by bowel gas. Only an anterior approach has been reported in the literature (Gimenez et al. 2003).

MRI (Hol et al. 2000): Near real-time imaging is possible with an optical tracking system and gradient echo scanning. This technique avoids vascular structures without contrast due to visualization of flow void. It may be helpful in the obese or post-surgical patient, or in anatomic distortion due to pathology. Both 2D and 3D reconstructions are possible with arbitrary orientation. One major weakness of this method is the lack of availability of a dedicated fixation device and optical tracking system in most health care facilities. In addition, it requires the use of an MRI-compatible needle and open MRI.

Endoscopic ultrasound (Gress et al. 1999, 2001): This technique is used by gastroenterologists and generally performed in specialized centers. It may offer some advantages including patient preference and lower cost.

4.1.5.2 Imaging Modalities for Diagnosis

CT is usually the favored procedure. The degree of pain relief can be correlated with tumoral invasion of the celiac ganglia preprocedure (Akhan et al. 2004).

MRI is helpful in indeterminate situations for malignancy of retroperitoneum or upper abdomen (pancreatic carcinoma). It may be useful for further characterization of acute and chronic pancreatitis including ductal abnormalities, fluid collections, and complications. In abdominal angina (chronic mesenteric vascular insufficiency), MRA can be useful when iodinated contrast CTA is contraindicated due to renal insufficiency or allergy.

Ultrasound may be helpful as the initial diagnostic modality with the clinical presentation of abdominal, flank, and back pain, while endoscopic ultrasound can be helpful in the upper abdomen. However, bowel gas can obscure pelvic organs.

4.1.6 Indications

The following are common indications for celiac plexus block and splanchnic nerve block:

- Diagnostic tool to determine whether flank retroperitoneal or upper abdominal pain is sympathetically mediated via the celiac plexus
- Acute pancreatitis**
- Palliation of the acute pain of chemoembolization**
- Abdominal angina**

The following are common indications for celiac plexus neurolysis:

- Malignancy of retroperitoneal** or upper abdomen** (especially pancreatic carcinoma, see Fig. 4.8)
- Chronic benign abdominal pain syndromes (chronic pancreatitis)**

4.1.7 Contraindications

The unique contraindications to celiac plexus block and splanchnic nerve block are aortic aneurysm, mural thrombus, and small bowel obstruction**

4.1.8 Complications

Multiple complications (Davies 1993; Fitzgibbon et al. 2001; Sett and Taylor 1991) have been reported, including:

- Hypotension
- Paresthesia of lumbar somatic verve
- Intravascular injection (venous or arterial)
- Deficit of lumbar somatic nerve
- Subarachnoid or epidural injection
- Diarrhea
- Renal injury: perinephric hematoma**, renal infarction** (intraparenchymal injection)
- Paraplegia (spinal cord infarction)** due to artery of Adamkiewicz injection
- Pneumothorax**
- Pleural effusion**
- Chylothorax**
- Vascular thrombosis** or embolism**
- Vascular trauma/pseudoaneurysm**
- Perforation of cysts** or tumors**
- Injection of the psoas muscle**
- Intradiscal injection**
- Abscess**
- Peritonitis**
- Retroperitoneal hematoma**
- Urinary tract abnormalities**

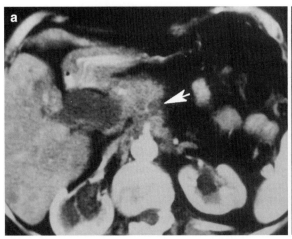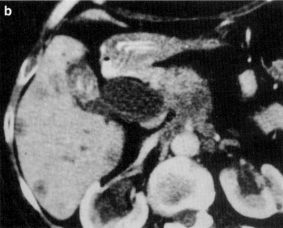

Fig. 4.8 (**a**) A 77-year-old woman with nonresectable adenocarcinoma of pancreatic head detected on dual-phase helical CT. Arterial phase CT image shows low-attenuation mass in the region of the pancreatic head and infiltration of the superior mesenteric artery (*arrow*). (**b**) Portal phase image obtained at same level as (**a**) shows presence of multiple liver metastases (Imbriaco et al. 2002)

- Failure of ejaculation
- Pain during and after procedure
- Failure to relieve pain

4.2 Lumbar Sympathetic Block

4.2.1 Anatomy

The lumbar sympathetic ganglia consist of a paravertebral trunk bilaterally extending from L1 through L5 which are variable in number. In addition, there is a prevertebral trunk of sympathetic ganglia at the midline. The paravertebral ganglia are located within the retroperitoneum under the crura of the diaphragm. They continue inferiorly along the anterolateral aspect of the vertebral bodies, medial to the psoas muscle to enter the pelvis at L5-S1. The aorta is anteromedial to the left trunk and the inferior vena cava (IVC) is anterior to the right trunk (Figs. 4.9–4.12).

The preganglionic fibers originate within the thoracolumbar spinal cord, which travel out of the cord with the spinal nerve into the white rami communicantes linking the spinal nerve with the sympathetic ganglion. Here the sympathetic fibers may or may not synapse within the ganglion. If they do not synapse they may continue into adjacent ganglia including the prevertebral ganglia supplying the pelvic viscera. Alternatively, the preganglionic fibers may synapse in the paravertebral ganglia and leave the ganglia via the gray rami communicantes to contribute to the lumbosacral plexus and all its branches.

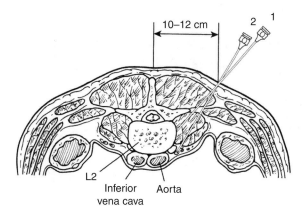

Fig. 4.9 Lumbar sympathetic block (Weiss 2007)

4.2.2 Function

The lumbar sympathetic trunk contains lumbar somatic afferents, visceral afferents, and postganglionic efferents, which provide innervation to the hip, lower limbs, and lower axial skeleton as well as their associated musculature. Functions include vasomotor (vasoconstriction), pilomotor (goose bumps), sudomotor (sweating).

4.2.3 Injection Site

The patient is placed prone and the L2 or L3 vertebral body transverse process is identified. The C-arm is rotated to superimpose the tip of the transverse process over the vertebral body. The needle puncture site is then determined in this projection over the tip of the transverse process. The needle is then advanced past the L2 or L3 transverse process superiorly or inferiorly until it reaches the anterolateral margin of the L2 or L3 vertebral body. This is the site of injection for the sympathetic ganglion (Figs. 4.11–4.12).

4.2.4 Cross-Sectional Anatomy

4.2.4.1 What Does the Needle Traverse?

The needle enters the skin and traverses the lumbodorsal fascia and the erector spinae muscle. It passes superior or inferior to the transverse process of the lumbar vertebra then traverses the psoas muscle and the sympathetic ganglion adjacent to the lateral margin of the lumbar vertebral body (Fig. 4.14).

4.2.4.2 Which Structures the Needle Should Avoid

It is advisable that the needle avoid the following structures: renal arteries at the level of L1; aorta on the left side; inferior mesenteric artery on the left side; inferior vena cava on the right side; kidney and ureter (avoid by not starting too far laterally); anterior spinal nerve root

Fig. 4.10 Abdominal portion of the sympathetic trunk, with the celiac plexus and hypogastric plexus (sympathetic trunk labeled at *center left*) (Gray 1918)

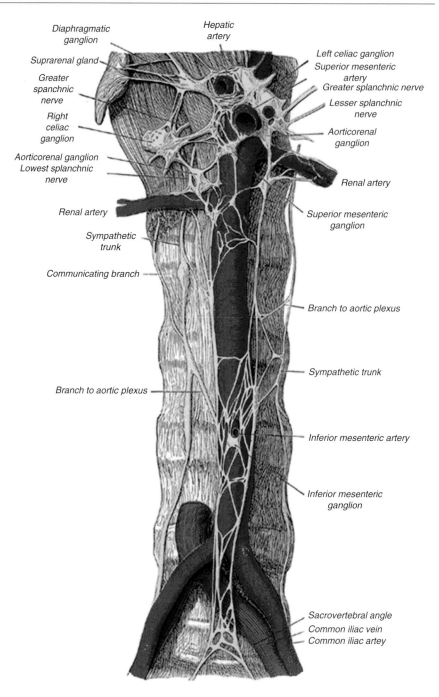

4.2.5 Imaging/Radiology

4.2.5.1 Image Guidance Modalities

(avoid going too far lateral (greater than 7–8 cm from the midline) and posterior); lumbar segmental artery and its divisions (spinal branch, anterior ramus and posterior ramus branches); artery of Adamkiewicz ((a) to the left 71% of the time, (b) between L1 and L3 65% of the time, (c) as high as T9 and as low as L5)) (Biglioli et al. 2004; Uotani et al. 2008).

These are similar to the modalities discussed in the section on thoracic sympathetic block. Fluoroscopy is well accepted and available. Cross-sectional techniques

Fig. 4.11 Anatomy of the lumbar sympathetic chain. The lumbar sympathetic ganglia are variable in number and location from one individual to another. Most commonly, the ganglia lie over the anteromedial surface of the vertebral bodies between L2 and L4. Temporary lumbar sympathetic block using local anesthetic is best performed by advancing a single needle cephalad to the transverse process of L2 or L3 to avoid exiting the nerve root. The needle tip is placed adjacent to the superior portion of the anteromedial surface of the L2 or L3 vertebral body. Use of 15–20 mL of local anesthetic solution will spread to cover multiple vertebral levels (*shaded region*) (Rathmell 2006)

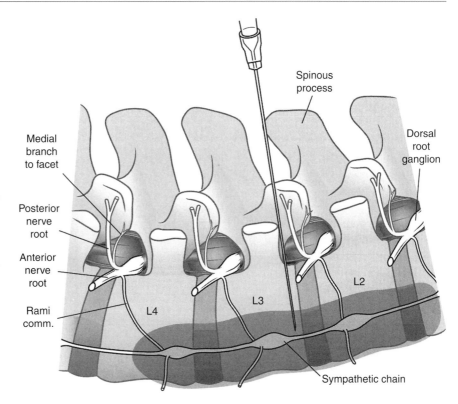

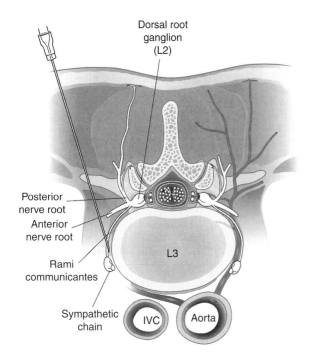

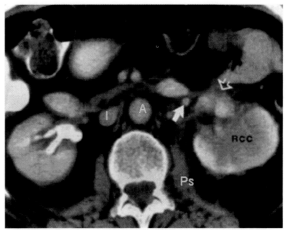

Fig. 4.12 Axial diagram of lumbar sympathetic block. A single needle passes over the transverse process, and the tip is in position adjacent to the lumbar sympathetic ganglia over the anteromedial surface of the L2 or L3 vertebral body (Rathmell 2006)

Fig. 4.13 CT scans demonstrate a renal cell carcinoma (*Rcc*) of the left kidney involving the renal vein (*open arrow*), with collateral retrograde flow down an enlarged left gonadal vein (*arrow*) coursing along the psoas muscle (*Ps*). *I* inferior vena cava; *A* aorta (Stallard et al. 1994)

(CT, ultrasound, MRI) may be useful in high risk patients. Of these, ultrasound (Kirvelä et al. 1992) and MRI (Sze and Mackey 2002) use have both been described.

4.2.5.2 Imaging for Diagnosis

CT is the procedure of choice for the evaluation of abdominal or pelvic pathology (malignancy (Fig. 4.13), nephroureteral calculi and for most visceral complications).

CTA is suitable for the evaluation of arterial pathology including complications (Fig. 4.15).

MRI is useful for imaging spinal complications.

MRA may be helpful in the evaluation of arterial pathology when iodinated contrast is contraindicated.

Angiography is more invasive, but may be useful if CTA or MRA is suboptimal or contraindicated.

Nuclear medicine imaging is able to provide three-phase bone scans and may be useful for reflex sympathetic dystrophy.

4.2.6 Indications

The following represent common indications for lumbar sympathetic block:

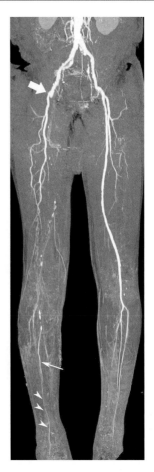

Fig. 4.15 Rutherford and Becker grade III (category 5) (refer to Table 4.1) disease and cutaneous trophic lesions in a 57-year-old man. Coronal MIP image from multi-detector row CT angiography with bone segmentation depicts occlusion of the right superficial femoral artery (*thick arrow*), reconstitution of the peroneal artery via collateral vessels, and patency of the distal anterior tibial (*thin arrow*) and dorsal pedal (*arrowheads*) arteries. In the left leg, below the knee, the patency of the anterior tibial artery and peroneal artery and occlusion of the posterior tibial artery also are depicted (Catalano et al. 2004)

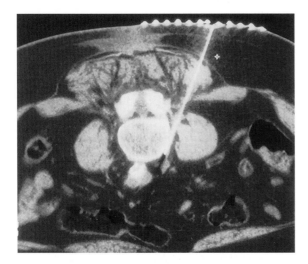

Fig. 4.14 Spinal sympathetic block. Axial CT scan shows the position of a 22-gauge spinal needle tip relative to the right lumbar sympathetic chain and adjacent vessels (Zinreich et al. 2001)

- Arterial insufficiency due to small vessel occlusion (Fig. 4.15; Table 4.1)
  - Diabetic gangrene**
  - Buerger's disease**
  - Raynaud's phenomenon and disease**
  - Failed vascular bypass surgery** or inoperable patient

- Renal colic due to renal calculi**
- Reflex sympathetic dystrophy (CRPS 1 and 11)**
- Intractable urogenital pain

Table 4.1 Clinical categories of chronic limb ischemia (Wright et al. 2004 and Rutherford et al. 1997)

Grade	Category	Clinical findings	Objective criteria
0	0	Asymptomatic	ABI = 1.0, normal treadmill test[†]
	1	Mild claudication	ABI = 1.0–0.8, treadmill test completed, AP after exercise <50 mmHg but ≥20 mmHg lower than BP
I	2	Moderate claudication	ABI = 0.8–0.6, symptoms between categories 1 and 3
	3	Severe claudication	ABI = 0.3–0.5, treadmill test cannot be completed, AP after exercise <50 mmHg
II	4	Ischemic rest pain	ABI ≤0.3, resting AP <40 mmHg, TP <30 mmHg
III	5	Minor tissue loss	ABI <0.3, resting AP <60 mmHg, TP <40 mmHg
	6	Major tissue loss	ABI <0.3, resting AP <60 mmHg, TP <40 mmHg

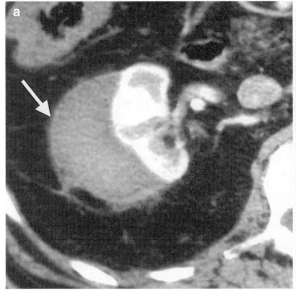

Fig. 4.16 Perinephric hematoma after renal radiofrequency (RF) ablation. (**a**, **b**) Unenhanced (**a**) and contrast material-enhanced (**b**) CT scans obtained shortly after RF ablation demonstrate a large perinephric hematoma (*arrow*) (Rhim et al. 2004). A similar complication may occur after a lumbar sympathetic block

- Cancer pain of the pelvic viscera**
- Amputation stump
- Phantom pain and frostbite
- Hyperhidrosis
- Phlegmasia alba dolens**
- Acrocyanosis
- Trench foot
- Erythromelalgia

4.2.7 Contraindications

The main contraindication to lumbar sympathetic block is anatomic anomalies.

4.2.8 Complications

Complications infrequently encountered in lumbar sympathetic block include the following:

- Intravascular injection can be significant if it results in injury to the renal artery, the inferior mesenteric artery or the artery of Adamkiewicz with resulting end organ injury**
- Intradiscal/intravertebral injection
- Subarachnoid injection
- Neuralgia of the genitofemoral nerve (post-sympathectomy pain in L1-2 distribution (over the anterior thigh) following neurolytic block)

- Necrosis of psoas**
- Sloughing of the ureter due to intra-ureteral injection**
- Bleeding/retroperitoneal hematoma**
- Hypotension
- Impotence or failure of ejaculation
- Hematuria/perinephric hematoma** due to renal puncture (Fig. 4.16).

References

Ugur F, Gulcu N, Boyaci A. Celiac plexus block with the long stylet needle technique. Adv Ther. 2007;24(2):296-301

Romanelli DF, Beckmann CF, Heiss FW. Celiac plexus block: efficacy and safety of the anterior approach. AJR Am J Roentgenol. 1993;160(3):497-500

Marra V, Debernardi F, Frigerio A, Menna S, Musso L, Di Virgilio MR. Neurolytic block of the celiac plexus and splanchnic nerves with computed tomography. The experience in 150 cases and an optimization of the technic. Radiol Med (Torino). 1999;98(3):183-8 [Italian]

Hol PK, Kvarstein G, Viken O, Smedby O, Tønnessen TI. MRI-guided celiac plexus block. J Magn Reson Imaging. 2000; 12(4):562-4

Gress F, Schmitt C, Sherman S, Ikenberry S, Lehman G. A prospective randomized comparison of endoscopic ultrasound- and computed tomography-guided celiac plexus block for managing chronic pancreatitis pain. Am J Gastroenterol. 1999;94(4):900-5

Gress F, Schmitt C, Sherman S, Ciaccia D, Ikenberry S, Lehman G. Endoscopic ultrasound-guided celiac plexus block for managing abdominal pain associated with chronic pancreatitis: a prospective single center experience. Am J Gastroenterol. 2001;96(2):409-16

Akhan O, Ozmen MN, Basgun N, Akinci D, Oguz O, Koroglu M, Karcaaltincaba M. Long-term results of celiac ganglia block: correlation of grade of tumoral invasion and pain relief. AJR Am J Roentgenol. 2004;182(4):891-6

Davies DD. Incidence of major complications of neurolytic coeliac plexus block. J R Soc Med. 1993;86(5):264-6

Fitzgibbon DR, Schmiedl UP, Sinanan MN. Computed tomography-guided neurolytic celiac plexus block with alcohol complicated by superior mesenteric venous thrombosis. Pain. 2001;92(1-2):307-10

Sett SS, Taylor DC. Aortic pseudoaneurysm secondary to celiac plexus block. Ann Vasc Surg. 1991;5(1):88-91

Biglioli P, Roberto M, Cannata A, Parolari A, Fumero A, Grillo F, Maggioni M, Coggi G, Spirito R. Upper and lower spinal cord blood supply: the continuity of the anterior spinal artery and the relevance of the lumbar arteries. J Thorac Cardiovasc Surg. 2004;127(4):1188-92

Uotani K, Yamada N, Kono AK, Taniguchi T, Sugimoto K, Fujii M, Kitagawa A, Okita Y, Naito H, Sugimura K. Preoperative visualization of the artery of Adamkiewicz by intra-arterial CT angiography. AJNR Am J Neuroradiol. 2008;29(2):314-8

Kirvelä O, Svedström E, Lundbom N. Ultrasonic guidance of lumbar sympathetic and celiac plexus block: a new technique. Reg Anesth. 1992;17(1):43-6

Sze DY, Mackey SC. MR guidance of sympathetic nerve blockade: measurement of vasomotor response initial experience in seven patients. Radiology. 2002;223(2):574-80

Rathmell JP. Atlas of image-guided intervention in regional anesthesia and pain medicine. Philadelphia, PA: Lippincott Williams and Wilkins, 2006

Gangi A, Dietemann JL, Schultz A, Mortazavi R, Jeung MY, Roy C. Interventional radiologic procedures with CT guidance in cancer pain management. Radiographics. 1996;16(6): 1289-304; discussion 1304-6

Titton RL, Lucey BC, Gervais DA, Boland GW, Mueller PR. Celiac plexus block: a palliative tool underused by radiologists. AJR Am J Roentgenol. 2002;179(3):633-6

Giménez A, Martínez-Noguera A, Donoso L, Catalá E, Serra R. Percutaneous neurolysis of the celiac plexus via the anterior approach with sonographic guidance. AJR Am J Roentgenol. 1993;161(5):1061-3

Imbriaco M, Megibow AJ, Camera L, Pace L, Mainenti PP, Romano M, Selva G, Salvatore M. Dual-phase versus single-phase helical CT to detect and assess resectability of pancreatic carcinoma. AJR Am J Roentgenol. 2002;178(6): 1473-9

Weiss LD. Easy injections. Philadelphia, PA: Elsevier, 2007. NLM ID: 101308328

Gray H. Anatomy of the Human Body. 20th ed. Thoroughly revised and re-edited by Warren H. Lewis. Philadelphia: Lea & Febiger, 1918.

Stallard DJ, Tu RK, Gould MJ, Pozniak MA, Pettersen JC. Minor vascular anatomy of the abdomen and pelvis: a CT atlas. Radiographics. 1994;14(3):493-513

Zinreich SJ, Murphy, K, Silbergleit, R. Invited commentary. Author's response. Radiographics. 2001;21:940

Catalano C, Fraioli F, Laghi A, Napoli A, Bezzi M, Pediconi F, Danti M, Nofroni I, Passariello R. Infrarenal aortic and lower-extremity arterial disease: diagnostic performance of multi-detector row CT angiography. Radiology. 2004;231(2): 555-63

Rhim H, Dodd GD, III, Chintapalli KN, Wood BJ, Dupuy DE, Hvizda JL, Sewell PE, Goldberg SN. Radiofrequency thermal ablation of abdominal tumors: lessons learned from complications. Radiographics. 2004;24:41-52

Wright LB, Matchett WJ, Cruz CP, James CA, Culp WC, Eidt JF, McCowan TC. Popliteal artery disease: diagnosis and treatment. Radiographics. 2004;24(2):467-79. Review

Rutherford RB, Baker JD, Ernst C, Johnston KW, Porter JM, Ahn S, Jones DN. Recommended standards for reports dealing with lower extremity ischemia: revised version. J Vasc Surg. 1997;26(3):517-38

Pelvis

Below we examine the strengths and weaknesses of imaging modalities for diagnosis in the pelvis.

Ultrasound: Among its strengths, transvaginal ultrasound has high diagnostic accuracy for pelvic pathology. It is the first-line imaging modality for pelvic pain, dysmenorrhea, and follow-up for previously detected abnormality (e.g., hemorrhagic cyst). If the study is negative in the setting of pelvic pain, the yield of further diagnostic studies is low, but definitive diagnosis can be made in a minority of patients (Harris et al. 2000). Transpelvic ultrasound is less sensitive than transvaginal ultrasound, but is also a first line imaging modality.

Indications (ACR Practice Guideline for the Performance of Pelvic Ultrasound in Females) for ultrasound include:

- Pelvic pain
- Dysmenorrhea (painful menses)
- Menorrhagia (excessive menstrual bleeding)
- Metrorrhagia (irregular uterine bleeding)
- Menometrorrhagia (excessive bleeding irregularly)
- Follow-up of previously detected abnormality (e.g., hemorrhagic cyst)
- Evaluation and/or monitoring of infertile patients
- Delayed menses or precocious puberty
- Postmenopausal bleeding
- Abnormal pelvic examination
- Further characterization of a pelvic abnormality noted on another imaging study (e.g., CT or MR)
- Evaluation of congenital anomalies
- Excessive bleeding, pain, or fever after pelvic surgery or delivery
- Localization of intrauterine contraceptive device
- Screening for malignancy in high-risk patients

Ultrasound's main *weakness* lies in the fact that bowel gas can obscure the pelvic organs.

CT: The main *indications* (ACR Practice Guideline for the Performance of Computed Tomography CT of the Abdomen and Computed Tomography of the Pelvis) for CT include the following:

- Evaluation of abdominal, flank, or pelvic pain
- Evaluation of known or suspected abdominal or pelvic masses or fluid collections
- Evaluation of primary or metastatic malignancies
- Evaluation of abdominal or pelvic inflammatory processes
- Assessment of abnormalities of abdominal or pelvic vascular structures
- Evaluation of abdominal or pelvic trauma
- Clarification of findings from other imaging studies or laboratory abnormalities
- Evaluation of known or suspected congenital abnormalities of abdominal or pelvic organs
- Guidance for interventional or therapeutic procedures within the abdomen or pelvis
- Treatment planning for radiation therapy
- Noninvasive angiography of the aorta and its branches

MRI: The major strength of *MRI* (Hubert and Bergin 2008) over ultrasound is that no limitation is imposed by bowel gas.

The principal *indications* (ACR Practice Guidelines for the Performance of Magnetic Resonance Imaging MRI of the Soft Tissue Components of the Pelvis) for MRI include the following:

- Evaluation of pelvic pain or masses (adenomyosis, ovarian cysts, torsion, tuboovarian abscess, solid masses, obstructed fallopian tubes, endometrioma, and fibroids), especially when ultrasound is not definitive.
- Assessment of pelvic floor pathology (superior to CT and ultrasound).

M.I. Syed and A. Shaikh, *Radiology of Non-Spinal Pain Procedures*, DOI: 10.1007/978-3-642-00481-0_5, © Springer-Verlag Berlin Heidelberg 2011

- Detection and staging of gynecologic malignancy (e.g., cervical and endometrial carcinoma). MRI is superior to CT and ultrasound.
- Evaluation of congenital anomalies of Müllerian duct development (embryologic origin of fallopian tubes, uterus, cervix, and upper part of vagina).
- More sensitive than CT for peritoneal implants.
- Pre-surgical/laparoscopic evaluation.
- Pre- and post-uterine artery embolization for fibroids.
- MRV (magnetic resonance venography) with dynamic imaging may be helpful in the non-invasive diagnosis and assessment of pelvic congestion syndrome.

The main *weakness* of MRI over ultrasound is that it may require intravenous contrast for assessment of pathology.

5.1 Hypogastric Plexus Block

5.1.1 Anatomy

The superior hypogastric plexus is a complex of nerve fibers situated ventral to L5 and S1 adjacent to the branching of the aorta and common iliac vasculature. This plexus is formed by contributions from the celiac, lumbar sympathetic chain, inferior mesenteric plexuses, and aortic plexus. Furthermore, it receives parasympathetic fibers from S2-S4 in the form of the pelvic splanchnic nerves. They course through the inferior hypogastric plexus into the superior hypogastric plexus. The superior hypogastric plexus splits into the right and left hypogastric nerves on either side, which course inferiorly at the outer aspect of the sigmoid colon and rectosigmoid junction to join with the inferior hypogastric plexuses. The superior plexus provides supply to the ureter, testicles/ovaries, the sigmoid colon, and the plexus at the iliac arteries. Lateral to the rectum, bladder, and reproductive organs is the inferior hypogastric plexus that forms bilaterally (Figs. 5.1 and 5.2).

5.1.2 Function

This plexus has both motor and sensory components. It provides vascular smooth muscle visceral pelvic sympathetic innervation. It also receives sensory innervation from the pelvic viscera including the bladder, rectum, perineum, vulva, prostate, ovary/testicle, and uterus.

5.1.3 Injection Site

A lateral and slightly cephalad approach is used to direct the needle tip posteromedially and inferiorly toward the midline, just anterior to the L5-S1 junction or inferior half of L5 (Figs. 5.1–5.2).

5.1.4 Radiologic Anatomy

The hypogastric plexus lies posterior to the left iliac vein and inferior to the aortic bifurcation.

5.1.5 Cross-Sectional Anatomy

5.1.5.1 What Does the Needle Traverse?

The needle traverses the lateral margin of the erector spinae muscles or the muscle itself. It passes adjacent to the iliac crest (superior medial aspect), as well as adjacent to the transverse process of L5. It also traverses the psoas muscle (Fig. 5.3).

5.1.5.2 Which Structures the Needle Should Avoid

Care should be taken to avoid the aorta, the common iliac arteries, the inferior mesenteric artery, and the median sacral artery. In addition, the inferior vena cava and the common iliac veins, ureters, as well as the ventral nerve roots, should be avoided.

5.1.6 Imaging/Radiology

The main modalities used for guidance include fluoroscopy and CT (Fig. 5.4).

Fig. 5.1 Axial diagram of superior hypogastric plexus block. Needles are advanced from either side over the junction between the sacral ala and the superior articular process of S1 to position the needle tips over the anterolateral surface of the L5/S1 disc space. Note the close proximity of the iliac vessels. The *inset* shows the plane and orientation of the axial diagram (Rathmell 2006)

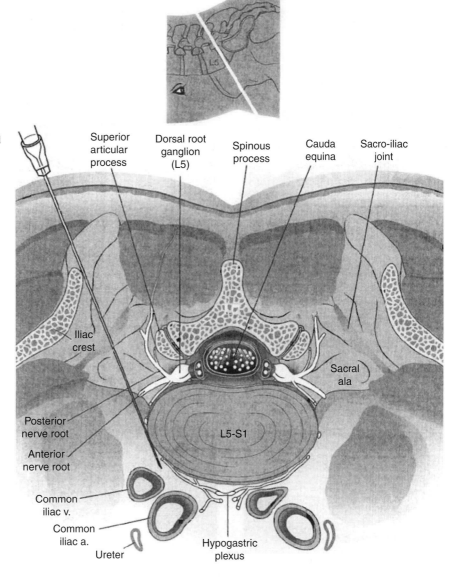

5.1.7 Indications

The principal indications for hypogastric plexus block include the following:

- Intractable chronic pelvic pain
- Malignant etiologies
  - Cervical cancer**
  - Prostate cancer**
  - Testicular cancer**
  - Radiation enteritis**
  - Ovarian cancer**
- Benign etiologies (Kuligowska et al. 2005)
  - Endometriosis (Fig. 5.5)**
  - Chronic PID**
  - Fibroids**
  - Adenomyosis**
  - Adhesions

Fig. 5.2 Anatomy of the superior hypogastric plexus. The superior hypogastric plexus is comprised of a loose, weblike group of interlacing nerve fibers that lie over the anterolateral surface of the L5 vertebral body and extend inferiorly over the sacrum. Needles are positioned over the anterolateral surface of the L5/S1 intervertebral disc or the inferior aspect of the L5 vertebral bodies to block the superior hypogastric plexus. Use of 8–10 mL of local anesthetic solution will spread along the anterior surface of the L5 vertebral body and the sacrum (*shaded area*) (Rathmell 2006)

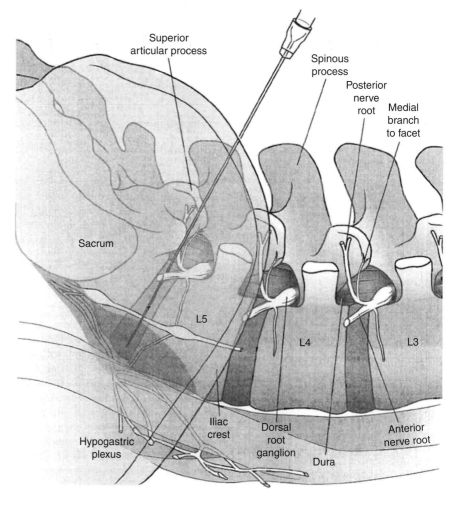

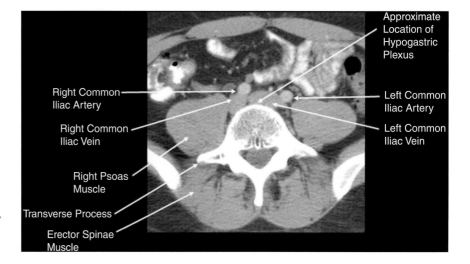

Fig. 5.3 Cross-sectional CT anatomy of hypogastric plexus region

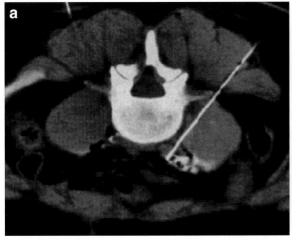
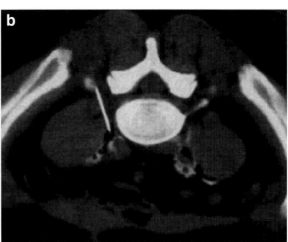

Fig. 5.4 CT scans show a bilateral needle posterior superior hypogastric plexus block in a 29-year-old woman with a 9-year history of pelvic pain. (**a**) Left needle is in a good position ante-rior to L4. (**b**) Right needle is in a good position anterolateral to L5. Note air and anesthetic that extend around the iliac vessels (Wechsler et al. 1995)

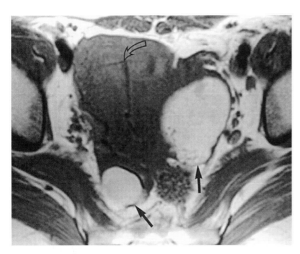

Fig. 5.5 Bilateral endometriomas in a 27-year-old woman. Axial T1-weighted MR image shows bilateral high-signal-intensity adnexal masses (*solid arrows*). An intrauterine device is seen within the uterus (*open arrow*) (Woodward et al. 2001)

- Inflammatory bowel disease**
- Hernia**
- Urinary tract disease**
- Pelvic congestion syndrome**
- Laceration of uterine support
- Nerve entrapment
- Oophoritis**

5.1.8 Contraindications

The main (relative) contraindication to hypogastric plexus block is atherosclerotic disease of the iliac arteries to avoid dislodging a plaque and producing a distal embolism**. Use CT guidance if a horseshoe or pelvic kidney is near the potential injection site.

5.1.9 Complications

The five principal complications associated with hypogastric plexus block are: (1) Vascular puncture: hemorrhage and hematoma (common iliac artery)**; (2) intramuscular and intraperitoneal injection; (3) subarachnoid and epidural injection; (4) renal hematoma** (of a pelvic kidney** or horseshoe kidney**), or (5) ureter puncture (urinoma)**.

5.2 Ganglion Impar Block

5.2.1 Anatomy

The ganglion impar is a lone retroperitoneal meshwork of nerves ventral to the sacrococcygeal spinal junction. It is formed by the fusion terminal confluence of the bilateral pelvic sympathetic trunks at their inferior aspect (Figs. 5.6–5.7).

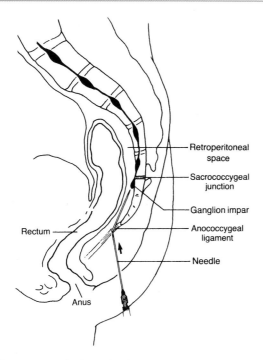

Fig. 5.6 Lateral schematic view demonstrates correct needle placement for blockade of ganglion impar and anatomic relations (Plancarte et al. 1993)

5.2.2 Function

The ganglion impar provides visceral sympathetic sensory supply to the rectum, perineum, vagina, and coccyx.

5.2.3 Injection Site

The needle is directed at the midline via a posterior approach at the upper margin of the inner gluteal crease over the anococcygeal ligament. A curved or angulated needle may be useful to position the needle tip anterior to the coccyx. Alternatively, a transsacrococcygeal or far lateral CT approach may be utilized.

5.2.4 Cross-Sectional Anatomy

5.2.4.1 What Does the Needle Traverse?

Using an anococcygeal approach, the needle traverses the anococcygeal ligament and the presacral space at the sacrococcygeal junction. A transcoccygeal approach has also been described (Hubert and Bergin 2008).

5.2.4.2 Which Structures the Needle Should Avoid

The needle should avoid the rectum and ideally the periosteum of the sacrum or coccyx.

5.2.5 Imaging/Radiology

Fluoroscopic guidance is the most widely reported mechanism of performing this procedure. A curved or bent needle is needed for an anococcygeal approach. The Trans-sacrococcygeal joint or transcoccygeal approach allows straight needles to be used (Fig. 5.8).

CT guidance is a safe method and can avoid rectal perforation and bleeding. In addition, it limits the risk of needle breakage. A lateral approach is facilitated through the gluteus maximus muscle (Fig. 5.9).

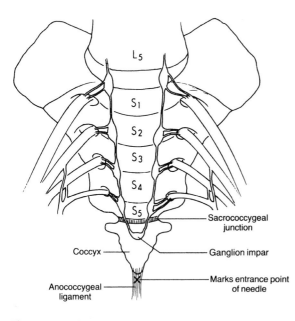

Fig. 5.7 Anterior schematic view through pelvis demonstrating location of ganglion impar and pertinent regional anatomy (Plancarte et al. 1993)

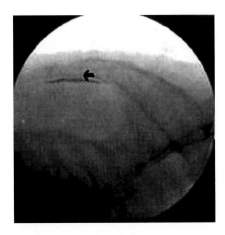

Fig. 5.8 View of spread of dye (*arrow*) in transsacrococcygeal approach (Toshniwal et al. 2007)

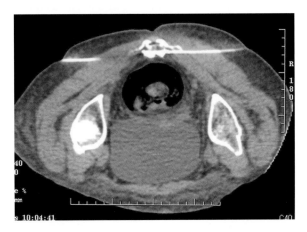

Fig. 5.9 Injection of contrast dye to confirm correct placement of the needle tip anterior to the sacrococcygeal junction (Ho et al. 2006)

MRI guidance has been reported (Mackey et al. 1999) (Fig. 5.10).

5.2.6 Indications

Principle indications (vague burning and localized perineal pain) for ganglion impar block include: (1) Pain arising from disorders from the viscera; (2) disorders from the viscera sympathetic structures in the pelvis and perineum especially in women; (3) advanced cancer of the cervix (Fig. 5.10), vulva, bladder, rectum, and endometriosis**; (4) intractable neoplastic

perineal pain of sympathetic origin; (5) postradiation proctitis**; (6) coccydynia.

5.2.7 Complications

The range of complications associated with ganglion impar block include: (1) Perforation of the rectum**; (2) periosteal injection; (3) impotence; (4) bladder incontinence/dysfunction; (5) neurolytic injection into nerve roots and rectal cavity; (6) neuritis/nerve root injection: (7) cauda equina syndrome**.

5.3 Sciatic Nerve Block

5.3.1 Anatomy

The sciatic nerve, the largest nerve in the body, originates from the L4-S3 nerve roots. It is formed from the anterior and posterior divisions of the lumbosacral plexus. It travels along at the anterior surface of the piriformis muscle past its inferior aspect as it leaves the pelvis below the greater sciatic notch at the greater sciatic foramen. At this point it lies between the greater trochanter and ischial tuberosity. It courses dorsal to the gemelli, obturator internus, and quadriceps femoris and anterior to the gluteus maximus. The sciatic artery, inferior gluteal artery, and the inferior gluteal veins travel with the sciatic nerve. The posterior femoral cutaneous branch innervating the posterior thigh is inconsistent in its anatomy. It may travel next to the sciatic or may be a separate entity from it superiorly (Fig. 5.11).

5.3.2 Function

The sciatic nerve (L4-S3 nerve roots) provides motor supply to the hamstrings, which are involved in hip extension and leg flexion (biceps femoris, semitendinosus, and semimembranosus). It also provides motor supply to flex and extend the ankle. Furthermore, it provides sensory supply to the posterolateral aspect of the thigh, knee, as well as the entire lower leg, toes, foot, and knee.

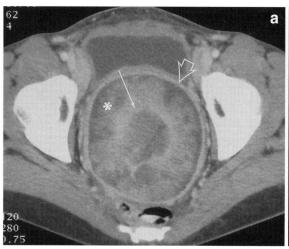
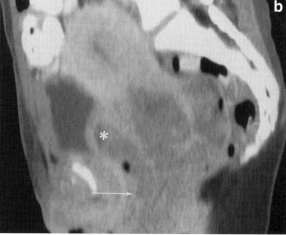

Fig. 5.10 Tumor extension into the vagina in a 50-year-old woman with clinical stage IIIB and imaging stage IIIA cervical cancer. Axial (**a**) and sagittal (**b**) CT images of the pelvis obtained with oral and intravenous contrast material show a low-attenuation mass in the cervix (*solid arrow*), which represents the primary tumor. The vagina (*open arrow*) is expanded by the tumor (*asterisk*) growing into it from the cervix. The tumor involves the lower one-third of the vagina, a finding consistent with stage III disease (Pannu et al. 2001)

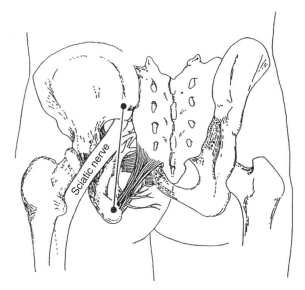

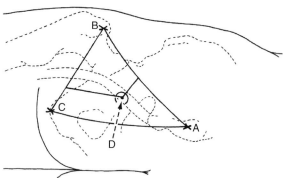

Fig. 5.12 Surface landmarks and entry point of the needle: *A*, posterior superior iliac spine; *B*, greater trochanter; *C*, ischial tuberosity; *D*, insertion site (Raj 2003b)

Fig. 5.11 The landmarks to be identified by fluoroscopy. *A*, posterior superior iliac spine; *B*, greater trochanter; *C*, ischial tuberosity. Refer to Fig. 5.12 (Raj 2003a)

5.3.3 Injection Site

Between a line segment connecting the posterior iliac spine and the greater trochanter the center point is localized. An orthogonal line segment is then drawn in an inferior direction from this center point. A third line segment is connected between the greater trochanter and the ischial tuberosity. This line segment is trisected. Another line is drawn vertically at the junction of the inner and middle third mark cephalad to intersect the first orthogonal line segment. The puncture site is where the lines meet (Fig. 5.12). The needle is advanced using a direct perpendicular approach to the piriformis muscle. The piriformis muscle is crossed until the sciatic nerve is reached. If a catheter is to be placed for continuous infusion analgesia, the catheter is advanced from this point along the nerve to the level of the lesser trochanter.

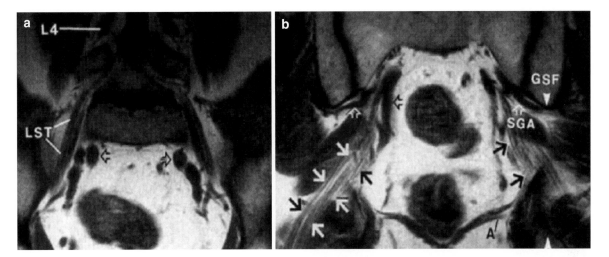

Fig. 5.13 Direct coronal images obtained (**a**) at the level of the sacral promontory and (**b**) through the greater sciatic foramen (*GSF*). This imaging plane optimally displays the L4 and L5 ventral rami, the LST (lumbosacral trunk), and the S1 contributions to the SN. The SN in the GSF is easily demonstrated in (**b**) (*solid arrows*). *A* levator ani; *SGA* superior gluteal artery. *Open arrows*, vessels; *arrowheads* in (**b**), superior and inferior boundaries of the GSF (Blake et al. 1996)

5.3.4 Cross-Sectional Anatomy

5.3.4.1 What Does the Needle Traverse?

The needle traverses the gluteus maximus and the subgluteal space, which contains the sciatic nerve (anterior to the quadratus femoris muscle) (Figs. 5.16–5.17).

5.3.4.2 Which Structures the Needle Should Avoid

It is advisable that the needle avoid the superior and inferior gluteal artery and vein as well as the ascending circumflex femoral artery (Figs. 5.13 and 5.16).

5.3.5 Imaging/Radiology

Fluoroscopy: This technique is based on anatomic landmarks, which sometimes may be inaccurate.

CT: This method is useful for the evaluation of bony pathology (fractures) or tumor. It has not yet been described in the medical literature for guidance of sciatic nerve block (Figs. 5.14 and 5.15).

Ultrasound: The subgluteal space is targeted between the greater trochanter and ischial tuberosity. This

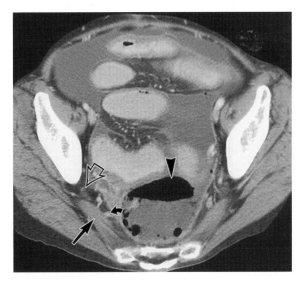

Fig. 5.14 CT depiction of sciatic nerve anatomy. CT scan shows the piriformis muscle (*straight solid arrow*), which underlies the gluteus maximus muscle and crosses the center of the greater sciatic foramen. Anterior to the piriformis muscle lie the inferior gluteal vessels (*curved arrow*). The sciatic nerve (*open arrow*) is seen along the anterolateral aspect of the piriformis muscle. Also identified is a deep pelvic abscess (*arrowhead*) and ascites (Harisinghani et al. 2002)

technique allows direct visualization of the sciatic nerve within the subgluteal space and vascular structures. Ultrasound is useful for the diagnosis of both vascular and soft tissue pathology (Figs. 5.16 and 5.17).

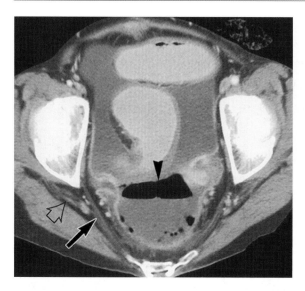

Fig. 5.15 CT depiction of sciatic nerve anatomy. CT scan obtained 1.5 cm inferior to Fig. 5.21 in the same patient. The sacrospinous ligament (*solid arrow*) forms the inferior margin of the greater sciatic foramen. Posterolateral to the ligament and adjoining the acetabulum is the sciatic nerve (*open arrow*). The presacral abscess (*arrowhead*) is again seen (Harisinghani et al. 2002)

MRI: This method is the study of choice for the diagnosis of lower extremity pathology after preliminary plain film radiographs have been obtained (Fig. 5.18).

5.3.6 Indications

The following are common indications (Gaertner et al. 2004) for sciatic nerve block:

- Sciatic nerve blocks with saphenous nerve blocks is indicated for surgery and analgesia of the ankle, foot and leg**
- Sciatic nerve blocks with femoral, obturator, and lateral femoral cutaneous nerve block is indicated for surgery and analgesia of the knee**
- Continuous infusion sciatic nerve block is indicated for:
  - Complex regional pain syndrome type one or two**
  - Vascular insufficiency**
  - Unilateral leg edema**
  - Cancer pain**
  - Severe acute or chronic pain
  - Total knee arthroplasty for arthritis/degenerative conditions (TKA)**
  - TKA replacement
  - Major trauma of leg or foot**
  - Above the knee Amputation **
  - Osteosarcoma of the knee**
  - Osteotomy of the tibia combined with a hallux**
  - Valgus osteotomy

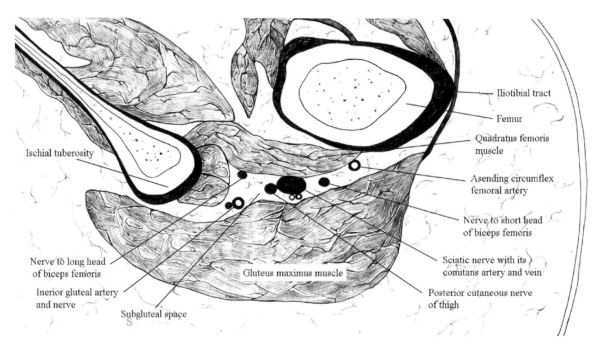

Fig. 5.16 Transverse section through the gluteal region at the level of the quadratus femoris muscle showing the subgluteal space and its contents (Karmakar et al. 2007)

Fig. 5.17 Transverse sonogram between the greater trochanter and ischial tuberosity showing the hypoechoic subgluteal space between the hyperechoic perimysium of the gluteus maximus and the quadratus femoris muscle. The sciatic nerve is seen as a hyperechoic nodule in the medial aspect of the subgluteal space (Karmakar et al. 2007)

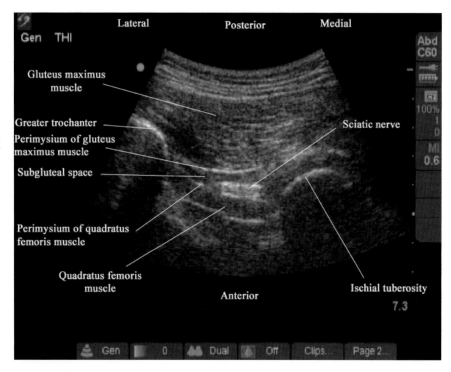

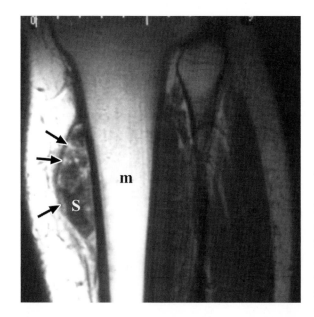

Fig. 5.18 Periosteal osteosarcoma involving anteromedial part of proximal portion of tibial diaphysis in a 34-year-old woman who presented with a progressive, painful mass. Coronal T1-weighted MR image (500/20) obtained after administration of intravenous gadolinium chelate demonstrates the well-defined juxtacortical soft-tissue mass (*S*) and normal marrow (*m*). Mild thick peripheral and septal enhancement with nodularity (*arrows*) is seen after contrast agent administration. T2-weighted MR images (not shown) revealed high signal intensity in the soft-tissue mass (Murphey et al. 2004, 1997)

– Physiotherapy
– Arthrolysis of the knee
– Anterior cruciate ligament repair**
– Arthrodesis of the ankle

5.4 Piriformis Muscle Injection

5.4.1 Anatomy

Piriformis syndrome is due to compression of the sciatic nerve within the piriformis muscle. The piriformis muscle has its origin at the anterolateral sacrum below the sacroiliac joint as well as the upper edge of the sciatic notch. It then traverses the superior portion of the greater sciatic foramen. The muscle then inserts at the superomedial aspect of the greater trochanter. Usually, the sciatic nerve courses inferiorly from the anterior aspect of the piriformis toward the piriformis lower margin to leave the pelvis through the sciatic notch. Sometimes, however, the nerve penetrates the piriformis itself in 15% of the population. This results in compression or entrapment of the sciatic nerve during overuse or injury (Fig. 5.19).

Fig. 5.19 Anterior (**a**) and posterior (**b**) views of the piriformis muscle (Raj 2003c)

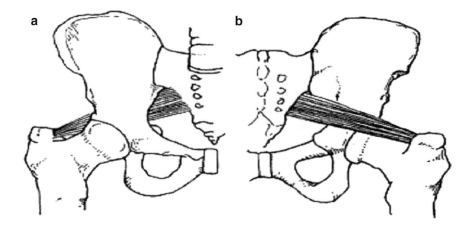

5.4.2 Function

The piriformis muscle is one of the external rotators of the hip that turns the lower extremity outward. The sciatic nerve (L4-S3 nerve roots) provides motor supply to the hamstrings, which are involved in hip extension and leg flexion (biceps femoris, semitendinosus, and semimembranosus). It also provides motor supply to flex and extend the ankle. Furthermore, it provides sensory supply to the posterolateral aspect of the knee, as well as the entire lower leg, toes, foot, and knee.

5.4.3 Clinical Presentation

Piriformis syndrome presents as pain in the sciatic nerve distribution. This involves the lower extremity and/or buttock region. There is also tenderness in the sciatic notch at the site of the sciatic nerve. This syndrome is distinguished from simple sciatica clinically by the pain being worse with sitting. On physical exam, the Pace Abduction test, Freiberg sign, and Bonnet's sign, among others, may be positive. Symptoms may be worsened by a prolonged combination of hip flexion, adduction, and medial rotation.

5.4.4 Etiology

Etiologies include anatomic variation, piriformis hypertrophy, trauma, overuse (bicycling or other athletic activities), and sacroiliac joint hypomobility.

5.4.5 Differential Diagnosis

Differential diagnoses include lumbar radiculopathy, facet arthropathy, and spinal stenosis.

5.4.6 Injection Site

Fluoroscopic guidance: Needle entry is just above the hip joint perpendicular to the skin at the midpoint between the trochanter and the sacrum.

CT guidance: Transgluteal puncture site chosen at mid piriformis level.

22-Gauge spinal needle advanced to anterior margin of piriformis adjacent to sciatic nerve (Fig. 5.20).

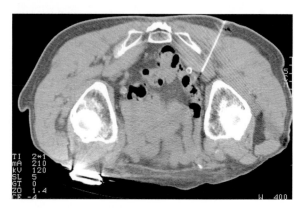

Fig. 5.20 CT of the piriformis muscle during image-guided injection. (Image courtesy of Keith E. Kortman, MD)

5.4.7 Cross-Sectional Anatomy

5.4.7.1 What Does the Needle Traverse?

Initially, the needle traverses the gluteus maximus, followed by the piriformis muscle.

5.4.7.2 Which Structures the Needle Should Avoid

It is advisable that the needle avoid the sciatic nerve as well as the inferior gluteal artery.

5.4.8 Imaging/Radiology

Fluoroscopy (Fishman et al. 1998) can be combined with EMG for enhanced accuracy.

Ultrasound (Peng and Tumber 2008) can directly visualize the muscle for guidance. Ultrasound use has also been reported for the diagnosis of piriformis syndrome (Broadhurst et al. 2004).

CT is able to directly visualize the muscle for guidance (Fanucci et al. 2001). In addition, it can characterize the enlarged piriformis muscle and sciatic nerve enlargement associated with piriformis syndrome (Jankiewicz et al. 1991). CT cannot assess pathological muscle edema, which MRI can do.

MRI (Lee et al. 2004) is the study of choice for the diagnosis of piriformis syndrome. It is able to exclude lumbar spine pathology (disc herniation or spinal stenosis). It also excludes pelvic masses. MRI evaluates the piriformis muscle for pathology (edema, hematoma, and size variation). Anatomic relationship of the sciatic nerve/sacral nerve roots to the piriformis can be assessed. MRI can show compression of the sciatic nerve at the sciatic notch, where the nerve courses inferior to the piriformis. It also allows better characterization of sciatic nerve pathology based on size and signal intensity (Fig. 5.21).

5.4.9 Indications

The indication for piriformis muscle injection is piriformis muscle syndrome**.

5.4.10 Complications

The unique complication associated with piriformis muscle injection is sciatic neuropathy**.

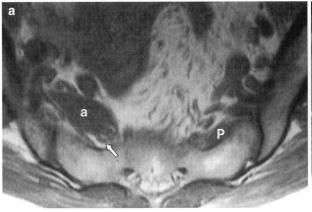
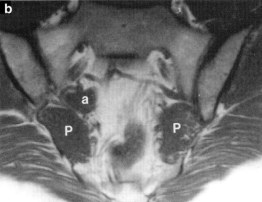
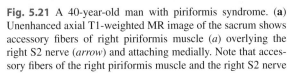

Fig. 5.21 A 40-year-old man with piriformis syndrome. (**a**) Unenhanced axial T1-weighted MR image of the sacrum shows accessory fibers of right piriformis muscle (*a*) overlying the right S2 nerve (*arrow*) and attaching medially. Note that accessory fibers of the right piriformis muscle and the right S2 nerve are of normal signal intensity. *P*, normal left piriformis muscle at sacral attachment. (**b**) Unenhanced oblique coronal T1-weighted MR image shows accessory fibers of right piriformis muscle (*a*) anterior to and obscuring right S2 nerve. *P*, normal right and left piriformis muscles (Lee et al. 2004)

5.5 Internal Pudendal Nerve Block

5.5.1 Anatomy

The internal pudendal nerve originates from the sacral plexus (S2-S4 ventral rami). It exits the pelvis through the inferior portion of the greater sciatic foramen (formed by the greater sciatic notch of the ilium, sacrotuberous ligament, sacrospinous ligament, and anterior sacroiliac ligament (below the piriformis and above the coccygeus muscle). It then drapes over the sacrospinous ligament and ischial spine to enter back into the pelvis via the lesser sciatic foramen (formed by the spine of the ischium/sacrospinous ligament, sacrotuberous ligament, and the ischial tuberosity) (Fig. 5.22). It then forms a neurovascular bundle with the internal pudendal artery and vein. It is enveloped in the pudendal canal (Alcock's canal) formed by the obturator fascia and travels adjacent to the lateral wall of the ischiorectal fossa. The inferior rectal nerve emanates from the internal pudendal nerve. The internal pudendal nerve itself then divides into the perineal nerve and the dorsal nerve of the penis or clitoris.

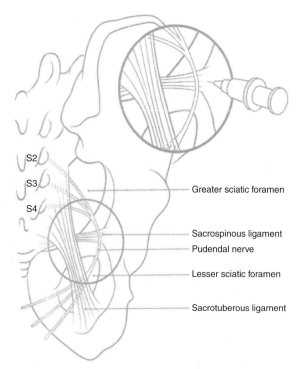

S2
S3
S4
Greater sciatic foramen
Sacrospinous ligament
Pudendal nerve
Lesser sciatic foramen
Sacrotuberous ligament

Fig. 5.22 The tract of the pudendal nerve and needle placement for the block (Choi et al. 2006)

5.5.2 Function

The internal pudendal nerve supplies the penis and clitoris. It provides sensation of the scrotum, perineum, and anus. It provides motor supply to the bulbospongiosus and ischiocavernosus muscle. It is responsible for ejaculation and orgasm as well as control of the external anal sphincter.

5.5.3 Clinical Presentation

Pudendal nerve entrapment syndrome presents as chronic perineal pain involving the genitalia, anorectal region, or perineum. It is worsened by sitting and relieved by standing. There is no pain, however, when sitting on a toilet seat. Symptoms of urinary hesitancy, urinary frequency, urinary urgency, painful bowel movements, and sexual dysfunction may also be present.

5.5.4 Etiology

- Entrapment of the pudendal nerve at the ischial spine between the sacrospinous and sacrotuberous ligament.
- Entrapment of the pudendal nerve within the pudendal canal flattened by the falciform process of the sacrotuberous ligament. The syndrome may also be associated with bicycling, chronic constipation, vaginal delivery, repetitive motion injury (dancers), sports, heavy lifting, squatting, gymnastics, and jogging etc. It may also be seen in metabolic diseases.
- Post hemorrhoidectomy pain.
- Transrectal biopsy of the prostate (Adsan et al. 2004).

5.5.5 Differential Diagnosis

Differential diagnosis includes chronic nonbacterial prostatitis.

5.5.6 Injection Site

Two injection sites can be used: (1) The transvaginal approach towards the ischial spine using manual palpation of the ischial spine through the vaginal wall with the patient in the lithotomy position. The needle is advanced using the finger for guidance. (2) The transperineal approach in males is directed just medial to the ischial tuberosity to the depth of 2–3 cm. The needle is advanced to the ischial spine using manual palpation through the rectum for guidance. The transgluteal approach is described for fluoroscopy, ultrasound, and CT below.

5.5.7 Cross-Sectional Anatomy

5.5.7.1 What Does the Needle Traverse? (Transgluteal Approach)

The needle traverses the gluteus maximus, the sacrotuberous ligament and the interligamentous space (between the sacrospinous ligament and the sacrotuberous ligament). The needle should stay posterior to the sacrospinous ligament and medial to the obturator fascia. The needle is adjacent to the pudendal neurovascular bundle (Fig. 5.25).

5.5.7.2 Which Structures the Needle Should Avoid

It is advisable that the needle avoid the internal pudendal artery and vein, the inferior gluteal artery (Gupta et al. 2004); (Peng and Tumber 2008), and the sciatic nerve.

5.5.8 Imaging/Radiology

Fluoroscopy (Abdi et al. 2004): A transgluteal approach is used in the prone position with ipsilateral oblique angulation of the c-arm to visualize the tip of the ischial spine (falciform process). This is less accurate than ultrasound or CT because the target is the ischial spine and there may be a failure of dispersal of injectate to the pudendal nerve. Furthermore, the interligamentous space cannot be visualized. However, fluoroscopy is readily available (Fig. 5.23).

Ultrasound (Kovacs et al. 2001): Using ultrasound guidance, the internal pudendal artery can be visualized reliably in its arch around the ischial spine. The sacrospinous and sacrotuberous ligaments can also be detected reliably. The pudendal nerve adjacent to the ischial spine can also be directly visualized in approximately 30–50% of cases via the transgluteal approach. The site of injection should be 8 mm medial to the tip of the ischial spine or 5 mm medial to the pudendal artery in the interligamentous plane between the sacrospinous and sacrotuberous ligaments (Fig. 5.24).

CT: The ischial spine (where the pudendal nerve wraps around it) is targeted via a posterior transgluteal approach (Thoumas et al. 1999); (McDonald and Spigos 2000). The pudendal canal is another target at a point between the neurovascular bundle and the obturator muscle (Fig. 5.25).

MRI is useful in pelvic floor evaluation for the diagnosis of etiologies of pudendal neuralgia.

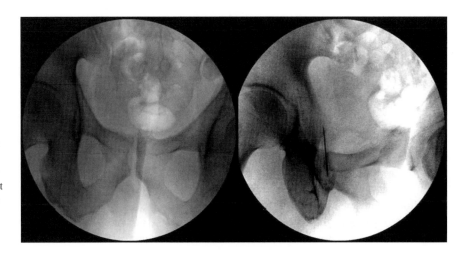

Fig. 5.23 (*Left*) Straight AP radiograph of the pelvic bones. (*Right*) Oblique view of the ischial spine. Note that the tip of the needle is at the falciform process of the ischial bone (Abdi et al. 2004)

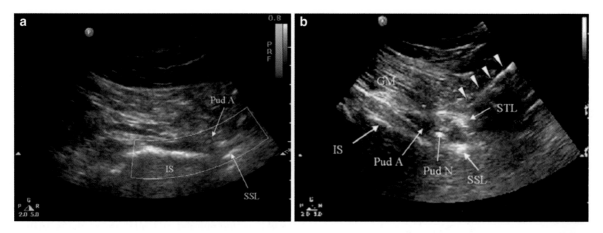

Fig. 5.24 Ultrasound picture of the pudendal nerve before and during injections. (**a**) Color Doppler showing the pudendal artery at the level of the ischial spine. (**b**) Ultrasound picture showing the interligamentous plane and the needle insertion following injection of local anesthetic and steroid. *STL* sacrotuberous ligament; *SSL* sacrospinous ligament; *Pud A* pudendal artery; *Pud N* pudendal nerve, *IS* ischium at ischial spine level; *GM* gluteus maximus. The needle was outlined by the *solid arrows* (Peng and Tumber 2008)

5.5.9 Indications

The most frequent indication for pudendal nerve block is chronic anoperineal pain or pelvic pain from pudendal neuralgia. Another common indication is labor pain during vaginal delivery.

5.5.10 Complications

A unique complication of pudendal nerve block is retroperitoneal hematoma** (Fig. 5.26).

5.6 Iliohypogastric–Ilioinguinal Nerve Block

5.6.1 Iliohypogastric Nerve Injection

5.6.1.1 Anatomy

The iliohypogastric nerve has its origin at L1 primarily with minor supply from T12. The superior branch is the iliohypogastric nerve and the inferior branch is the ilioinguinal nerve. The iliohypogastric nerve crosses through the psoas muscle and passes the lateral margin to travel anteriorly adjacent to the quadratus

lumborum. It then courses behind the kidney into the lateral abdominal wall. At the iliac crest region, it travels between the transversus abdominis and internal oblique muscles. The nerve has an anterior cutaneous branch and a lateral cutaneous branch (Figs. 5.27–5.29).

5.6.1.2 Function

The iliohypogastric nerve supplies the inferior portion of the transversus abdominis and internal oblique muscles. The anterior cutaneous branch supplies sensation to the skin just above the pubic region.

5.6.1.3 Clinical Presentation

Iliohypogastric nerve injury causes suprapubic and inguinal pain with extension to the genital region. There is minimal sensory loss due to the small area of skin supplied by this nerve. The iliohypogastric nerve shares in providing sensation to areas also supplied by either the genitofemoral or ilioinguinal nerves.

5.6.1.4 Etiology

The main cause of iliohypogastric nerve damage is surgical injury. This can be seen following abdominal,

Fig. 5.25 Cadaver of a 77-year-old man with diabetes mellitus. CT scans were obtained with cadaver prone. (**a, b**) Thin-slice CT scans obtained at level of ischial spine show sacrospinous (*short arrows*, **a**) and sacrotuberous (*long arrows*, **a**) ligaments and calcified internal pudendal artery (*arrowhead*, **a**) marking location of pudendal bundle. (**b**) Transgluteal needle is visible, and injected contrast agent is seen filling interligamentous space. (**c–e**) In thin-section CT scans obtained at level of pudendal canal, calcified internal pudendal artery (*arrowhead*, **c**) marks site of pudendal bundle in canal, and fat plane between neurovascular bundle and obturator internus muscle is clearly seen (*arrow*, **c**) and (**d**) obtained 2.5 mm caudal to (**c**) shows transgluteal needle in fat plane lateral relative to neurovascular bundle. Contained medially by obturator fascia, injected contrast agent fills pudendal canal, obliterating fat plane (**e**) (Hough et al. 2003)

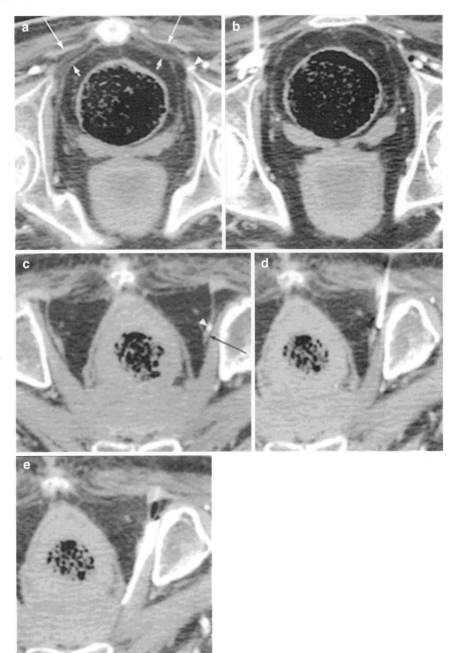

or pelvic surgery (hernia repair, nephrectomy**, appendectomy**, suture/staple placement**), spontaneous development during pregnancy or post partum, neuroma, psoas abscess/mass **, or blunt trauma to the groin (Shadbolt et al. 2001).

5.6.1.5 Differential Diagnosis

Differential diagnoses include upper lumbar radiculopathy** and other etiologies for inferior pelvic/inguinal pain**.

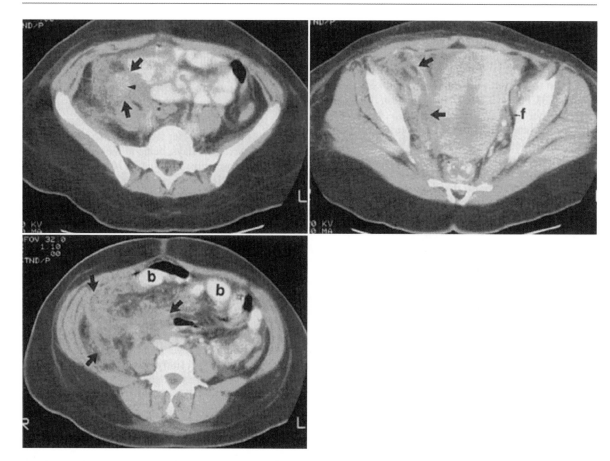

Fig. 5.26 Retroperitoneal hematoma after pudendal nerve block. Routine axial CT scan images after the intravenous administration of contrast media, at the pelvic rim (*top*) and lower pelvis (*middle*) show abnormal heterogeneous fluid and soft tissue densities in the right retroperitoneal space (retroperitoneal hematoma) along the right iliac and psoas muscles (*arrows*). The area of high density (*arrowhead*) within the lesion is consistent with hemorrhage. The enlarged postpartum uterus is slightly deviated to the left. The normal fat planes along the right pelvic sidewall are obliterated compared with the normal fat plane (*f*) on the left side. *Bottom*: An Axial CT scan taken below the right renal fossa shows heterogenous fluid and soft tissue densities (*arrow*) in the right retroperitoneal compartment along the right psoas muscle. The normal bowel loops (*b*) are displaced anteriorly and to the left (Kurzel et al. 1996). (Reproduced from West J of Med, Kurzel et al, vol. 164, pp 523-5, 1996 with permission from BMJ Publishing Group Ltd.)

5.6.1.6 Injection Site

The site of iliohypogastric nerve injection is 3 cm medial to the anterior superior iliac spine between the anterior superior iliac spine and the umbilicus (Fig. 5.27).

5.6.2 Ilioinguinal Nerve Injection

5.6.2.1 Anatomy

The ilioinguinal nerve is formed by the combination of the T12 and L1 anterior rami. It travels just below the iliohypogastric nerve in a similar course through the psoas. The ilioinguinal nerve then travels along the lateral abdominal wall to the anterior abdominal wall. As it reaches the iliac crest at its ventral aspect, it courses between the transversus abdominis and internal oblique muscles (see Figs. 5.28–5.30).

5.6.2.2 Function

The ilioinguinal nerve supplies motor function to the transversus abdominis and internal oblique muscles in their inferior portion. It supplies sensation to the pubic symphysis. It also supplies sensation to the upper and medial portion of the femoral triangle (formed by the inguinal ligament superiorly, adductor magnus medially,

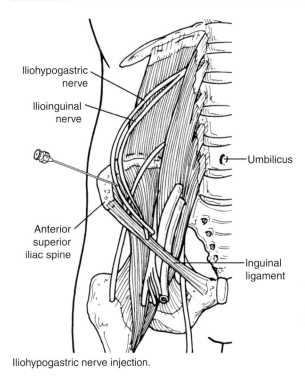

Iliohypogastric nerve injection.

Fig. 5.27 Iliohypogastric nerve injection (Weiss 2007a; p. 129, Fig. 6-17)

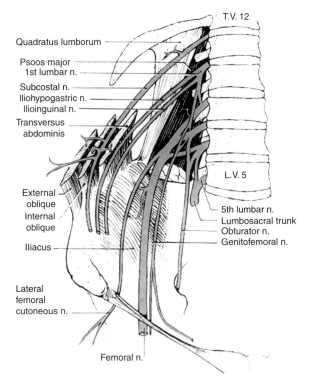

Fig. 5.28 Origin, course, and relations of ilioinguinal, iliohypogastric, and genitofemoral nerves (Waldman 2001)

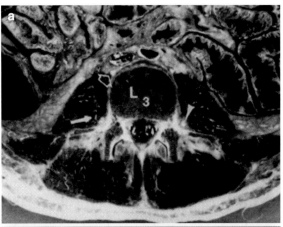

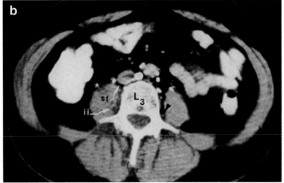

Fig. 5.29 (**a**) Normal anatomic section. (**b**) Normal CT section. At the level of L3, the L2 spinal nerve is seen posterior to the psoas muscle. The iliohypogastric and ilioinguinal nerves pierce the psoas fasciculi. The *arrowhead* indicates the L2 spinal nerve; the *arrow* indicates the iliohypogastric and ilioinguinal (*ii*) nerves, and the *open arrow* indicates the sympathetic trunk. *Curved arrows* indicate the regions of the above nerves not actually identified in the CT sections. *Asterisk* indicates genitofemoral nerve located on the surface of the psoas muscle (Gebarski et al. 1986)

and the sartorius laterally). Furthermore, it supplies sensation to the anterior scrotum and base of the penis in men as well as the mons pubis and labia majora in women.

5.6.2.3 Clinical Presentation (Ilioinguinal Nerve Injury)

In ilioinguinal nerve injury there is often pain in the inner groin and thigh as well as the genital region that can extend into the inferior abdominal region. There may be hypersensitivity or decreased sensation of the skin overlying the inguinal ligament.

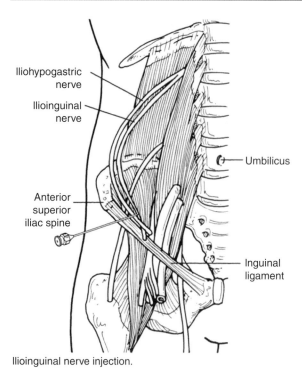

Iliohypogastric nerve

Ilioinguinal nerve

Anterior superior iliac spine

Umbilicus

Inguinal ligament

Ilioinguinal nerve injection.

Fig. 5.30 Ilioinguinal nerve injection (Weiss 2007b; p. 130, Fig. 6-19)

5.6.2.4 Etiology

Common causes of ilioinguinal nerve injury include: Lower abdominal**, pelvic** or inguinal surgery**, femoral catheterization, pregnancy, and traumatic injury to the lower external oblique aponeurosis**.

5.6.2.5 Differential Diagnosis

The differential diagnoses include upper lumbar radiculopathy**, obturator neuropathy**, femoral neuropathy**, lateral femoral cutaneous neuropathy, iliohypogastric neuropathy, genitofemoral neuropathy, other etiologies of inferior pelvic/inguinal pain.

5.6.2.6 Injection Site

The site of injection is 2–3 cm medial and inferior to the anterosuperior iliac spine (Figs. 5.30–5.32).

5.6.3 Cross-Sectional Anatomy (Iliohypogastric–Ilioinguinal Nerve)

5.6.3.1 What Does the Needle Traverse?

The needle first traverses the external oblique superior to the iliac crest, followed by the transverse abdominis. It is important to stay superficial to the internal oblique muscle.

5.6.3.2 Which Structures the Needle Should Avoid?

The needle ought to avoid the peritoneum and the femoral nerve.

5.6.4 Imaging/Radiology

- CT, ultrasound, or MRI maybe useful only to exclude pathologies other than ilioinguinal or iliohypogastric nerve entrapment/neuroma. (Vervest et al. 2006) (Fig. 5.31)
- Anatomic landmark guidance
  - Most commonly performed

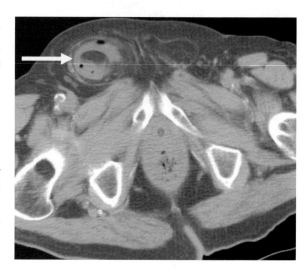

Fig. 5.31 Direct inguinal hernia in a 57-year-old man. Axial unenhanced reformatted CT image of the abdomen shows a direct inguinal hernia (*arrow*) medial to the inferior epigastric vessels on the right side of the groin. Note the presence of bowel loops in the hernia sac. If this patient underwent a hernia repair he would be at risk for iliohypogastric nerve entrapment (Aguirre et al. 2005)

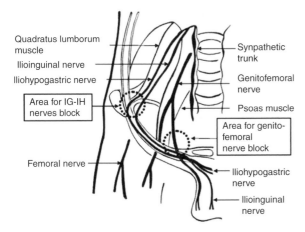

Quadratus lumborum muscle
Ilioinguinal nerve
Iliohypogastric nerve
Area for IG-IH nerves block
Femoral nerve
Synpathetic trunk
Genitofemoral nerve
Psoas muscle
Area for genito-femoral nerve block
Iliohypogastric nerve
Ilioinguinal nerve

Fig. 5.32 Course of the ilioinguinal, iliohypogastric, and genitofemoral nerves. The *circle* indicates area infiltrated with local analgesic for each block. The center of the circle (*dotted line*) indicates the point of insertion of the needle for each nerve block (Sasaoka et al. 2005)

- Ultrasound guidance
  - Can directly visualize the ilioinguinal and iliohypogastric nerves (Fig. 5.33).

- May allow one to avoid adjacent vessels and the peritoneal cavity
- Can avoid femoral nerve

5.6.5 Indications

The following are common indications for ilioinguinal–iliohypogastric plexus block:

- Injury to the ilioinguinal–ilioinguinal injury to the nerve
  - Suture or staple placement
  - Fibrous adhesions or neuroma
- Surgical procedures
  - Laparoscopy
  - Needle bladder suspension
  - Open and laparoscopic hernia repair
  - Cesarean section**
  - Nephrectomy**
  - Appendectomy**

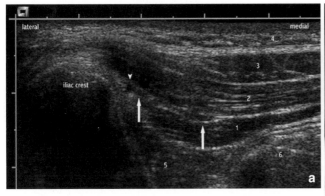

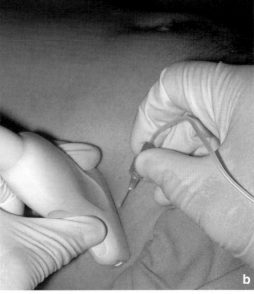

Fig. 5.33 Inguinal sonoanatomy (**a**) obtained by the transducer position as shown in (**b**). The *lateral arrow* points to the ilioinguinal nerve. The medial arrow points to the iliohypogastric nerve. Both are lying between the transverse abdominal (*1*) and internal oblique abdominal muscle (*2*). The *arrowhead* points to a small vessel next to the ilioinguinal nerve. In contrast to the nerves, the vessel appears completely dark (hypoechogenic). The nerves appear dark with a white horizon and white spots inside (typical sonographic morphology of a peripheral nerve). *3*, External oblique muscle; *4*, subcutaneous tissue. *5*, iliac muscle; *6*, intraperitoneal space. (**b**) Transducer and needle position to perform a block of the inguinal nerves. The lateral edge of the transducer is in contact with the iliac crest about 5 cm cranial and lateral (posterior) to the anterior superior iliac spine (Curatolo and Eichenberger 2007)

– Abdominoplasty
– Anterior superior iliac crest bone graft
• Spontaneous development of ilioinguinal-iliohypogastric neuropathy during pregnancy or post partum
• Post-operative pain
  – Inguinal hernia repair**
  – Appendectomy** or caesarian
  – Orchiopexy
• Psoas abscess/mass**
• Blunt trauma to the groin (Shadbolt et al. 2001)
• To diagnose and treat chronic pain from nerve entrapment, neuroma, and neuralgia

5.7 Genitofemoral Nerve Block

5.7.1 Anatomy

The genitofemoral nerve originates from the L1 and L2 anterior rami. It forms in the psoas muscles. It traverses the psoas to its ventral surface and continues inferiorly. In the vicinity of the inguinal ligament, it divides into genital and femoral branches (Figs. 5.29 and 5.34).

The femoral branch courses along the anterior surface of the psoas and travels below the inguinal ligament lateral to the common femoral artery. It then extends into the upper thigh.

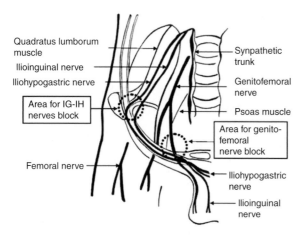

Fig. 5.34 Course of the ilioinguinal, iliohypogastric, and genitofemoral nerves. The *circle* indicates area infiltrated with local analgesic for each block. The center of the circle (*dotted line*) indicates the point of insertion of the needle for each nerve block (Sasaoka et al. 2005)

The genital branch courses medial to the femoral branch and travels through the deep inguinal ring to enter the inguinal canal.

5.7.2 Function

The genitofemoral nerve has two main branches. The genital branch supplies the scrotum, spermatic cord, and cremaster muscles. The femoral branch supplies sensation to the anterior proximal thigh.

5.7.3 Clinical Presentation

Genitofemoral nerve injury/entrapment typically presents with groin pain worse with ambulation and rotation of the hip. It may also result in decreased sensation within the anterior proximal thigh lateral to the ilioinguinal nerve distribution.

5.7.4 Etiology

Causes of genitofemoral nerve injury include: Lower abdominal**/pelvic**/inguinal surgery**, blunt or penetrating trauma**, iliopsoas mass/hemorrhage**, or pregnancy**.

5.7.5 Differential Diagnosis

Differential diagnoses include upper lumbar radiculopathy, obturator neuropathy, femoral neuropathy, lateral femoral cutaneous neuropathy, ilioinguinal neuropathy, and iliohypogastric neuropathy.

5.7.6 Injection Site

The injection site is usually at or below the inguinal ligament adjacent to the saphenous nerve (Fig. 5.34).

5.7.7 Cross-Sectional Anatomy

5.7.7.1 What Does the Needle Traverse?

The needle traverses the rectus abdominis (inferior aspect), the aponeurosis of the external oblique, and passes just superior and lateral to the pubic tubercle (see Fig. 5.36).

5.7.7.2 Which Structures the Needle Should Avoid?

It is advisable that the needle avoid the testicular artery and vas deferens within the spermatic cord (Peng and Tumber 2008) the femoral nerve, artery, and vein, the peritoneum, and the bladder.

5.7.8 Imaging/Radiology

Imaging is commonly performed for the purposes of anatomic landmark guidance.

Fluoroscopy may be used in obese patients to locate the pubic tubercle between the anterior superior iliac spine and the pubic symphysis.

Ultrasound may be useful for guidance and for the diagnosis of testicular pathology (Fig. 5.35).

CT/MRI are useful in the diagnosis to exclude other causes of pelvic pathology.

5.7.9 Indications

The following are common indications (Trescot 2003) for genitofemoral nerve block:

- In conjunction with ilioinguinal and iliohypogastric nerve blocks for:
- Inguinal hernia repair** (indications of surgery can be imaged)
- Orchiopexy** (indications of surgery can be imaged)
- Hydrocelectomy** (indications of surgery can be imaged)
- In conjunction with femoral nerve block for long saphenous vein stripping
- To diagnose and treat genitofemoral neuralgia
- To investigate chronic testicular pain
- Post radiofrequency ablation of renal tumors (may not be treatable with percutaneous genitofemoral nerve block and may require laparoscopic visualization to isolate and treat the proximal genitofemoral nerve) (Boss et al. 2005).

5.7.10 Complications

The following complications are encountered in both ilioinguinal-iliohypogastric and genitofemoral nerve blocks: (1) Hemorrhage**; (2) peritoneal puncture**; (3) local hematoma**; (4) undesired motor blockade of the femoral nerve; (5) colonic puncture** during ilioinguinal nerve block in a child (Fig. 5.37).

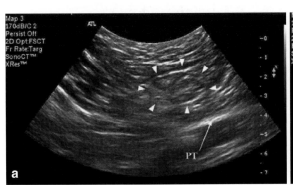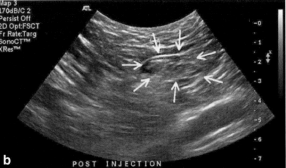

Fig. 5.35 Ultrasound pictures showing pre- and post-injection into spermatic cord during genitofemoral nerve block. (**a**) Spermatic cord before injection (*arrowheads*). (**b**) Spermatic cord (*arrows*) after injection (Peng and Tumber 2008)

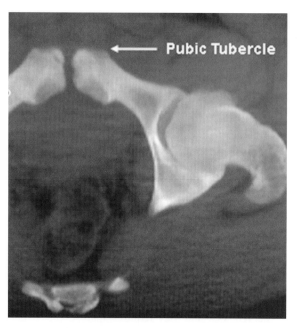

Fig. 5.36 CT axial anatomy with bone algorithm at the level of the genitofemoral nerve, which lies just superior and lateral to the pubic tubercle

5.8 Lateral Femoral Cutaneous Nerve Block

5.8.1 Anatomy

The lateral femoral cutaneous nerve originates from the anterior rami of L2-L4. The lateral femoral cutaneous nerve is formed in the psoas muscle and extends inferiorly and laterally beyond this muscle. It traverses anterior to the iliacus muscle in the direction of the anterior superior iliac spine. It then courses below the inguinal ligament laterally and splits into the anterior and posterior branches (Fig. 5.38 and 5.39).

5.8.2 Function

The lateral femoral cutaneous nerve provides sensation to the anterior lateral thigh above the knee.

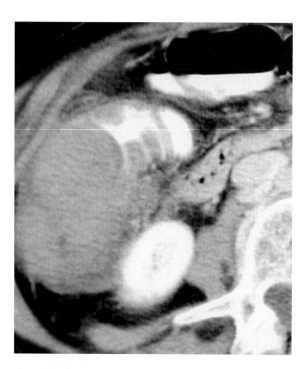

Fig. 5.37 Intramural hematoma. Contrast-enhanced CT image from a patient with melanoma shows an extensive submucosal hemorrhage that occurred during a biopsy performed at colonoscopy (Pickhardt et al. 2007)

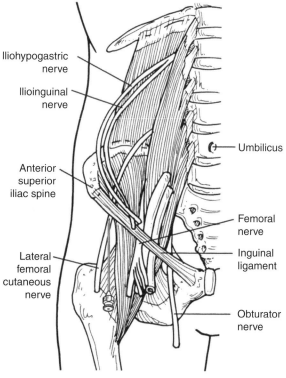

Fig. 5.38 Lateral femoral cutaneous nerve injection (Weiss 2007c; p. 133, Fig. 6-21)

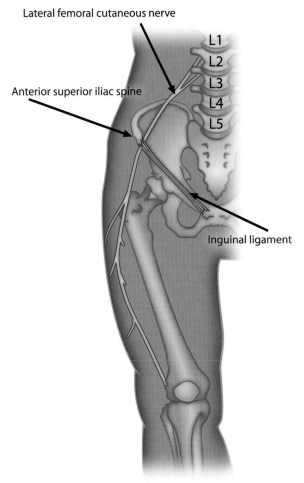

Fig. 5.39 Lateral femoral cutaneous nerve block

5.8.3 Clinical Presentation

The clinical syndrome is known as meralgia paresthetica. It causes burning/paresthesia in the proximal and anterolateral thigh, which is worsened with weight-bearing, hip extension, or the prone position. Entrapment/injury to the nerve usually occurs at the inguinal ligament.

5.8.4 Etiology

Etiologies include trauma** to the region of the anterior superior iliac spine, seatbelt injury, tight garments, belt, or girdles; previous surgery**, pregnancy**, tumor**, uterine fibroids**, diverticulitis**, appendicitis**, and abdominal aortic aneurysm**; obesity/ascites**; prolonged sitting/standing; pelvic tilt due to leg length inequality**, entrapment by fascia related to the anterior superior iliac spine, and encasement of the nerve within the bone by the anterior superior iliac spine apophysis; Perthes disease**, abduction splints, and diabetes.

5.8.5 Differential Diagnosis

The differential diagnosis includes upper lumbar radiculopathy**, obturator neuropathy**, femoral neuropathy**, ilioinguinal neuropathy, iliohypogastric neuropathy, and genitofemoral neuropathy.

5.8.6 Injection Site

The injection site lies 2–3 cm medial and inferior to the anterior superior iliac spine (ASIS) just below the inguinal ligament (Fig. 5.38).

5.8.7 Imaging/Radiology

Ultrasound can be used for guidance (Tumber et al. 2008); (Hurdle et al. 2007). The nerve can be identified in the inguinal region in 70% of cases (Damarey et al. 2009).

5.8.8 Indications

The two principal indications for lateral femoral cutaneous block are:

- Meralgia paresthetica syndrome
- Post-operative (appendectomy, laparotomy, iliac harvesting, etc.)**
- Post traumatic**
- Compression or injury to the LFCN near the ASIS through or under the inguinal ligament**
- Rarely compression of the nerve due to neoplasm** (see Fig. 5.40), abdominal aortic aneurysm** (should be evaluated for prior to block), or contained iliopsoas hemorrhage**.

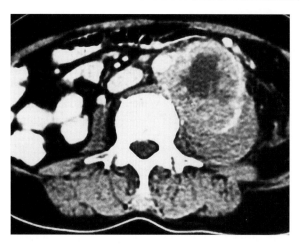

Fig. 5.40 Primary iliopsoas involvement by tumor in a 46-year-old woman with carcinoma of the cervix. Contrast-enhanced CT scan shows a heterogeneous necrotic tumor in the left psoas muscle (Muttarak and Peh 2000)

5.8.9 Complications

The two main complications associated with femoral cutaneous block are: (1) Neuritis secondary to needle trauma or drug toxicity, (2) inadvertent femoral nerve block.

References

Harris RD, Holtzman SR, Poppe AM. Clinical outcome in female patients with pelvic pain and normal pelvic US findings. Radiology. 2000;216(2):440-3

ACR Practice Guideline for the Performance of Pelvic Ultrasound in Females. http://www.acr.org/SecondaryMainMenu Categories/quality_safety/guidelines/us/us_pelvic.aspx

ACR Practice Guideline for the Performance of Computed Tomography (CT) of the Abdomen and Computed Tomography of the Pelvis). http://www.acr.org/Secondary MainMenu Categories/quality_safety/guidelines/dx/gastro/ct_abdomen_pelvis.aspx

Hubert J, Bergin D. Imaging of the female pelvis: when should MRI be considered. Appl Radiol. 2008;37(1):9-24

ACR Practice Guidelines for the Performance of Magnetic Resonance Imaging (MRI) of the Soft Tissue Components of thePelvis.http://www.acr.org/SecondaryMainMenuCategories/quality_safety/guidelines/dx/gastro/mri_pelvis.aspx

Kuligowska E, Deeds L III, Lu K III. Pelvic pain: overlooked and underdiagnosed gynecologic conditions. Radiographics. 2005;25(1):3-20. Review

Plancarte R, Arnescua C, Patt RB: Sympathetic neurolytic blockade. In Patt RB (ed): Cancer Pain. Philadelphia, JB Lippincott, 1993, pp 377-425.

Mackey S, Sze D, Gaeta R. Magnetic resonance therapy guided regional blockade for pain management (abstr). Anesthesiology. 1999;91:968

Gaertner E, Lascurain P, Venet C, Maschino X, Zamfir A, Lupescu R, Hadzic A. Continuous parasacral sciatic block: a radiographic study. Anesth Analg. 2004;98(3):831-4

Fishman SM, Caneris OA, Bandman TB, Audette JF, Borsook D. Injection of the piriformis muscle by fluoroscopic and electromyographic guidance. Reg Anesth Pain Med. 1998;23(6):554-9

Peng PW, Tumber PS. Ultrasound-guided interventional procedures for patients with chronic pelvic pain – a description of techniques and review of literature. Pain Physician. 2008;11 (2):215-24

Broadhurst NA, Simmons DN, Bond MJ. Piriformis syndrome: correlation of muscle morphology with symptoms and signs. Arch Phys Med Rehabil. 2004;85(12):2036-9

Fanucci E, Masala S, Sodani G, Varrucciu V, Romagnoli A, Squillaci E, Simonetti G. CT-guided injection of botulinic toxin for percutaneous therapy of piriformis muscle syndrome with preliminary MRI results about denervative process. Eur Radiol. 2001;11(12):2543-8

Jankiewicz JJ, Hennrikus WL, Houkom JA. The appearance of the piriformis muscle syndrome in computed tomography and magnetic resonance imaging. A case report and review of the literature. Clin Orthop Relat Res. 1991;(262):205-9

Adsan O, Inal G, Ozdo an L, Kaygisiz O, U urlu O, Cetinkaya M. Unilateral pudendal nerve blockade for relief of all pain during transrectal ultrasound-guided biopsy of the prostate: a randomized, double-blind, placebo-controlled study. Urology. 2004;64(3):528-31

Gupta S, Nguyen HL, Morello FA Jr, Ahrar K, Wallace MJ, Madoff DC, Murthy R, Hicks ME. Various approaches for CT-guided percutaneous biopsy of deep pelvic lesions: anatomic and technical considerations. Radiographics. 2004;24 (1):175-89

Kovacs P, Gruber H, Piegger J, Bodner G. New, simple, ultrasound-guided infiltration of the pudendal nerve: ultrasonographic technique. Dis Colon Rectum. 2001;44(9):1381-5

Thoumas D, Leroi AM, Mauillon J, Muller JM, Benozio M, Denis P, Freger P. Pudendal neuralgia: CT-guided pudendal nerve block technique. Abdom Imaging. 1999;24(3): 309-12

McDonald JS, Spigos DG. Computed tomography-guided pudendal block for treatment of pelvic pain due to pudendal neuropathy. Obstet Gynecol. 2000;95(2):306-9

Shadbolt CL, Heinze SB, Dietrich RB. Imaging of groin masses: inguinal anatomy and pathologic conditions revisited. Radiographics. 2001;21 Spec No:S261-71. Review

Vervest HA, Bongers MY, van der Wurff AA. Nerve injury: an exceptional cause of pain after TVT. Int Urogynecol J Pelvic Floor Dysfunct. 2006;17(6):665-7

Trescot AM. Cryoanalgesia in interventional pain management. Pain Physician. 2003;6(3):345-60

Boss A, Clasen S, Kuczyk M, Anastasiadis A, Schmidt D, Claussen CD, Schick F, Pereira PL. Thermal damage of the genitofemoral nerve due to radiofrequency ablation of renal cell carcinoma: a potentially avoidable complication. AJR Am J Roentgenol. 2005;185(6):1627-31

Tumber PS, Bhatia A, Chan VW. Ultrasound-guided lateral femoral cutaneous nerve block for meralgia paresthetica. Anesth Analg. 2008;106(3):1021-2

Hurdle MF, Weingarten TN, Crisostomo RA, Psimos C, Smith J. Ultrasound-guided blockade of the lateral femoral cutaneous nerve: technical description and review of 10 cases. Arch Phys Med Rehabil. 2007;88(10):1362-4

Damarey B, Demondion X, Boutry N, Kim HJ, Wavreille G, Cotten A. Sonographic assessment of the lateral femoral cutaneous nerve. J Clin Ultrasound. 2009;37(2):89-95

Rathmell JP. Atlas of image-guided intervention in regional anesthesia and pain medicine. Philadelphia, PA: Lippincott Williams and Wilkins, 2006

Wechsler RJ, Maurer PM, Halpern EJ, Frank ED. Superior hypogastric plexus block for chronic pelvic pain in the presence of endometriosis: CT techniques and results. Radiology. 1995;196(1):103-6

Woodward PJ, Sohaey R, Mezzetti TP Jr. Endometriosis: radiologic-pathologic correlation. Radiographics. 2001;21(1): 193-216; questionnaire 288-94

Waldman SD. Interventional pain management, 2nd ed. Philadelphia, PA: Saunders, 2001

Toshniwal GR, Dureja GP, Prashanth SM. Transsacrococcygeal approach to ganglion impar block for management of chronic perineal pain: a prospective observational study. Pain Physician. 2007;10(5):661-6

Ho KY, Nagi PA, Gray L, Huh BK. An alternative approach to ganglion impar neurolysis under computed tomography guidance for recurrent vulva cancer. Anesthesiology. 2006; 105(4):861-2

Pannu HK, Corl FM, Fishman EK. CT evaluation of cervical cancer: spectrum of disease. Radiographics. 2001;21(5): 1155-68. Review

Raj PP. Radiographic imaging for regional anesthesia and pain management. New York: Churchill Livingstone, 2003a:247-8

Raj PP. Radiographic imaging for regional anesthesia and pain management. New York: Churchill Livingstone, 2003b

Blake LC, Robertson WD, Hayes CE. Sacral plexus: optimal imaging planes for MR assessment. Radiology. 1996;199(3): 767-72

Harisinghani MG, Gervais DA, Hahn PF, Cho CH, Jhaveri K, Varghese J, Mueller PR. CT-guided transgluteal drainage of deep pelvic abscesses: indications, technique, procedure-related complications, and clinical outcome. Radiographics. 2002;22(6):1353-67

Karmakar MK, Kwok WH, Ho AM, Tsang K, Chui PT, Gin T. Ultrasound-guided sciatic nerve block: description of a new approach at the subgluteal space. Br J Anaesth. 2007;98(3): 390-5

Murphey MD, Jelinek JS, Temple HT, Flemming DJ, Gannon FH. Imaging of periosteal osteosarcoma: radiologic-pathologic comparison. Radiology. 2004;233(1):129-38

Murphey MD, Robbin MR, McRae GA, Flemming DJ, Temple HT, Kransdorf MJ. The many faces of osteosarcoma. Radiographics. 1997;17(5):1205-31

Raj PP. Radiographic imaging for regional anesthesia and pain management. New York : Churchill Livingstone, 2003c:250

Lee EY, Margherita AJ, Gierada DS, Narra VR. MRI of piriformis syndrome. AJR Am J Roentgenol. 2004;183(1):63-4

Choi SS, Lee PB, Kim YC, Kim HJ, Lee SC. C-arm-guided pudendal nerve block: a new technique. Int J Clin Pract. 2006;60(5):553-6

Abdi S, Shenouda P, Patel N, Saini B, Bharat Y, Calvillo O. A novel technique for pudendal nerve block. Pain Physician. 2004;7(3):319-22

Hough DM, Wittenberg KH, Pawlina W, Maus TP, King BF, Vrtiska TJ, Farrell MA, Antolak SJ Jr. Chronic perineal pain caused by pudendal nerve entrapment: anatomy and CT-guided perineural injection technique. AJR Am J Roentgenol. 2003;181(2):561-7

Kurzel RB, Au AH, Rooholamini SA. Retroperitoneal hematoma as a complication of pudendal block. Diagnosis made by computed tomography. West J Med. 1996; 164(6):523-5

Weiss LD. Easy injections. Philadelphia, PA: Elsevier, 2007a:129, Figure 6-17. NLM ID: 101308328

Waldman SD. Interventional pain management, 2nd ed. Philadelphia, PA: W.B Saunders Company, 2001:509. ISBN 0-7216-8748-2

Gebarski KS, Gebarski SS, Glazer GM, Samuels BI, Francis IR. The lumbosacral plexus: anatomic-radiologic-pathologic correlation using CT. Radiographics. 1986;6(3):401-25

Weiss LD. Easy injections. Philadelphia, PA: Elsevier, 2007b:130, Figure 6-19. NLM ID: 101308328

Aguirre DA, Santosa AC, Casola G, Sirlin CB. Abdominal wall hernias: imaging features, complications, and diagnostic pitfalls at multi-detector row CT. Radiographics. 2005; 25(6): 1501-20. Review

Sasaoka N, Kawaguchi M, Yoshitani K, Kato H, Suzuki A, Furuya H. Evaluation of genitofemoral nerve block, in addition to ilioinguinal and iliohypogastric nerve block, during inguinal hernia repair in children. Br J Anaesth. 2005;94(2):243-6

Curatolo M, Eichenberger U. Ultrasound-guided blocks for the treatment of chronic pain. Tech Reg Anesth Pain Manag. 2007;11:95-102

Pickhardt PJ, Kim DH, Menias CO, Gopal DV, Arluk GM, Heise CP. Evaluation of submucosal lesions of the large intestine: part 2. Nonneoplastic causes. Radiographics. 2007;27(6): 1693-703. Review

Weiss LD. Easy injections. Philadelphia, PA: Elsevier, 2007c:133, Figure 6-21. NLM ID: 101308328

Muttarak M, Peh WC. CT of unusual iliopsoas compartment lesions. Radiographics. 2000;20 Spec No:S53-66

Extremities: General Overview

6

6.1 Radiology of the Extremities

Radiology is not usually necessary unless the clinical diagnosis is not straightforward, or the patient is not responding to initial treatment of the originally diagnosed pathology. It may also be necessary prior to intervention, especially surgery. Guidance is also a major indication for imaging.

6.1.1 Plain Film Radiographs

Plain film radiographs are the first line of imaging and may be the only imaging required in many situations. This modality has the highest spatial resolution for fine cortical and trabecular definition. It is useful for elucidating bone and joint pathology such as fractures/dislocations, tumor, and arthritis including septic arthritis, as well as radiodense foreign bodies. Plain film radiography is sensitive for osteopenia, bone resorption, soft tissue calcification and is superior to MRI in identifying these findings in relevant clinical scenarios such as hyperparathyroidism, renal osteodystrophy, CPPD, etc.

The drawback of plain film radiography is its poor visualization of soft tissues and its inability to perform cross-sectional imaging resulting in an inherent limitation in diagnostic capability.

Flouroscopy is the use of continuous real-time radiographic imaging and is helpful for guidance during injections.

6.1.2 Ultrasound

Ultrasound is to be compared with other cross-sectional imaging modalities such as CT and especially MRI, which it rivals in soft tissue resolution.

Ultrasound is fast, more readily available, and has better spatial resolution than CT or MRI (with high resolution transducers). This spatial resolution allows definition of collagen fibril microanatomy of soft tissues such as tendons, ligaments and muscles, and the fascicular microanatomy of peripheral nerves.

Ultrasound permits real-time or dynamic scanning combined with immediate patient feedback. In other words, it demonstrates pathology in different relevant anatomical positions to reproduce the clinical symptoms. Examples include dynamic compression of the median nerve in the carpal tunnel by a ganglion cyst during flexion.

Dynamic scanning is very useful in conditions such as snapping hip, snapping triceps, nerve compression, ligament or tendon injuries where certain motions elicit pain, numbness or weakness, or other physical exam findings.

Ultrasound can assess vascularity with power Doppler in real-time without contrast which can be correlated with the exact point of tenderness. Hypervascularity associated with inflammation can be assessed. It may thus discern acute vs. chronic injury in some situations and can also assess soft tissue tumor vascularity.

It is easier to perform at the bedside and is often preferred by and more comfortable for patients. In addition, it is less expensive than CT or MRI. Unlike CT, there is no ionizing radiation.

M.I. Syed and A. Shaikh, *Radiology of Non-Spinal Pain Procedures*,
DOI: 10.1007/978-3-642-00481-0_6, © Springer-Verlag Berlin Heidelberg 2011

Overall, ultrasound is very useful at evaluating tendons, nerves, muscles, ligaments, soft tissue masses, joint effusion, bursal fluid, and synovial hypertrophy. It is tremendously useful as a real-time guidance modality.

Its disadvantage is that it is operator dependent. There are numerous artifacts associated with scanning that need to be accounted for which could result in false negatives or false positives. A drawback is that, outside of academic subspecialty departments, most radiologists are unfamiliar with the modality of musculoskeletal ultrasound.

Another disadvantage is that it can only image joints serially rather than simultaneously as can CT or MRI. This disadvantage is pertinent in closely spaced joints such as in the hand or wrist. Ultrasound is limited in its evaluation of bone beyond the cortex including marrow. It is also less capable at assessing central joint cartilage and intraarticular ligaments (cruciate ligaments of the knee).

6.1.3 Computed Tomography

CT is a cross-sectional imaging modality using X-rays, but has a much higher soft tissue contrast resolution than plain film radiography (though less spatial resolution). CT, like plain film, has the strength of being able to demonstrate exquisite cortical and trabecular bone detail. It can therefore be very useful in revealing complex fracture through multiplanar reconstruction such as triplane fractures of the distal tibia (presurgical evaluation). It can demonstrate soft tissue calcifications superior to MRI such as in dialysis-dependent end-stage renal disease or amyloidosis. It is also readily available and scans can be performed relatively quickly and reproducibly. CT is also very useful for guidance, but the guidance is usually not real time as with ultrasound or fluoroscopy. Real-time guidance can be performed with CT fluoroscopy.

CT has less spatial resolution compared to high resolution ultrasound and less soft tissue resolution than MRI. A significant disadvantage is relatively high dosage of ionizing radiation to the patient. Contrast, if needed, can help define pathology including its relative vascularity. However, it can be nephrotoxic in renally compromised patients and can cause rare but serious contrast reactions.

6.1.4 Magnetic Resonance Imaging

MRI has the highest soft tissue contrast resolution of any of the modalities in use today. It is superior at defining the presence and extent of soft tissue pathology, as well as its relationship to adjacent structures including vasculature. MR angiography can further elucidate this. MRI is sensitive for articular cortex and articular cartilage and is the only modality capable of adequately assessing the bone marrow.

The MRI evaluation of bone marrow is not specific, but can be useful in identifying insufficiency fractures and avascular necrosis. It is superior to arthrography, CT arthrography, and ultrasound for evaluation of the articular cartilage. Furthermore, MR arthrography has the highest specificity and sensitivity for many conditions including rotator cuff tendon tear. It is the gold standard for erosions and for evaluating the intraarticular portion of large joints. MRI should be obtained if joint instability is present.

It is usually obtained when preoperative planning is required by surgeons. When combined with plain film radiographs, the specificity of MRI increases since it is relatively insensitive for calcification. MRI is reproducible and not operator dependent. Furthermore, it does not utilize ionizing radiation.

Its disadvantage is that its contrast agent (gadolinium) can induce nephrogenic systemic fibrosis in patients with renal insufficiency. It cannot be performed in the setting of pacer implantable cardiac defibrillators, aneurysm clips, or drug-eluting stents for the first 6 months to 1 year. It requires a cooperative patient who does not have claustrophobia. Furthermore, it is the most expensive modality.

6.1.5 Bone Scan

This technique is performed using nuclear medicine scintigraphy. It is sensitive for pathology, but very nonspecific and vague in localizing the exact anatomic site. However, it can be useful in the evaluation of radiographically occult fractures (stress fractures), osteomyelitis/septic arthritis, and reflex sympathetic dystrophy (complex regional pain syndrome).

6.2 Structures

General structures include tendons, nerves, bursa, and joints.

6.2.1 Joints

In evaluating joints, the major pathology besides facture is that of arthritis. Plain films should be obtained prior to any joint injection. MRI or MR arthrography should be performed if joint instability is present.

6.2.1.1 Osteoarthritis

In osteoarthritis with plain film radiographs, specific findings include osteophyte formation with joint space narrowing, and subchondral cyst formation, as well as subchondral sclerosis. CT reveals similar findings to plain films. On ultrasound, effusions, synovial thickening, and cysts may be identified. Power Doppler is useful in assessing hypervascularity reflective of the intensity of inflammation. On MRI, synovial thickening, effusions, and destructive cartilage changes may be identified as well as cyst. Adjacent bone marrow edema with areas of remodeling may also be seen. Furthermore, ligament injury may be identified.

6.2.1.2 Rheumatoid Arthritis

In rheumatoid arthritis using plain film radiographs, marginal erosions are the hallmark of diagnosis. Joint space narrowing and soft tissue swelling may be seen. Periarticular osteopenia may also be identified. Erosions are usually marginal. Joint alignment deformity occurs as the disease progresses. On ultrasound, effusions, synovial thickening, and cysts may be identified. Adjacent soft tissue pathology involving the ligament or tendons may also be seen. Power Doppler is useful in assessing hypervascularity reflective of the intensity of inflammation. On MRI, erosions, synovial thickening, effusions, and destructive cartilage changes may be identified. Cyst as well as bone marrow edema with areas of remodeling may be seen. Adjacent soft tissue pathology involving the ligament or tendons may also be seen.

Rheumatoid arthritis typically affects the following joints: proximal interphalangeal (finger), metacarpophalangeal, wrist, metatarsophalangeal, knee, shoulder, and less frequently the hip.

6.2.1.3 Calcium Pyrophosphate Deposition Disease

Calcium pyrophosphate deposition disease (CPPD) should be considered if plain film osteoarthritic (joint space loss, subchondral sclerosis, subchondral cysts and osteophytes) changes are noted within the elbow, shoulder, wrist (radiocarpal joint), metacarpophalangeal joint or isolated to the patellofemoral joint. Chondrocalcinosis (cartilage calcification) is the hallmark of this disease and is seen commonly in the knee, wrist, hip, shoulder (glenoid labrum and acromioclavicular joint) and pubic symphysis. A subtype of CPPD (pseudorheumatoid) is characterized by marginal erosions similar to rheumatoid arthritis with articular bone cortex indistinctness in the interphalangeal and metacarpophalangeal joints. Radiocarpal joint indentation may also be seen. Calcification may also be seen of the joint capsule or synovium and can also involve extraarticular soft tissue structures such as tendons, ligaments, and bursae.

CT can easily identify the pathology of CPPD but is usually not used clinically. MRI can detect chondrocalcinosis as areas of low signal intensity in the articular cartilage but may need to be correlated with plain films. Calcification within the meniscus can result in a false positive for a meniscal tear. Ultrasound may visualize synovitis and calcifications. Power Doppler can be helpful in assessing the extent of hypervascularity of the synovium.

6.2.1.4 Septic Arthritis

Septic arthritis is manifested by indistinctness of the cortex on plain films with severe joint space loss/erosions and periarticular osteopenia with associated soft tissue swelling. CT may better delineate these findings. Joint effusion with synovial thickening (synovitis) may be seen on ultrasound, CT, or MRI with extensive soft tissue swelling. Marrow edema is seen in the adjacent bone with MRI. Extensive enhancement is also seen within the joint and soft tissues on MRI. Findings seen on imaging are not specific for septic arthritis. Joint aspiration is therefore still critical in making the diagnosis.

Septic arthritis should be excluded in any monoarticular arthritis. It is seen more frequently in children than adults and tends to involve the knee or hip. In adults the joints more commonly involved include the sacroiliac joint, symphysis pubis, sternoclavicular joint, spine, and acromioclavicular joint.

Lyme disease is another form of infectious arthritis that should be suspected in the setting of a tick bite followed by the typical bull's-eye shaped rash (erythema migrans).

6.2.1.5 Gout

Gout is manifested by erosions at the joint margin with characteristic overhanging edges and soft tissue swelling with soft tissue deposition of urate crystals (tophi). Joint space loss occurs in later stages of the disease. It occurs in a nonuniform manner. Using ultrasound in gouty arthritis in small joints, there may be visualization of the deposition of monosodium urate crystal on the cartilaginous surface as well as tophaceous material within the joint. In addition, erosions, effusions, and synovial hypertrophy with hypervascularity on power Doppler imaging may be seen. The findings can be specific for gout and provide a noninvasive means of diagnosis. With experienced operators ultrasound is more sensitive than plain films to diagnose gouty arthritis.

CT can identify the erosions and soft tissue calcifications as well as intraarticular joint space loss. MRI can reveal erosions, joint effusion, soft tissue edema, and soft tissue tophi, which have variable signal intensity depending on the density of calcification and water content. Gout typically affects the first metatarsophalangeal joint, ankle, knee, finger joints, wrist, elbow, and sacroiliac joint.

6.2.1.6 Seronegative Inflammatory Arthropathy (Psoriatic Arthritis)

Psoriatic arthritis is manifested by surface erosions (at the joint margin and articular surface), enthesitic erosions (at the joint capsule extending away from the joint), as well as bone proliferative changes including enthesophytes on plain films. Osteoporosis is not usually seen,

unlike rheumatoid arthritis. Soft tissue swelling is seen with joint space loss in large joints and joint space increase in small joints (due to osteolysis). Periosteal reaction may be present, adjacent to the shaft of the phalanges. Ultrasound is more sensitive than plain films in detecting effusion, synovitis, and enthesitis (inflammation at the tendon attachment). Power Doppler can be help in assessing the intensity of hypervascularity. Ultrasound is limited, however, to assessment of small joints, as in other forms of arthritis. CT is useful in evaluating the spine but not in the peripheral joints. MRI is superior at detecting synovitis, effusions, and bone edema. It can demonstrate enthesitis manifest by tendon attachment and adjacent increased signal intensity in the bone marrow. If seen at numerous sites, this is specific for seronegative spondyloarthropathy such as psoriatic arthritis to distinguish it from rheumatoid arthritis. Psoriatic arthritis involves the finger, wrist, and feet, most commonly followed by the sacroiliac joints and spine.

Ankylosing spondylitis is another inflammatory seronegative spondyloarthropathy which has similar findings of erosions, osseous proliferative changes, and nonuniform joint involvement. It is predisposed to involve the axial skeleton including spine and sacroiliac joint, but can also involve the knees, shoulders, and hips. Fusion or ankylosis of the spine, sacroiliac joint, and hips occur in advanced stages. It involves the hands and feet much less frequently.

6.2.2 Tendons

Pathology of the tendons can also be identified. This is usually seen with ultrasound or MRI. The classes of pathology of the tendon include tendinosis (degenerative change), partial tear, full thickness tear, and tenosynovitis. It is usually diagnosed clinically by physical examination findings, including elicitation of pain during movement of the muscle against resistance.

The normal anatomy of the tendon on ultrasound is that of a hyperechoic structure with fibrils identified within the tendon (Figs. 6.1–6.2). This is better delineated with high-resolution ultrasound (9–16 MHz). An artifact called anisotropy may artifactually result in the hypoechogenicity of tendinopathy if the transducer is not carefully aligned along the long axis of the tendon. This is distinguished from true pathology since the artifact disappears with proper alignment.

Fig. 6.1 Biceps tendon, longitudinal view. The biceps tendon (*arrows*) is seen as an echogenic structure with an internal fibrillar pattern (Papatheodorou et al. 2006)

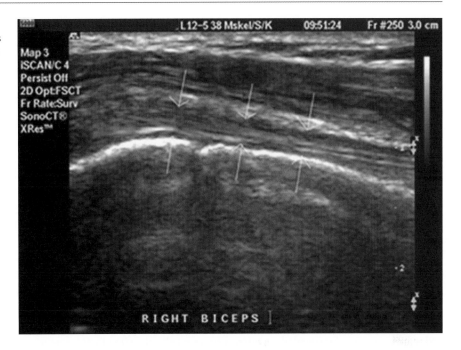

Fig. 6.2 Biceps tendon, transverse view. The biceps tendon (*arrows*) lies within the bicipital groove, between the lesser (*LT*) and greater (*GT*) tuberosities and below the deltoid muscle (Papatheodorou et al. 2006)

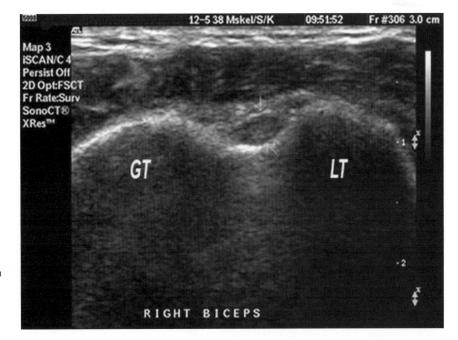

On MRI, the normal tendon is uniformly dark (low signal intensity) on T1- and T2-weighted imaging. An artifact called the magic angle is known to occur during T1-weighted imaging when the tendon is imaged 55° to the angle of the dominant magnetic field. This causes the tendon to artifactually appear bright. T2-weighted images, however, are normal and this distinguishes the artifact from pathology.

In the setting of tendinosis, with ultrasound, a hypoechoic swollen tendon (with loss of its normal fibrillar structure) may be identified. On MRI, there is an enlarged tendon with abnormal inhomogeneous signal intensity within the tendon, which is nonuniform.

In the setting of the partial thickness tear on ultrasound, there is thinning or thickening of the tendon as well as altered echogenicity. On MRI, a partial thickness tear is manifested as increased signal intensity, which may not reach that of fluid when the signal intensity does not extend through the full width of the tendon.

A full thickness tear on ultrasound demonstrates a hypoechoic enlarged tendon at the fragment ends. There is hyperemia on color Doppler imaging at the ends of the tendon. The tendon is surrounded by synovial fluid. On MRI, there is discontinuity of the tendon or increased signal intensity, which is isointense to fluid. The increased signal intensity extends through the full width of the tendon.

Tenosynovitis/stenosing tenosynovitis is usually diagnosed clinically through exam findings including tests and maneuvers. On ultrasound, the tendon is surrounded by sonolucent fluid collection or hyperechoic synovium/

pannus. On MRI, there is thickening of the tendon with a fluid-filled synovial sheath.

6.2.3 Nerves

A normal nerve manifests as a round structure with internal fascicles on axial and longitudinal imaging in both ultrasonography and MRI (Fig. 6.3). When there is nerve entrapment, clinically a Tinel's sign may be seen where tenderness is elicited over the nerve at the site of entrapment by gently tapping the site. The neurological exam may be compromised. An EMG may be the first-line diagnostic study.

Ultrasound may demonstrate a hypoechoic enlarged nerve or it may visualize the nerve being compressed by adjacent pathology. A sonographic Tinel's sign may be performed where direct transducer compression at the site of entrapment yields symptoms. This is useful in ulnar nerve dislocation with elbow flexion in cubital

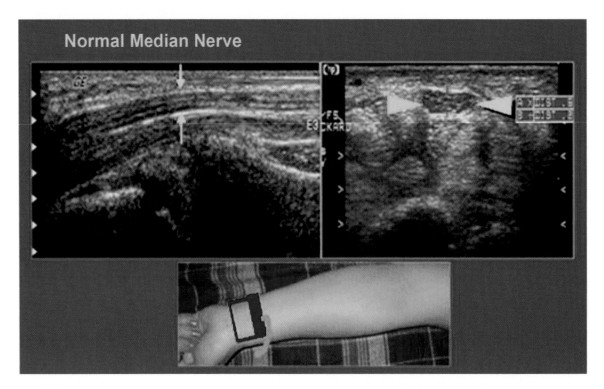

Fig. 6.3 Image (*bottom*) shows the normal median nerve. US scans show the normal median nerve as parallel echoic lines (*arrows*) in the sagittal section (*left*) and as a reticular pattern (*arrowheads*) in the transverse section (*right*) (Chiou et al. 2003)

syndrome. It is useful in Morton's neuroma with the sonographic Mulder's sign where medial and lateral compression of the foot causes plantar displacement of the neuroma resulting in symptoms. Ultrasound has higher resolution compared to MRI and allows dynamic imaging to elucidate nerve entrapment. MRI demonstrates enlargement and contrast enhancement of the nerve. Denervation edema within the innervated musculature may be seen as well as fatty replacement and atrophy of the muscles in advanced stages.

6.2.4 Bursae

Presentation of bursitis on physical exam includes a tender fluctuant mass as well as tests or maneuvers that reveal the pathology. On ultrasound, fluid-filled sonolucent structure is seen. The findings may be dynamic. For instance, iliopsoas bursitis is associated with snapping hip syndrome.

On MRI, there is enlargement of the fluid-filled sac with or without rim enhancement and with or without surrounding edema.

6.3 Contraindications

Contraindications to injection include infection, severe juxta-articular osteoporosis, intraarticular fracture, joint instability, and injection of the joint more than three times a year or within 6 weeks. Complications of injection include infection, tendon rupture, hematoma, intravascular injection, steroid post injection flare, calcification, local tissue necrosis, skin atrophy, depigmentation, and fat necrosis (MacMahon et al. 2008).

References

MacMahon PJ, et al. Injectable corticosteroids and local anesthetic preparation: a review for radiologist. Radiology. 2008;252(3)

Papatheodorou A, Ellinas P, Takis F, Tsanis A, Maris I, Batakis N. US of the shoulder: rotator cuff and non-rotator cuff disorders. Radiographics. 2006;26(1):e23

Chiou HJ, Chou YH, Chiou SY, Liu JB, Chang CY. Peripheral nerve lesions: role of high-resolution US. Radiographics. 2003;23(6):e15

Upper Extremity

7.1 Introduction

The main strengths and weaknesses of imaging modalities for diagnosis in the upper extremity are discussed below.

7.1.1 Plain Film Radiographs

This is the first-line modality in imaging for upper extremity pathology. This technique enables imaging of the bone, effusions, and any calcified pathology, as well as radiodense foreign bodies. It is also able to evaluate fractures/dislocations, arthritis, infection, and tumor.

7.1.2 Bone Scan

This technique is performed using nuclear medicine scintigraphy. It is sensitive for pathology, but very non-specific and vague in localizing the exact anatomic site. However, it can be useful in the evaluation of radiographically occult fractures (stress fractures), osteomyelitis/septic arthritis, and reflex sympathetic dystrophy (complex regional pain syndrome).

7.1.3 Ultrasound

This method is used more commonly outside the US. It is useful for evaluating soft tissue pathology such as joints, tendons, and ligaments. It can also be used complementary to MRI for assessing tendon and ligament pathology. Although it has real-time imaging capability, one disadvantage is its operator dependency. Ultrasound can also be used as an aid to guidance similar to flouroscopy.

7.1.4 CT

This technique enables cross-sectional imaging for the evaluation of bone and joint pathology. It is less useful for soft tissue pathology compared to MRI. It is available in acute or emergency settings in the hospital 24/7.

7.1.5 MRI

MRI is the modality of choice for musculoskeletal imaging for nearly all pathology due to its superior soft tissue contrast and its ability to image in any plane. However, it is poor in imaging cortical bone due to lack of signal in the cortical bone, although this is considered a relatively minor weakness. CT is superior to MRI in evaluating cortical bone. MRI is able to directly image the musculature, cartilage of joints, joint spaces, tendons, ligaments, bursae, and nerves. In addition, MR arthrography is useful in increasing the sensitivity of articular pathology. However, MRI's limitations include metal artifacts and calcified pathology.

M.I. Syed and A. Shaikh, *Radiology of Non-Spinal Pain Procedures*,
DOI: 10.1007/978-3-642-00481-0_7, © Springer-Verlag Berlin Heidelberg 2011

7.1.6 Major Pathology to Exclude (Contraindication to Injection)

- Joint infection (septic arthritis)**.
  - Cortical indistinctness
  - Periosteal reaction
  - Joint space loss
  - Periarticular osteopenia
  - Joint fluid or effusion
    Joint aspiration may be necessary for diagnosis prior to any steroid injection
  - MRI and CT are more sensitive in diagnosis than plain films
- Fracture**
  - Would show as cortical discontinuity
  - Periosteal reaction if subacute
  - Malalignment if fracture is complete
  - MRI and CT are more sensitive than plain film radiograph
- Bleeding diathesis
- Acute traumatic soft tissue injury**
- Maximum limit of steroid dose attained
- Joint prosthesis for joint injections only**
- Impending joint surgery (within days)

7.1.7 Complications in the Upper Extremity

The principal complications encountered in the upper extremity include:

- Hematoma/bleeding**
- Infection**
- Transient synovitis (post-injection steroid flare)**
- Transient or permanent upper extremity weakness and paresthesias (these can be seen in nerve injections or inadvertent ulnar nerve injection for medial epicondylitis)
- Radial artery injury for first carpometacarpal joint and de Quervain's injections**
- Injection into the tendon with possible rupture (elbow or first CMC injection)**
- Steroid arthropathy (questionable evidence)**

7.2 Upper Extremity Joints, Bursae, and Tendons

7.2.1 Shoulder

7.2.1.1 Glenohumeral Joint Injection
(Figs. 7.1 and 7.2)

Anatomy

The glenohumeral joint is a synovial line ball-and-socket articulation, which attaches the head of the humerus to the glenoid fossa of the scapula. The cartilaginous glenoid labrum broadens the extent of the glenoid fossa to increase stability. The joint is also supported mostly by the rotator cuff muscles since the ligaments are relatively weak and the joint capsule is a lax structure. The capsule of the joint is traversed by the long head of the biceps muscle. The associated bursae include the subacromial, subdeltoid, subcoracoid, coracobrachial, and subscapularis bursa. The ligaments include the superior middle and inferior glenohumeral ligaments as well as the coracohumeral and transverse humeral ligaments.

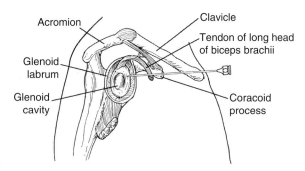

Fig. 7.1 Glenohumeral joint injection, anterior approach (Weiss 2007a, Fig. 3-1)

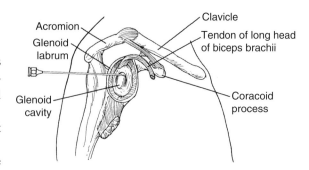

Fig. 7.2 Glenohumeral joint injection – posterior approach (Weiss 2007b, Fig. 3-3)

Function

This is the most mobile joint in the body. It is capable of flexion/extension and abduction/adduction as well as lateral/medial rotation and circumduction.

Clinical Presentations

Glenohumeral arthritis presents with pain and stiffness of the shoulder and loss of mobility. It affects 20% of the population. The symptoms are identical for rheumatoid arthritis or osteoarthritis and frozen shoulder [adhesive capsulitis] (fibrosis of the joint capsule). Rheumatoid arthritis tends to be polyarticular with the shoulder involved usually after at least several years of chronicity. Osteoarthritis may be relatively monoarticular. Frozen shoulder clinically has severely decreased passive range of motion on exam. It is associated with trauma or prolonged lack of shoulder usage.

Etiology

Glenohumeral arthritis may be caused by osteoarthritis/degenerative arthritis,** inflammatory arthritis (rheumatoid arthritis,** gout,** pseudogout/calcium pyrophosphate deposition disease**) systemic lupus erythematosus,** ankylosing spondylitis,** and psoriatic arthritis,** and infection.** Chronic rotator cuff tear may also result in glenohumeral arthritis, especially in the setting of calcium pyrophosphate deposition disease (Milwaukee shoulder).**

Differential Diagnosis

The differential diagnosis of glenohumeral arthritis includes:
- Rotator cuff impingement syndrome**
- Bursitis **involving the subacromial or subdeltoid bursae
- Fracture**
- Suprascapular neuropathy**
- Glenohumeral instability**
- Cervical radiculopathy (disk herniation,** spondylosis**)

- Adhesive capsulitis**
- Acromioclavicular joint arthritis**
- Calcific tendonitis**
- Biceps tendonitis**
- Reflex sympathetic dystrophy**
- Thoracic outlet syndrome**
- Avascular necrosis of the humeral head**

Injection Site

The arm needs first to be externally rotated. In the anterior approach the needle is advanced 1 cm lateral and inferior to the coracoid process. The needle is directed posterior and slightly superiorly and laterally. If the needle hits the bone it should be pulled back and redirected at a slightly different angle. In the posterior approach the needle should be inserted 2 cm under the posterolateral edge of the acromion. The needle is directed so as to target the coracoid process (ventrally and medially).

Imaging/Radiology

Fluoroscopy (Fig. 7.3).

CT (Fig. 7.4).

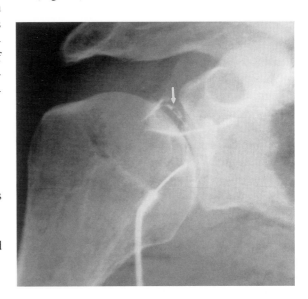

Fig. 7.3 Right shoulder in a 54-year-old man. Anteroposterior fluoroscopic image demonstrates intraarticular contrast material visualized between the glenoid and humerus (*arrow*) (Jacobson et al. 2003)

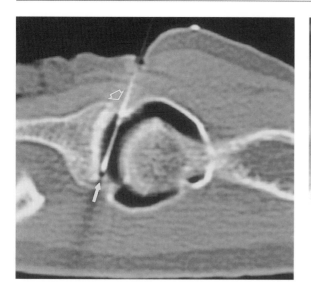

Fig. 7.4 Left shoulder in a 55-year-old man. With the shoulder placed in an oblique position to visualize the glenohumeral joint in profile, a 20-gauge spinal needle was inserted from an anterior approach directly into the joint without contact of the humeral head. Axial computed tomographic (CT) image obtained after injection of air and contrast agent demonstrates the path of the needle through the anterior labrum (*open arrow*) with its tip at the base of the posterior labrum (*solid arrow*) (Jacobson et al. 2003)

Ultrasound: Ultrasound can also be used as an aid to guidance.

Plain film radiographs: AP views as well as the axillary views obtained (to evaluate the glenoid).

In rheumatoid arthritis, there is osteopenia as well as marginal or juxta-articular erosions. There is associated uniform joint space loss, synovial cyst formation, and humeral head elevation. In osteoarthritis, there is asymmetric joint loss with osteophyte formation, subchondral sclerosis, and cyst formation. Erosions may also be seen (Fig. 7.5).

Ultrasound: In osteoarthritis, finding such as osteophyte, intraarticular loose bodies, bone cyst, joint effusions, and joint space narrowing may be identified.

In rheumatoid arthritis, synovial cyst hypertrophy, juxta-articular erosions, and joint effusions can be identified. There is also a high incidence of associated rotator cuff pathology in rheumatoid arthritis. Ultrasound is useful in assessing the rotator cuff tendon for tendinosis as well as a partial or complete tear. The tendon may demonstrate thickening as well as heterogeneous echogenicity or hypoechoic foci. There may also be associated findings of cortical irregularity involving the greater tuberosity and bursal fluid in this setting of rotator cuff pathology.

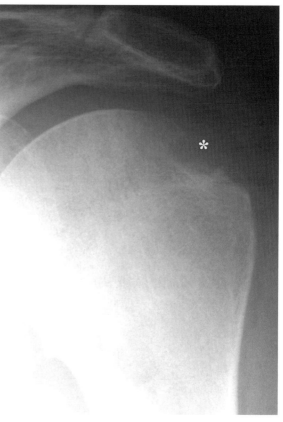

Fig. 7.5 Long-standing rheumatoid arthritis of the shoulder joint. Radiograph (detail view) of the left shoulder shows deep erosion (*asterisk*) at a typical site (Sommer et al. 2005)

In adhesive capsulitis, capsular thickening may be identified as well as decreased articular volume. Adhesions may also be seen. Furthermore, on dynamic scanning, there is abnormal supraspinatus tendon bulging below the acromion on dynamic scanning upon abduction of the arm (Papatheodorou et al. 2006a).

MRI: In addition to CT, MRI may be needed if surgery is contemplated (Fig. 7.6).

MRI can identify rotator cuff tears, which are also seen in rheumatoid arthritis. It is excellent at identifying previously described intraarticular pathology in all forms of arthritis. In adhesive capsulitis, standard MRI is not as reliable as MR arthrography.

MR arthrography in adhesive capsulitis demonstrates decreased joint volume, thickening of the joint capsule, and coracohumeral ligament. There is also obliteration of the fat triangle between the coracohumeral ligament and coracoid process (subcoracoid triangle sign) (Fig. 7.7). It is to be understood that MR

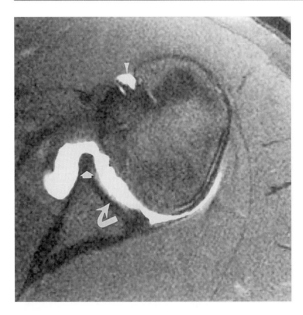

Fig. 7.6 Normal left shoulder in an 18-year-old man. MR image (400-ms repetition time, 21-ms echo time) obtained with fat saturation pulse sequences after intraarticular administration of gadolinium shows high-signal-intensity contrast material distending the glenohumeral joint and long head of the biceps brachii tendon sheath (*arrowhead*). Note the oblique orientation of the glenoid articular surface (*curved arrow*) and medial location of the anterior labrum (*straight arrow*) relative to the humerus (Jacobson et al. 2003)

arthrography is typically used for identification of loose bodies, chondral defects, supraspinatus tears, and labral/ligamentous pathology in the setting of injury/pain for athletes (pitchers, volleyball players, swimmers).

Indications

The two main indications include: (1) Adhesive capsulitis,** (2) arthritis,** including osteoarthritis,** rheumatoid arthritis,** and as well as other forms of arthritis.**

7.2.1.2 Acromioclavicular Joint Injection (Fig. 7.8)

Anatomy

This is the joint involving the junction between the acromion to the clavicle. There are three associated ligaments including the acromioclavicular ligament, coracoacromial ligament, and coracoclavicular ligament.

Function

The acromioclavicular joint permits the arm to be raised above the head by functioning as a pivot point.

Clinical Presentation

Arthritis of the acromioclavicular joint is manifested as pain and tenderness at the acromioclavicular joint, which worsens with the arm in front of the chest. The pain can radiate to the chest or neck. There may be prominence of the joint on exam.

Etiology

This constitutes a repetitive use injury. It may be seen in weight lifters or other athletes.

Acromioclavicular joint arthritis can be caused by osteoarthritis,** posttraumatic (prior clavicle fracture** or AC joint dislocation**), rheumatoid arthritis (rare),** CPPD, psoriatic arthritis,** ankylosing spondylitis,** and infection.**

Differential Diagnosis

The differential diagnosis includes distal clavicular osteolysis,** rotator cuff pathology,** fracture,** and acromioclavicular joint instability.**

Injection Site

A superior approach is utilized just over the gap between the distal clavicle and medial edge of the acromion.

Imaging/Radiology

Plain film radiographs: Plain films (Zanca view) demonstrate joint space narrowing, erosions, osteophyte formation, subchondral sclerosis, and cyst formation. Fluoroscopy can be used as guidance for injection.

Ultrasound: Joint effusions can be seen. Ultrasound can exclude inflammation at the joints if the capsule is visualized to be less than 3 mm in width (Alasaarela et al. 1997). Ultrasound can also provide guidance for injection and aspiration.

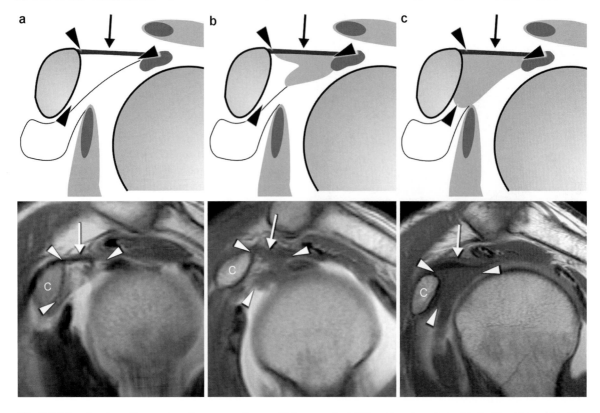

Fig. 7.7 Line drawings (*top row*) and corresponding sagittal oblique T1-weighted (600/12) images (*bottom row*) of subcoracoid fat triangle. Borders of the triangle (*arrowheads*) are defined anterosuperiorly by the coracoid process (*C*), superiorly by the coracohumeral ligament (*arrow*), and posteroinferiorly by the joint capsule. (**a**) Normal anatomy in a subject without frozen shoulder. (**b**) Partial obliteration of subcoracoid fat triangle in a 57-year-old patient with frozen shoulder. (**c**) Complete obliteration of subcoracoid fat triangle (i.e., subcoracoid triangle sign) in a 55-year-old patient with frozen shoulder (Mengiardi et al. 2004)

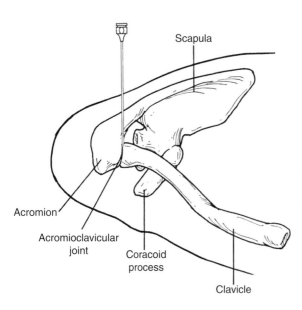

Fig. 7.8 Acromioclavicular joint injection (Weiss 2007c, Fig. 3-5)

CT: CT is best at visualizing the bony surface changes in arthritis (erosions, cysts, sclerosis, joint space narrowing).

MRI: MRI is more sensitive than ultrasound in detecting soft tissue abnormalities. Findings demonstrated include joint space narrowing, capsular hypertrophy, osteophytes, subchondral cyst, subchondral bone marrow edema, and joint effusion in the setting of arthritis. MRI can be predictive of pain relief after joint injection based on the presence of caudal osteophyte formation and hypertrophy/thickening of the joint capsule greater than or equal to 3mm (Figs. 7.9 and 7.10) (Strobel et al. 2003).

Indications

The three main indications for acromioclavicular joint injection include: (1) arthritis,** including osteoarthritis,** rheumatoid arthritis,** as well as other forms of

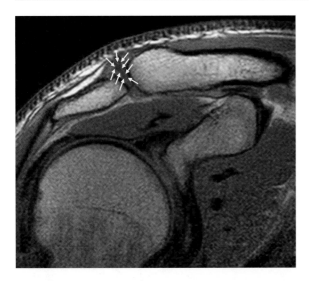

Fig. 7.9 Normal MRI in a 24-year-old asymptomatic male volunteer. Protocol was used in a manner identical to that used in an ex vivo study. A superficial coil was fixed directly anterior to the acromioclavicular joint. No evidence of major displacement due to respiration was observed. *Arrows* mark border between intraarticular disk and articular cartilage on lateral end of clavicle and acromion, respectively (Fialka et al. 2005)

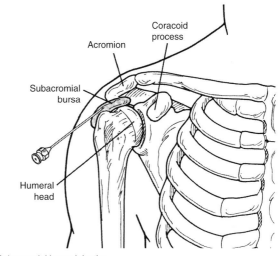

Subacromial bursa injection.

Fig. 7.11 Subacromial bursa injection (Weiss 2007d, Fig. 5-1)

arthritis;** (2) distal clavicular osteolysis;** (3) mild acromioclavicular ligament sprain (Alasaarela et al. 1997).

7.2.1.3 Subacromial Bursa Injection (Fig. 7.11)

Anatomy

The subacromial bursa is located below the acromion and coracoacromial ligament. It is superficial to the supraspinatus muscle. The subacromial bursa extends laterally below the deltoid and above the greater tuberosity of the humerus. The subdeltoid bursa is an extension of the subacromial bursa. Bursitis occurs due to impingement of the subacromial bursa by the acromion or its osteophyte. It is the most commonly inflamed shoulder bursa.

Function

The subacromial bursa prevents friction between the rotator cuff tendon (subscapularis, supraspinatus, infraspinatus, and teres minor) and the acromion/coracoacromial ligament.

Clinical Presentation

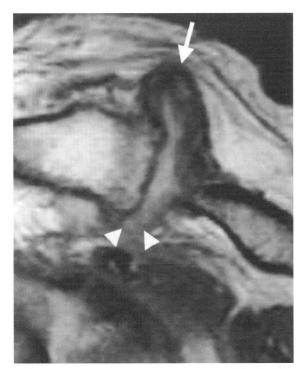

Fig. 7.10 Abnormal MRI in a 70-year-old woman with shoulder pain. Oblique sagittal T1-weighted spin-echo MRI (TR/TE, 600/12) shows severe acromioclavicular joint osteoarthritis with cranial (*arrow*) and caudal (*arrowheads*) osteophytes. Pain relief after selective injection of anesthetics was 50% (Strobel et al. 2003)

Subacromial bursitis is manifested by pain in the outer shoulder radiating down distally in the upper extremity. It worsens with elevation of the arm above the head. Pain may also occur at night when lying on the affected side.

Subacromial bursitis occurs due to repetitive overhead activity or trauma.

Differential Diagnosis

The differential diagnosis includes rotator cuff tear and cervical radiculopathy.

Injection Site

A lateral or posterior approach between the acromion and the humeral head parallel to the acromial angle can be used. The lateral approach is preferred (to avoid rotator cuff tendon injection).

Imaging/Radiology

Plain film radiographs: The outlet-Y or transscapular-Y view is helpful to visualize the subacromial space. Type II and type III acromions result in impingement of the subacromial bursa. The type II acromion is curved and slanted inferiorly at its anterior aspect. The type III acromion is beaked and slanted inferiorly at its anterior

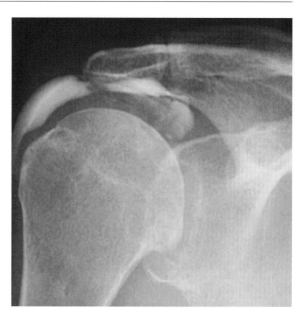

Fig. 7.13 A 56-year-old man with hypertrophic inflammatory change in the acromioclavicular joint with secondary impingement and tendinopathy and a partial-thickness tear at the insertion of the supraspinatus tendon (grade 4). Symptom duration was 8 months. After injection, the patient reported initial complete resolution of symptoms lasting 4 weeks with gradual return of symptoms. At 6-month follow-up evaluation, symptoms had not returned to baseline, and patient reported improvement in activities of daily living. The outcome was classified as a partial response to treatment. The subacromial bursogram shows partial-thickness tear at the insertion of the supraspinatus tendon [See Fig 7.15 for corresponding MRI] (Hambly et al. 2007)

aspect, while the type IV acromion is convex instead of concave at its inferior surface. The axillary view can demonstrate calcification within the coracoacromial ligament. The anterior and posterior views demonstrate the glenohumeral joint and subacromial spurring. It can also identify calcification in calcific tendinitis.

Fluoroscopy/arthrography(bursography):Fluoroscopy can be useful in diagnosing and guiding treatment of subacromial bursitis. Arthrography can be useful for diagnosing complete rotator cuff tendon tear (Figs. 7.12 and 7.13).

Ultrasound: Ultrasound is useful in identifying rotator cuff tendon pathology (tendinosis, partial tears, and full thickness tear as well as impingement). It can identify a fluid-filled bursa and subacromial bursitis. Ultrasound can be used for guidance in subacromial bursa injection.

CT: Usually CT is not utilized in favor of fluoroscopy or ultrasound.

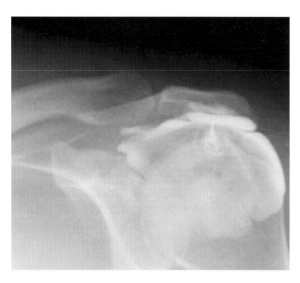

Fig. 7.12 A 30-year-old man with grade 1 findings of isolated subacromial bursitis and symptom duration of 1 month who reported complete resolution of symptoms after fluoroscopically guided subacromial steroid injection. Subacromial bursogram shows isolated subacromial bursitis [See Fig 7.14 for corresponding MRI] (Hambly et al. 2007)

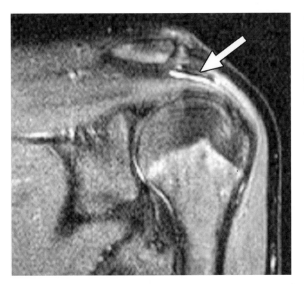

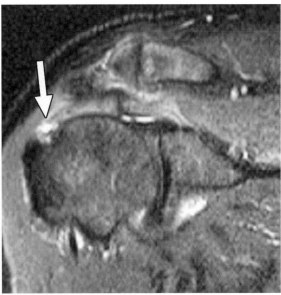

Fig. 7.14 (Same patient as in Fig. 7.12) A 30-year-old man with grade 1 findings of isolated subacromial bursitis and symptom duration of 1 month who reported complete resolution of symptoms after fluoroscopically guided subacromial steroid injection. Coronal oblique STIR MR image (TR/TE, 2,000/20; inversion time, 160 ms; echo-train length, 8) shows isolated subacromial bursitis (*arrow*) (Hambly et al. 2007)

Fig. 7.15 (Same patient as in Fig. 7.13) A 56-year-old man with hypertrophic inflammatory change in acromioclavicular joint with secondary impingement and tendinopathy and partial-thickness tear at the insertion of the supraspinatus tendon (grade 4). Symptom duration was 8 months. After injection, the patient reported initial complete resolution of symptoms lasting 4 weeks with gradual return of symptoms. At 6-month follow-up evaluation, symptoms had not returned to baseline, and the patient reported improvement in activities of daily living. The outcome was classified as a partial response to treatment. Coronal oblique STIR MR image (TR/TE, 2,000/20; inversion time, 160 ms; echo-train length, 8) shows partial-thickness tear (*arrow*) at insertion of supraspinatus tendon (Hambly et al. 2007)

MRI: This is the best modality in identifying rotator cuff pathology (Figs. 7.14 and 7.15). It can identify fluid in the subacromial bursa in the setting of bursitis and can exclude rotator cuff tear especially with MR arthrography.

7.2.1.4 Injection for Rotator Cuff Tendinopathy
(Fig. 7.16)

Anatomy

Indications

The six main indications for subacromial bursa injection are: (1) adhesive capsulitis,** (2) subacromial**/subdeltoid bursitis**; (3) rotator cuff impingement**: Injection of the subacromial bursa allows distinction of impingement syndrome from complete rotator cuff tear (weakness and loss of range of motion may not improve after injection in the setting of a complete tear); (4) rotator cuff tendinosis (supraspinatus tendonitis**/tendinosis**); (5) partial rotator cuff tear; and (6) subacromial spurs** (Tallia and Cardone 2003; Fongemie et al. 1998).

The rotator cuff is comprised of the supraspinatus, infraspinatus, subscapularis, and teres minor muscles. The muscles insert onto the proximal lateral humerus at either the greater or lesser tubercles as a conjoint tendon forming a single continuous linear attachment. The supraspinatus muscle originates from the supraspinous fossa of the scapula at its dorsal aspect above the spine of the scapula. The infraspinatus muscle originates from the infraspinous fossa along the dorsal aspect below the spine of the scapula. The subscapularis muscle originates from the subscapularis fossa at the ventral aspect of the scapula. The teres minor originates from the dorsal surface at the axillary margin of the scapula. The supraspinatus, infraspinatus, and teres minor insert at

Complications

Complications include myositis.**

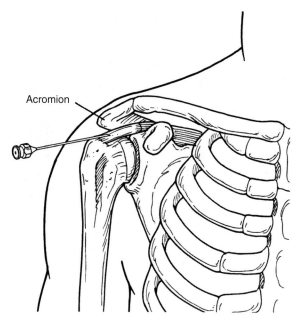

Acromion

Fig. 7.16 Rotator cuff tendon injection (Weiss 2007e, Fig. 4-11)

the greater tubercle humerus. The subscapularis inserts at the lesser tubercle of the humerus as well as the anterior aspect of the shoulder joint capsule.

The supraspinatus and subscapularis muscles surround the long head of the biceps tendon.

Function

The supraspinatus performs abduction of the shoulder or arm. The infraspinatus and teres minor perform external rotation of the arm or shoulder. The subscapularis muscle performs internal rotation of the arm or shoulder. It also brings the arm anteriorly and inferiorly when the upper extremity is elevated. The rotator cuff muscles are necessary to stabilize the glenohumeral joints due to the intrinsic laxity of the joint capsule and ligaments, which permit a wide range of motion.

Clinical Presentation

Rotator cuff tendon injury presents as shoulder pain in the anterolateral shoulder. There is pain when reaching forward and lifting, leaning forward, and inducing pressure on the shoulder, overhead activity, or abduction. There may also be loss of range of motion and weakness in advanced stages of abduction. There are

various signs on physical exam including the Neer impingement sign, Hawkins-Kennedy impingement sign, and painful arc sign. These may demonstrate pain with abduction to resistance.

Etiology

Possible etiologies include overuse, impingement** from the acromion vs. intrinsic tendon degeneration secondary to age, adhesive capsulitis,** glenohumeral instability,** and trauma including anterior dislocation.**

Differential Diagnosis

Differential diagnoses include quadrilateral space syndrome,** suprascapular neuropathy,** cervical radiculopathy (HNP,** spondylosis**), brachial plexopathy,** adhesive capsulitis,** musculocutaneous neuropathy, shoulder instability,** glenoid labral tear,** acromioclavicular joint pathology,** glenohumeral arthritis,** biceps rupture,** and avulsion fracture of the greater tuberosity.**

Injection Site

The needle is placed into the subacromial bursa similar to the previously discussed section on subacromial bursitis. The tendon sheath itself is usually not targeted.

Imaging/Radiology

On cross-sectional imaging (ultrasound, CT, and MRI) findings range from tendinosis to complete tear.

Plain film radiographs: In complete tears, there is superior subluxation of the humeral head against the acromion. There is decreased acromiohumeral distance on the AP view. If the distance is less than or equal to 7 mm, there is a full thickness tear of the supraspinatus in 90% of cases. There is also an associated tear of the infraspinatus in 67% of cases and a tear of the subscapularis in 43% of cases. When correlated with MRI, there is also likely to be atrophic fatty degeneration of the rotator cuff muscles especially the infraspinatus. Acromion morphology on plain films may also be identified (type I through type IV) (Saupe et al. 2006) (see Sect. 7.2.1.3). Calcific tendinitis is a

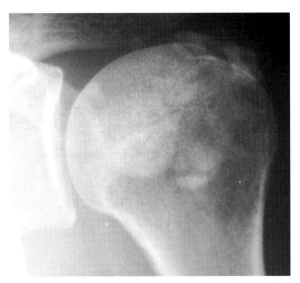

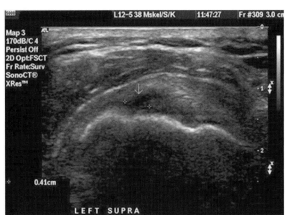

Fig. 7.19 Supraspinatus tendon, longitudinal view. An articular-side partial-thickness tear appears as a distinct hypoechoic defect (*arrow*) at the tendon's articular surface, abutting the articular cartilage (Papatheodorou et al. 2006b)

Fig. 7.17 A 56-year-old woman who had calcific tendinitis for 2 years. Anteroposterior radiograph of the shoulder shows large calcifications involving the supraspinatus and infraspinatus tendons (del Cura et al. 2007)

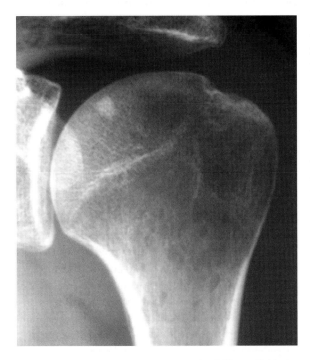

Fig. 7.18 A 56-year-old woman who had calcific tendinitis for 2 years. No calcification can be seen 1 year after treatment (del Cura et al. 2007)

condition due to deposition of hydroxyapatite in the rotator cuff tendons. This manifests on plain film as foci of calcified nodules or cloudy calcifications with indistinct margins (Figs. 7.17 and 7.18).

CT: CT is useful as guidance for MR arthrography (a rotator interval approach rather than anterior approach) (Mulligan 2008).

Ultrasound: Ultrasound has the advantage of dynamic imaging to evaluate for impingement of the rotator cuff tendon while the upper extremity is elevated. The normal appearance of the tendon on ultrasound is that of hyperechoic echotexture with multiple internal fibrils. The upper margin bows upward as it narrows towards the greater tuberosity. The greater tuberosity itself has a uniform margin. With a partial tear of the bursal surface, there is loss of the normal bulbous margin of the muscle such that it appears to have a flat margin. With a tear of the articular surface, there is hypoechoic and non-uniform echotexture. There is cortical irregularity at the greater tuberosity of the humerus where the insertion occurs (Fig. 7.19).

With a full thickness tear, there is a gap in the tendon or lack of visualization of the tendon on orthogonal views. A stump may be seen where the tendon is retracted. Cortical irregularity of the greater tuberosity may be seen. Fluid is seen in the joint space and in the subdeltoid-subacromial bursa. An uncovered cartilage sign may also be seen where there is a thin bright curvilinear margin at the junction of the humeral head articular cartilage and the joints fluid.

In calcific tendinitis, echogenic foci are seen with or without posterior shadowing within the tendon. Hyperemia can also be assessed in rotator cuff tears with power Doppler imaging. Ultrasound may direct needle lavage in the treatment of calcific tendinitis (Serafini et al. 2009) (Figs. 7.20 and 7.21).

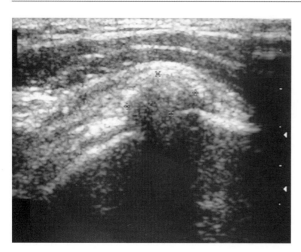

Fig. 7.20 A 39-year-old woman with calcific tendinitis of 6 months' standing. Note changes in sonogram of calcification after percutaneous treatment. Before treatment, longitudinal sonogram of supraspinatus tendon shows focus of calcification and acoustic shadow (del Cura et al. 2007)

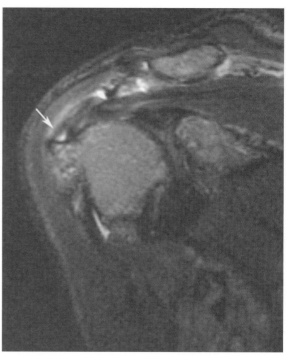

Fig. 7.22 A 62-year-old man with right shoulder pain. Coronal oblique modified inversion recovery (present figure) and coronal oblique fat-suppressed T2-weighted fast spin-echo (Fig. 7.23) MR images of shoulder obtained at same location both show fluid signal intensity within the articular surface of the supraspinatus tendon (*arrow*). Signal abnormality does not appear to extend through the bursal surface of the tendon. All three reviewers interpreted these findings as partial-thickness articular surface tear of supraspinatus tendon (Kijowski et al. 2005)

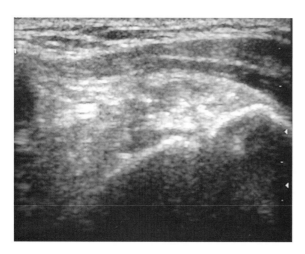

Fig. 7.21 Note changes in sonogram of calcification after percutaneous treatment. At 10 weeks after treatment, the volume of calcification has been considerably reduced and no acoustic shadow is seen (del Cura et al. 2007)

MRI: MRI is the most useful modality in shoulder pain due to subacromial impingement and rotator cuff pathology. It also diagnoses bursitis and the structural etiology of impingement. T1-weighted fat-saturated sagittal images as well as fat-suppressed oblique coronal, sagittal, and axial T2 and proton-density images are often obtained with the use of an extremity or dedicated shoulder coil.

In the setting of tendinosis or tendinopathy, tendon enlargement may be identified with increased signal intensity on both T2-weighted and STIR sequences. With

a partial rotator cuff tear, there is an interruption in the continuity of the tendon manifested by increased signal intensity on proton-density and T2-weighted sequences. This is seen at either the articular or bursal surface, but does not penetrate through the full width of the tendon (Figs. 7.22 and 7.23). In the setting of a full thickness tear, an interruption in the continuity of the tendon is seen with increased signal intensity on proton-density or T2-weighted sequences. This extends through the complete thickness of the tendon. It should be borne in mind that the full thickness tear may be a pinpoint tear or may extend throughout the entire tendon. When it does extend throughout the entire tendon, it would result in loss of function. Intramuscular cysts are associated with full and partial rotator cuff tears. These represent fluid collections in the sheath or substance of the rotator cuff muscles. They do not extend to the articular or bursal surface.

In the setting of tendinopathy as well as partial or full thickness tears, the degree of pathology correlates

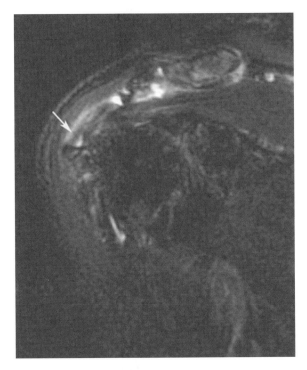

Fig. 7.23 A 62-year-old man with right shoulder pain. Coronal oblique modified inversion recovery (Fig. 7.22) and coronal oblique fat-suppressed T2-weighted fast spin-echo (present figure) MR images of shoulder obtained at the same location both show fluid signal intensity within the articular surface of the supraspinatus tendon (*arrow*). Signal abnormality does not appear to extend through the bursal surface of the tendon. All three reviewers interpreted these findings as partial-thickness articular surface tear of supraspinatus tendon (Kijowski et al. 2005)

inversely with improvement after subacromial bursa injection.

MRI is also useful in identifying rotator cuff impingement by identifying the morphology of the subacromial arch.

Magnetic resonance arthrography is the most sensitive and specific for rotator cuff tears. A partial thickness tear may be demonstrated involving the supraspinatus or infraspinatus. An articular surface tendon tear is revealed by contrast partially entering the articular surface of the tendon (on T1-weighted images). In a bursal surface partial tear, there is preexisting fluid entering this portion of the tendon. A partial tear of the subscapularis muscle may be demonstrated by a defect of the cranial third or less of the tendon.

In the setting of a full thickness tear of the supraspinatus or infraspinatus, contrast extends through the tendon or the tendon is not identified. Contrast may be seen within the subacromial or subdeltoid bursa on T1-weighted images. When a full thickness tear involves the subscapularis muscle, the defect is much more than involving the cranial one-third of the tendon.

Ultrasound and standard MRI are comparable in sensitivity and specificity for complete and partial rotator cuff tears, although ultrasound is more cost-effective though operator dependent. It requires the use of experienced practitioners.

MRI/MR arthrography can be very useful prior to surgery when repair is contemplated both for surgical planning based on the extent of pathology and to identify patients who are surgically irreparable. It is therefore preferred by most surgeons (de Jesus et al. 2009).

7.2.1.5 Injection for Bicipital Tendinopathy or Tendinitis (Fig. 7.24)

Anatomy

The long head of the biceps tendon originates from the supraglenoid tubercle of the scapula as well as the superior margin of the glenoid labrum. It travels through the shoulder joint capsule and then transverses between the greater and lesser tuberosities of the humeral head in the bicipital groove. It is stabilized in the bicipital groove by ligaments including the transverse humeral ligament, superior glenohumeral ligament, and the coracohumeral ligament, as well as the pectoralis major. The short head of the biceps originates from the

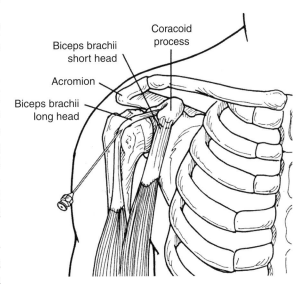

Fig. 7.24 Biceps tendon injection (Weiss 2007f, Fig. 4-5)

coracoid process of the scapula. The muscle inserts into the radial tuberosity. The biceps also attaches to the medial aspect of the forearm over the cubital fossa at the bicipital aponeurosis (lacertus fibrosis). This overlies the median nerve and brachial artery. The muscle is supplied by the musculocutaneous nerve (C5–C7).

Function

The biceps brachii muscle performs flexion at the elbow and supination of the forearm.

Clinical Presentation

Bicipital tendinitis presents as sharp shooting or burning pain in the anterior shoulder worsened with overhead anterior motion such as overhead reaching, throwing, lifting, or pulling. It is also worsened at night. There may be an associated reduction in range of motion.

If the tendon ruptures, pain is sudden and severe and a mass may form in the arm from the muscle fragment retracting. Tenderness is noted at the bicipital groove during various maneuvers with resisted arm motion.

Etiology

Possible etiologies include chronic repetitive motion, impingent syndrome,** rotator cuff tear** with associated lesions of the coracohumeral ligament** and superior glenohumeral ligament** (at the rotator cuff interval capsule), shoulder instability,** traumatic injury,** tight shoulder capsule, and osteoarthritis.**

Differential Diagnosis

Differential diagnoses include:

- Rotator cuff injury**
- Suprascapular neuropathy**
- Cervical radiculopathy**
- Brachial plexopathy**
- Adhesive capsulitis**
- Musculocutaneous neuropathy
- Shoulder instability**
- Glenoid labral tear**
- Acromioclavicular joint pathology**

- Arthritis of the glenohumeral joint**
- Biceps rupture**
- Avulsion fracture of the greater tuberosity**

Injection Site

The needle is placed in the front of the shoulder 3–4 cm caudal to the palpable acromion tip ventral outer aspect overlying the bicipital groove. Care is taken to inject into the tendon sheath and not the tendon itself. The injection is useful for confirming a diagnosis, as well as for relief of symptoms.

Imaging/Radiology

Radiology is useful if there is no improvement after treatment.

Plain film radiographs: Plain film radiographs may demonstrate calcification of the biceps tendon. Degenerative joint disease of the acromioclavicular or glenohumeral joint may be demonstrated. The Fisk view evaluates the biceps groove.

Ultrasound: Ultrasound may assess the biceps tendon during dynamic motion to assess the stability of the tendon. Dislocation may occur during external rotation. The morphology of the tendon can also be ascertained to evaluate for calcification or edema. Power Doppler imaging can reveal hyperemia within the biceps tendon. Normally, the biceps tendon has a hyperechoic echotexture with multiple internal fibrils. With the onset of tendinosis, the tendon may be swollen and hypoechoic with fluid at the tendon sheath. Increased blood flow on color Doppler may also be noted. The findings may be similar in the situation of a partial thickness tear. Ultrasound is not very sensitive for tendinosis/tendinopathy or partial thickness tear.

In the setting of a complete tear, there is an inhomogeneous appearance to the tendon. In the acute setting of a complete tear, the tendon is not seen inside the bicipital groove. There is also retraction of the muscle. In a chronic full thickness tendon tear, the upper portion of the tendon is not seen within the groove.

In chronic subluxation of the tendon, the tendon is noted to be outside the bicipital groove during external rotation (Papatheodorou et al. 2006b).

In biceps tendon tenosynovitis there is inflammation of the biceps tendon due to chronic repetitive motion injury or in inflammation/injury of adjacent

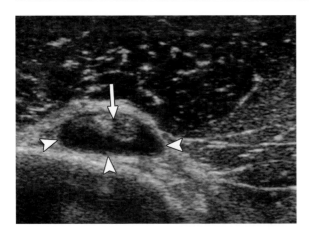

Fig. 7.25 A 39-year-old man with clinical findings of proximal biceps tenosynovitis. Transverse sonogram shows hypoechoic biceps tendinopathy (*arrow*) and marked tenosynovitis (*arrow heads*). No fluid was detected in joint or other recesses (Robinson 2009)

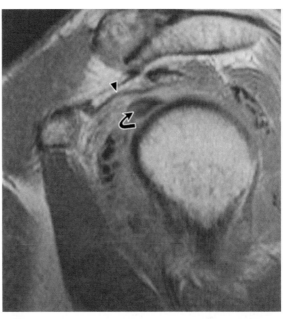

Fig. 7.26 A 61-year-old man with a superior labral anteroposterior (SLAP) tear and long head of biceps tendinopathy (anterior is to the reader's left). A contiguous oblique sagittal image shows a focus of increased signal intensity in the biceps tendon (*arrow*) just inferior to the coracohumeral ligament (*arrowhead*) (Tung et al. 2000)

shoulder structures. This is manifested by fluid accumulation in the tendon sheath (Fig. 7.25).

MRI: MRI of biceps tendinopathy may simulate that of a partial tear. This is manifested by abnormal signal intensity, which is not as intense as fluid and does not involve the entire thickness of the biceps tendon. In the setting of a full thickness tear or rupture, there is discontinuity of the tendon or increased signal intensity, which is isointense to fluid extending through the complete width of the tendon. MRI is also useful for excluding other shoulder or biceps abnormality. This includes associated glenoid labral tears (SLAP) (Fig. 7.26). There may also be associated rotator cuff tears with anterior extension of the tear from the supraspinatus tendon. This may involve the coracohumeral or superior glenohumeral ligament, which is known as the rotator cuff interval capsule (Krief 2005). The biceps is no longer covered by the coracohumeral ligament and may be compressed by the coracoacromial ligament. The anterior sling may then be released, which maintains the biceps tendon within the bicipital groove. This results in instability of the biceps tendon. The actual etiology of bicipital tendon instability may thus be revealed.

MRI can only provide static images of the biceps brachii tendon. Ultrasound can provide unique dynamic evaluation of the biceps tendon for intermittent subluxation when there is concurrent anterior supraspinatus or superior subscapularis tendon tears.

This is important since biceps tendon pathology is common in the setting of rotator cuff tear and is associated with a poorer surgical outcome after rotator cuff tendon repair.

MR arthrography has low sensitivity for biceps tendinopathy.

Complications

Complications may include tendon atrophy**/rupture** and inflammatory reaction.**

7.2.1.6 Injection for Scapulothoracic Bursitis (Snapping Scapula Syndrome)
(Fig. 7.27)

Anatomy

The scapulothoracic bursa is situated between the serratus anterior muscle and the ventral aspect of the scapula.

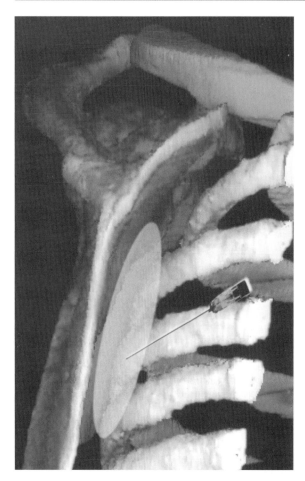

Fig. 7.27 A schematic drawing based on three-dimensional CT, posterior view, shows scapulothoracic bursa injection. A *gray oval* indicates the location of the bursa as expected from the literature. The bursa is commonly small and limited to one or two ribs. The needle was guided parallel to the tender rib until it reached the surface of the rib at the point reproducing the patient's pain (Hodler et al. 2003)

Function

The scapulothoracic bursa decreases friction between the scapula and posterior chest wall.

Clinical Presentation

Scapulothoracic bursitis results in shoulder/periscapular pain exacerbated by motion of the scapulothoracic joint with associated crepitus. Snapping scapula syndrome is movement of the scapulothoracic joint resulting in noise creation. It occurs as a result of chronic repetitive motion injury (this may be seen in baseball pitchers). Snapping scapula syndrome has a clinical overlap with scapulothoracic bursitis. Bursitis,

however, may not necessarily result in the sound generation (crepitus).

Etiology

Etiologies include ventral scapular osteochondromas,** malunion of the scapular** or rib fractures,** Sprengel's deformity, (rare congenital deformity where one scapula is positioned higher than the other)** severe scoliosis,** and congenital abnormality of the scapula.**

Differential Diagnosis

Differential diagnoses include thoracic outlet syndrome** and cervical spine radiculopathy.**

Injection Site

The needle is directed laterally towards the affected scapulothoracic bursa at the medial edge of the scapula until the point of tenderness is reached overlying the rib.

Imaging/Radiology

Fluoroscopy: Medial to lateral approach with the scapula winging away from the chest wall. Cranial-caudal angulation is performed to superimpose the anterior and posterior portions of the ribs. The needle is aimed toward the site of point tenderness. The injection may also be done without fluoroscopy using anatomic landmarks (Fig. 7.28).

Plain film radiographs: Plain films may demonstrate bony abnormalities (see Sect. 7.2.1.6.4) as described above.

C-arm fluoroscopy: Can be used as guidance for injection.

Ultrasound: There is a single case report of diagnosis made with ultrasound (Huang et al. 2005).

CT: CT demonstrates sensitivity for bony abnormalities as well as underlying etiologies (Fig. 7.29). CT can also be used for injection guidance.

MRI: MRI visualizes the bursa if bursitis is clinically suspected. It is seen as a thin-walled cystic mass.

Indications

Bursitis at the inferior medial scapular border (scapulothoracic bursitis) is the main indication.

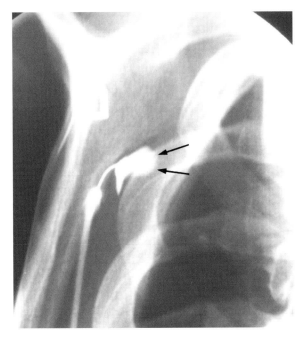

Fig. 7.28 A 41-year-old man who underwent mixed injection in the left shoulder. Tangential spot radiograph shows how part of the contrast medium is well contained in a defined space. Blurring of contrast medium (*arrows*), indicating partial intramuscular leakage, is minimal (Hodler et al. 2003)

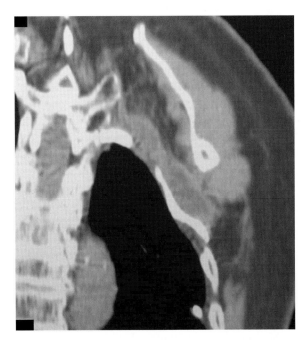

Fig. 7.29 A 74-year-old woman with scapulothoracic bursitis associated with thoracoplasty. A coronal multiplanar reformatted CT image shows ellipsoidal mass along left upper chest wall (Fujikawa et al. 2004)

7.2.2 Elbow and Surrounding Structures

7.2.2.1 Elbow Joint Injection (Fig. 7.30)

Anatomy

The elbow joint involves articulation between the humerus proximally and the radius and ulna distally. The elbow joint is surrounded by a single synovial lining. There are three components: (1) the humeroulnar joint between the trochlea of the humerus and olecranon of the ulna; (2) the humeroradial joint between the capitulum of the humerus and the head of the radius; and (3) the proximal radioulnar joint. Ligaments include the ulnar collateral, radial collateral, and annular ligaments.

Function

The elbow joint permits flexion and extension as well as pronation/supination.

Clinical Presentation

Arthritis of the elbow joint is manifested by pain and stiffness, which is worsened with flexion or extension. There may also be decreased range of motion. The most common cause is rheumatoid arthritis. Rheumatoid arthritis usually involves both elbows and may include the shoulders, wrists, and hands. Symptoms start at the

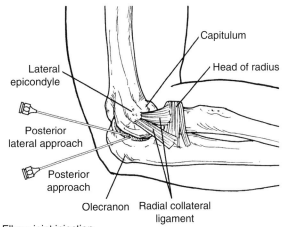

Elbow joint injection.

Fig. 7.30 Elbow joint injection (Weiss 2007g, Fig. 3-9)

lateral or radial side of the elbow resulting in pain with pronation/supination. There is often associated swelling and rheumatoid arthritis. In osteoarthritis, pain with extension can be seen. Locking of the joint or sudden halts in movement may be noted.

Etiology

Etiologies include rheumatoid arthritis,** osteoarthritis,** posttraumatic arthritis,** gout,** and CPPD.**

Differential Diagnosis

Differential diagnoses include synovial osteochondromatosis,** pigmented villonodular synovitis** septic arthritis,** occult fractures,** osteochondritis dissecans,** epicondylitis,** and cubital tunnel syndrome.**

Injection Site

Using the landmarks of the radial head, the olecranon tip, and the lateral epicondyle of the distal humerus, a triangle is formed. The needle is then advanced using a posterolateral approach into the center of the triangle. For the posterior approach, the needle is advanced to the superior lateral edge of the olecranon.

Imaging/Radiology

Plain film radiographs: Plain films demonstrate joint space narrowing in the setting of arthritis and should be obtained prior to joint injection. In rheumatoid arthritis, effusion may be manifested as elevation of the posterior and anterior fat pads. Erosions, osteopenia, and soft tissue swelling may be noted. In osteoarthritis, there is osteophyte formation, subchondral sclerosis, and subchondral cyst. Joint bodies may be seen as calcified. In primary osteoarthritis, the joint space and articular cartilage is relatively preserved with narrowing more commonly seen at the radiocapitellar joint. Advanced rheumatoid arthritis may also have deformity and secondary osteophyte formation (Fig. 7.31).

Fluoroscopy: This may be useful for guidance and arthrography. Arthrography can demonstrate synovial

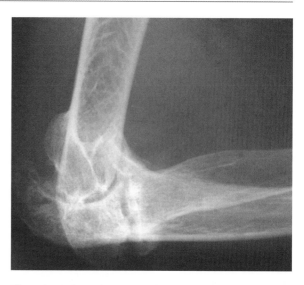

Fig. 7.31 Advanced rheumatoid arthritis. Radiograph (detail view) shows mutilation and deformity of the left elbow. Secondary degenerative osteophytes are seen (Sommer et al. 2005)

pathology including intraarticular loose bodies, as well as capsular/ligamentous intactness.

Ultrasound: Ultrasound is superior to plain films for detecting tiny erosions and soft tissue abnormalities of the bursae, tendons, and ligaments. It can also detect radiographically occult fractures, osteophytes, and intraarticular loose bodies. It is also able to assess the joint capsule and synovium. In trained hands, some authors believe it to be an excellent and efficient alterative to MRI in evaluating the elbow (Martinoli et al. 2001).

CT: CT is useful for bony pathology including visualizing the articular cartilage.

MRI: This modality is more sensitive in early rheumatoid arthritis at characterizing synovitis and bone changes. It is also very sensitive for intraarticular osteochondral joint bodies in osteoarthritis and calcium pyrophosphate deposition disease (CPDD), as well as synovial osteochondromatosis. It can visualize synovial membrane thickening in rheumatoid arthritis, gout, and crystal arthritides. It is also excellent at detecting joint effusion and synovial cyst around the joint (usually in the antecubital fossa). Gadolinium enhancement distinguishes synovial membrane thickening from fluid since they otherwise appear similar. Erosions are seen as bright lesion at the joint margins. MR arthrography is useful for direct visualization of ligament tears (Bhutani et al.).

MRI or MR arthrography should be performed in the setting of joint instability (Fig. 7.32).

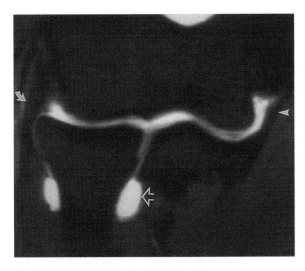

Fig. 7.32 Normal elbow. Direct coronal oblique fat-suppressed T1-weighted MR arthrographic image demonstrates the anterior band of the UCL as a linear low-signal intensity area (*arrowhead*), as well as the RCL (*curved arrow*). The anterior band of the UCL extends from the medial humeral epicondyle to the sublime tubercle of the ulna. The contrast material normally pools around the radial neck (*open arrow*) (Steinbach et al. 2002)

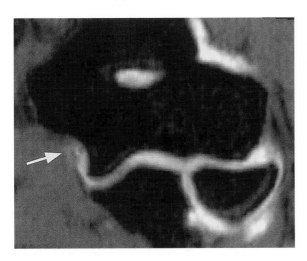

Fig. 7.33 Full-thickness tear of the UCL. Direct coronal oblique fat-suppressed T1-weighted MR arthrographic image of the elbow demonstrates complete ligamentous disruption at the humeral attachment (*arrow*) (Example of joint instability as a contraindication to injection.) (Steinbach et al. 2002)

Indications

The four principal indications for injection of the elbow are: (1) osteoarthritis,** (2) rheumatoid arthritis,** (3) crystal arthritides,** (4) radial head fractures (aspirate for blood or fat globulins in this setting of suspected fracture, rather than for injection).

Contraindications

The chief contraindication to elbow injection is joint prosthesis.** Other contraindications include infection** and joint instability** (Fig. 7.33).

Complications

Complications encountered in elbow injection include steroid arthropathy (although there is questionable evidence to support this)** and injection into the tendon with possible rupture.**

7.2.2.2 Lateral and Medial Epicondyle Injection

Anatomy-General anatomy of the epicondyles (Figs. 7.34 and 7.35)

Injection for Lateral Epicondylitis (Tennis Elbow) (Fig. 7.36)

Anatomy

The lateral epicondyle of the humerus is the point of origin for the muscles of extension and supination in the forearm

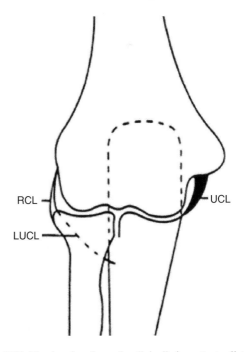

Fig. 7.34 The drawing shows the clinically important collateral ligaments of the elbow: the anterior bundle of the UCL, the RCL, and the lateral UCL (*LUCL*) (Cotten et al. 1997)

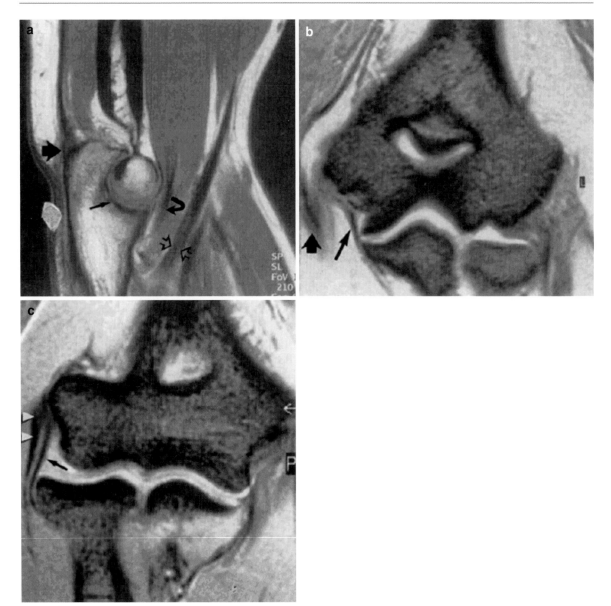

Fig. 7.35 (**a**) Anatomy of the normal elbow. Sagittal T1-weighted MR image shows an apparent defect in the articular surface of the olecranon seen as an interruption of the normal cortical signal void (*small arrow*); this is a normal groove and should not be mistaken for a pathologic entity. The triceps tendon is attached to the proximal olecranon (*large arrow*), the distal biceps tendon courses anterior to the radial tuberosity (*open arrows*), and the brachial muscle inserts on the ulna (*curved arrow*). (**b**) Normal ulnar collateral ligament (UCL) and flexor tendon bundle. Coronal T2-weighted MR image shows the intact UCL extending from the medial humeral epicondyle to the proximal ulna (*long arrow*). The flexor tendons arise more superficially on the medial humeral epicondyle (*short arrow*). (**c**) Normal radial collateral ligament (RCL) (*arrow*) and extensor tendon bundle. Coronal T2-weighted MR image shows the RCL as a linear band of signal void just deep to the extensor tendon groups (*arrowheads*) which originates on the lateral humeral epicondyle (Sonin et al. 1996)

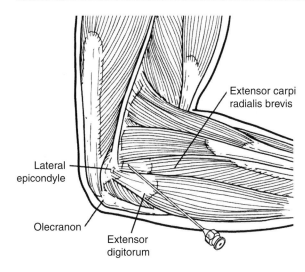

Fig. 7.36 Lateral epicondylitis injection (Weiss 2007h, Fig. 4-7)

(extensor carpi radialis brevis). This muscle tendon is therefore usually involved in the lateral epicondylitis. There is less often involvement of the extensor carpi radialis longus, extensor digitorum, and extensor carpi ulnaris. There may be associated entrapment of a small branch of the radial nerve (radial tunnel syndrome).

Function

The lateral epicondyle is the site of attachment for muscles performing extension and supination.

Clinical Presentation

Lateral epicondylitis presents with pain and tenderness over the lateral epicondyle exacerbated by extension or supination.

Etiology

Repetitive stress and overuse injuries with acute and chronic forms. It is seen in up to 50% of tennis players. It is also seen in recreational athletes, especially in racket sports.

Differential Diagnosis

Differential diagnoses include fracture,** osteochondritis dissecans,** intraarticular osteochondral fragments,** and arthritis (radiocapitellar degenerative joint disease**), radial tunnel syndrome,** entrapment of the musculocutaneous nerve, entrapment of the median nerve,** tumor,** cervical radiculopathy,** and complete tear of the tendon at the lateral epicondyle.**

Injection Site

The lateral approach is utilized just distal to the lateral epicondyle superficial to the tendon (avoiding intratendon injection).

Imaging/Radiology

Imaging is not usually needed unless symptoms are refractory to medical management.

Plain film radiographs: Calcification may be seen adjacent to the lateral epicondyle. Plain films are useful to exclude degenerative joint disease and osteochondritis dissecans, as well as joint bodies (intraarticular osteochondral fragments).

Ultrasound: Ultrasound can be useful for guidance of injection. It is sensitive, but has low specificity in diagnostic evaluation. Findings include intratendinous calcification, tendon hypertrophy, adjacent cortical irregularity, focal hypoechoic areas, and widespread heterogeneity of the tendon (Levin et al. 2005a) (Fig. 7.37).

CT: CT is useful to exclude fracture or osteochondritis dissecans if it is suspected.

MRI: MRI is more sensitive than ultrasound (Miller et al. 2002). The main findings include increased signal intensity within the extensor tendon adjacent to the insertion at the lateral epicondyle. There may be associated abnormality of the lateral collateral ligament including thickening, partial tear, and complete tear (Figs. 7.38 and 7.39).

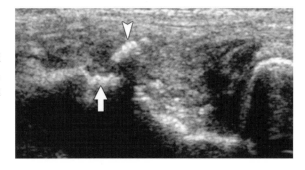

Fig. 7.37 Longitudinal US scan of the common extensor tendon of the symptomatic right elbow in a 37-year-old man with lateral epicondylitis. The tendon is thickened and diffusely heterogeneous, with a calcification (*arrowhead*) and markedly irregular adjacent bone (*arrow*) (Levin et al. 2005b)

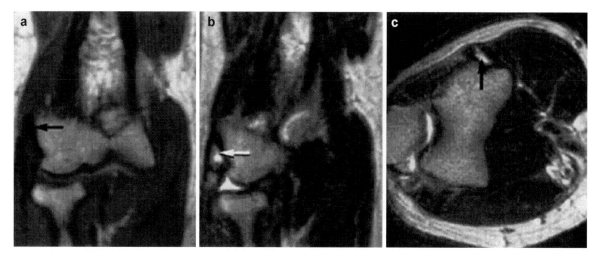

Fig. 7.38 Lateral epicondylitis. (**a**) Coronal T1-wieghted (600/15) MR image demonstrates subtle intermediate signal intensity at the origin of the extensor tendon group (*arrow*). Normally, this area is devoid of signal, but edema can be poorly seen on T1-weighted images. (**b**) T2-weighted (3,800/90) turbo MR image of the same region demonstrates obvious high signal intensity (*arrow*), denoting extensive edema. (**c**) Axial T2-weighted (3,800/90) turbo MR image also shows high signal intensity in the extensor tendon (*arrow*), indicating severe inflammation (Sonin et al. 1996)

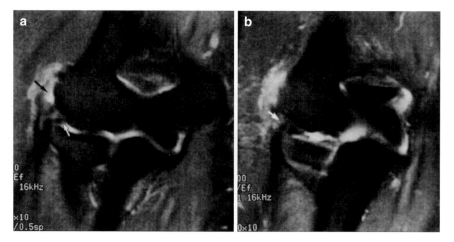

Fig. 7.39 Coronal T2 weighted fast spin-echo images with fat saturation (TR/TE 3,000/60) in a 56-year-old woman with lateral elbow pain. (**a**) MR image shows surgically proven complete tear (*long arrow*) of the common extensor tendon consistent with severe epicondylitis. Origin of lateral ulnar collateral ligament is thickened, with mildly increased signal intensity (*short arrow*). (**b**) Image reveals thickening and increased signal intensity at origin of lateral ulnar collateral ligament (*arrow*). Thickening of the ligament was found at surgery (Bredella et al. 1999)

Injection for Medial Epicondylitis (Golfer's Elbow) (Fig. 7.40)

Anatomy

The anterior medial epicondyle of the humerus serves as the origin for the muscles of flexion and pronation in the forearm (flexor carpi radialis, pronator teres, and palmaris longus). These muscles are therefore usually involved in medial epicondylitis. The flexor carpi ulnaris and flexor digitorum superficialis are less frequently involved. Up to 50% of patients may have evidence of ulnar nerve compression in the medial epicondylar groove.

Function

The medial epicondyle is the site of attachment for muscles performing flexion and pronation.

Clinical Presentation

Medial epicondylitis presents with pain and tenderness over the medial epicondyle exacerbated by flexion or pronation.

Etiology

Etiologies include repetitive stress or overuse injury with acute and chronic forms. Activities such as golfing, pitching, or serving are implicated.

Differential Diagnosis

Differential diagnoses include ulnar collateral ligament injury,** stress fracture,** osteochondritis dissecans,** ulnar neuropathy,** elbow arthritis,** complete tendon tear** with valgus instability (requires surgery), pronator teres syndrome,** and cervical radiculopathy.**

Injection Site

A medial approach is utilized just distal to the medial epicondyle superficial to the tendon avoiding intratendon injection.

Imaging/Radiology

Plain film radiographs: AP, lateral, and oblique views are helpful to exclude pathology (fractures, intraarticular osteochondral body, and arthritis). Calcification may be seen adjacent to the medial epicondyle in up to one-third of patients.

Ultrasound: Ultrasound can accurately diagnose medial epicondylitis. In experienced hands, it is reliable, more readily available, and more cost effective than MRI (Park et al. 2008). It may be useful for the evaluation of tendinosis and partial thickness tears. This is seen as a focal hypoechoic and anechoic abnormality. Tendon non-visualization may be present in the setting of complete tear. Intratendon calcification and cortical bone irregularity may be identified.

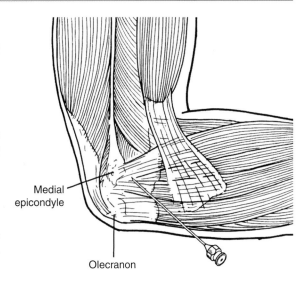

Fig. 7.40 Medial epicondylitis injection (Weiss 2007i, Fig. 4-9)

CT: CT is useful if fracture or osteochondritis dissecans are suspected.

MRI: MRI is usually not needed except for ambiguous clinical presentation or if the patient is refractory to medical therapy. MRI is reliable for medial epicondylitis. It demonstrates thickening and increased signal intensity on T1- and T2-weighted sequences of the common flexor tendon. There is also soft tissue edema surrounding this tendon. This finding is specific for medial epicondylitis (Fig. 7.41). MRI is also useful for the diagnosis of the associated ulnar nerve entrapment. It may also demonstrate osteochondritis dissecans, fractures, or other forms of soft tissue injury. MR arthrography is useful to demonstrate ulnar collateral ligament rupture (Kijowski 2005).

Indications

The two main indications (Genovese 1998) for lateral and medial epicondyle injection are: (1) lateral epicondylitis (tennis elbow),** and (2) medial epicondylitis (golfer's elbow).**

Complications

Complications (Cotten et al. 1997) frequently encountered in lateral and medial epicondyle injection include: (1) steroid arthropathy (although there is questionable evidence to support this)**; (2) ulnar nerve injection

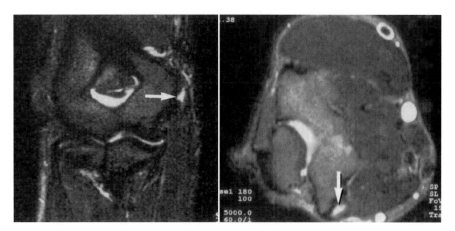

Fig. 7.41 (**a**, **b**) Medial epicondylitis. (**a**) Coronal fat-suppressed T2-weighted (2,550/90) turbo MR image demonstrates high signal intensity equivalent to that of fluid at the origin of the flexor tendon group (*arrow*). (**b**) Axial turbo STIR (repetition time ms/inversion time ms = 5,000/60/120) MR image shows high signal intensity adjacent to normal marrow in the medial epicondyle (*arrow*). Partial avulsion of the tendon can be difficult to differentiate from severe tendonitis (Sonin et al. 1996)

for medial epicondylitis; (3) injection into the tendon with possible rupture.**

7.2.2.3 Injection for Olecranon Bursitis (Fig. 7.42)

Anatomy

The olecranon bursa is located adjacent to the proximal ulna extensor aspect.

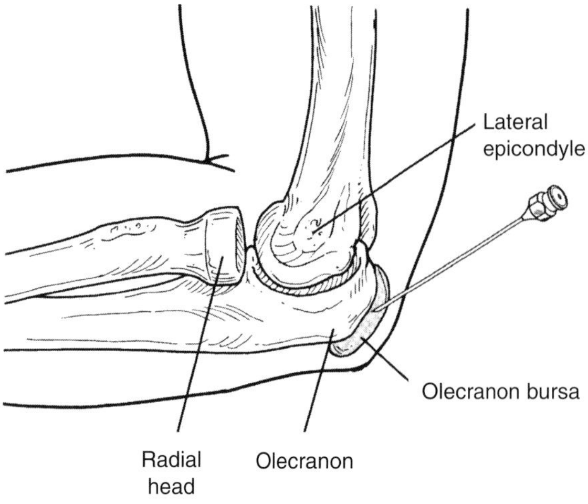

Function

The olecranon bursa serves to decrease friction over the extensor surface of the proximal elbow (olecranon) with the adjacent skin.

Clinical Presentation

Olecranon bursitis presents with painful swelling at the posterior elbow with associated tenderness. There is normal range of motion.

Etiology

Etiologies include repetitive trauma** or infection** (one third of cases are septic), rheumatoid arthritis,** gout,** and calcium pyrophosphate deposition disease.**

Injection Site

With flexion of the elbow a posterior approach is utilized over the palpable olecranon bursa. It is important to avoid the ulnar nerve within the ulnar groove medially.

Imaging/Radiology

Plain film radiographs: Plain films are useful to evaluate for fracture. They are also able to demonstrate calcifications.

Fig. 7.42 Olecranon bursa injection (Weiss 2007j, Fig. 5-3)

Ultrasound: This modality is considered a very effective means for diagnosis. Findings include fluid, synovial membrane thickening, loose bodies, hypervascularity, and rheumatoid nodules in rheumatoid arthritis (Blankstein et al. 2006).

MRI: MRI is usually not needed unless for evaluation of osteomyelitis or abscess formation. MRI of aseptic olecranon bursitis demonstrates a complex fluid collection (hypointense on T1-weighted images and variable signal intensity on T2-weighted sequences) with rim enhancement (Fig. 7.43). There is soft tissue edema with contrast enhancement. There may be thickening of the triceps tendon. Bone marrow edema may be seen within the olecranon. However, this finding is more commonly seen in septic bursitis. Lobulation of the margin, septations within the bursa, soft tissue edema, and thickening of the triceps tendon are more commonly seen in septic bursitis. A large number of overlapping MRI findings, however, are noted with septic bursitis and aseptic bursitis. Bursal aspiration is still the gold standard when infection is suspected (Floemer et al. 2004).

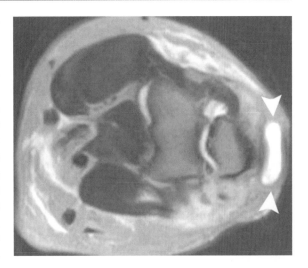

Fig. 7.43 A 61-year-old man with surgically confirmed rupture of the triceps tendon at the insertion of the olecranon and concomitant nonseptic effusion of the olecranon bursa. Axial T2-weighted fat-suppressed image (4,050/70) shows homogeneous hyperintense signal in well-defined collection (*arrowheads*) without lobulation (Floemer et al. 2004)

Indications

The four principal indications for olecranon bursa injection are: (1) Olecranon bursitis (noninfectious), (2) gout, (3) rheumatoid arthritis, (4) trauma. Aspiration only is performed for an infectious bursitis.

Contraindications

The main contraindication to olecranon bursa injection is joint prosthesis** and infection** (see (Fig. 7.44).

Complications

Injection into the triceps tendon with possible rupture** is the chief complication encountered in olecranon bursa injection.

7.2.3 Wrist, Hand, and Fingers

7.2.3.1 Injection of the Radiocarpal Joint and the Intercarpal Joints (Figs. 7.45 and 7.46)

Anatomy

The wrist is the most complex joint within the body. It is composed of numerous bones and joints. The bones include the distal radius and ulna as well as the eight carpal bones and five metacarpal bones. The joints include the distal radioulnar, radiocarpal, and intercarpal joints, as well as the carpometacarpal joints. The triangular-fibrocartilage complex separates the distal ulna and the proximal carpal row (scaphoid, lunate, and triquetrum). It attaches the distal radius to the ulnar styloid. The distal carpal row is formed by the trapezium, trapezoid, capitate, and hamate bone (radial to ulnar). The pisiform bone lies adjacent to the triquetrum.

The wrist joint is divided into the radiocarpal, distal radioulnar, and midcarpal joints. In addition, there is a common carpometacarpal, first carpometacarpal joint, and pisiform-triquetral joint. The most important is the radiocarpal compartment. This is formed by the distal radius and triangular fibrocartilage complex proximally as well as the proximal carpal row distally. Proximal to the triangular fibrocartilage complex lies the distal radioulnar joint. The scapholunate and lunate triquetral ligaments and the corresponding bones of the proximal carpal row separate the radiocarpal joint from the mid carpal compartment. The mid carpal joint separates the proximal and distal rows of the carpal bones.

In addition to the scapholunate and lunate triquetral ligaments, numerous other ligaments form attachments between the rest of the carpal bones. These are known as the interosseous ligaments. Furthermore, the intercarpal joints are reinforced by the radiate carpal and

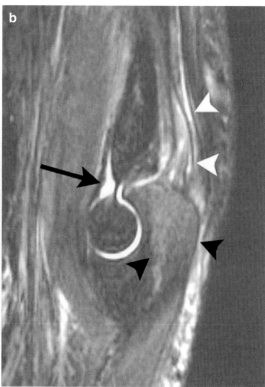

Fig. 7.44 (a) A 26-year-old woman with culture-proven septic olecranon bursitis. Axial T2-weighted fat-suppressed fast spin-echo image (TR/TE, 4,500/35; inversion time, 60 ms) of the right elbow reveals effusion (*arrow*) in the olecranon bursa with marked hypointense signal complexity of collection. (b) Sagittal T2-weighted fat-suppressed image (5,735/90) reveals moderate joint effusion (*arrow*) of elbow and hyperintense thickening (*white arrowheads*) of insertion of triceps. Note also the hyperintense signal of olecranon bone marrow (*black arrowheads*) (Floemer et al. 2004)

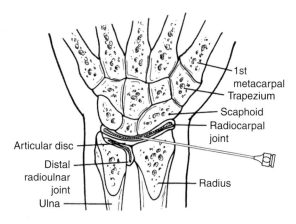

Fig. 7.45 Wrist joint (radiocarpal) injection (Weiss 2007k, Fig. 3-11)

pisohamate ligaments as well as the palmar and dorsal intercarpal ligament.

The distal row carpal bones are attached to the metacarpal bone by the dorsal carpometacarpal and pisometacarpal ligaments. The lateral and medial aspect of the joint is supported by the radial and ulnar collateral ligaments, respectively.

The flexor retinaculum is a fibrous structure that prevents the tendons of the extrinsic flexor hand muscles from stretching away from the wrist. The extensor retinaculum forms a similar row for the extrinsic extensor hand muscles. The extensor retinaculum subdivides the tendons into six dorsal compartments whereas the flexor retinaculum has no similar subdivisions.

Function

The wrist performs pronation and supination at the distal radioulnar joint. It performs radial and ulnar deviation via the radiocarpal and mid carpal joint. It also performs dorsiflexion and palmar flexion.

Radial deviation is performed by the extensor carpi radialis longus, abductor pollicis longus, extensor

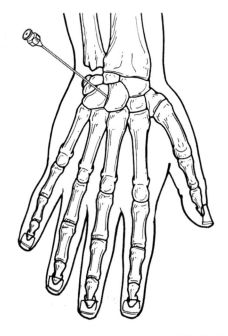

Fig. 7.46 Intercarpal joint injection (Weiss 2007l, Fig. 3-13)

pollicis longus, flexor carpi radialis, and flexor pollicis longus. Ulnar deviation is performed by the extensor carpi ulnaris, flexor carpi ulnaris, extensor digitorum, and extensor digiti minimi. Dorsiflexion is performed by the extensor digitorum, extensor carpi radialis longus, extensor carpi radialis brevis, extensor indicis, extensor pollicis longus, and extensor digitorum minimi.

Palmar flexion is performed by the flexor digitorum superficialis, flexor digitorum profundus, flexor carpi ulnaris, flexor pollicis longus, flexor carpi radialis, and abductor pollicis longus.

Clinical Presentation

Arthritis of the wrist presents as severe pain with progressive loss of range of motion at either the radiocarpal or intercarpal joints.

Etiology

Osteoarthritis may be primary.** It also may be secondary** to trauma as well as fracture/dislocation** of the distal radius or scaphoid. Chronic scapholunate dissociation** and lunate dislocation** may also result in osteoarthritis, as may avascular necrosis** and carpal

instability.** Other forms of arthritis include rheumatoid arthritis** as well as gout.** Calcium pyrophosphate deposition disease,** psoriatic arthritis,** and Lyme disease** are also seen within the wrist.

Differential Diagnosis

Differential diagnoses include scaphoid fracture,** de Quervain's tenosynovitis,** scapholunate dissociation,** Kienböck's disease (avascular necrosis of the lunate),** distal radius fracture,** Preiser disease** (avascular necrosis of the scaphoid), scaphotrapezoid-trapezial joint arthritis,** and tendonitis.**

Injection Site

For the radiocarpal joint, a dorsal approach is used between the extensor indicis and extensor pollicis longus tendon while the wrist is pronated and resting slightly flexed on a towel. Fluoroscopy or ultrasound may be helpful.

For the intercarpal joint, a dorsal approach is utilized. Fluoroscopy or ultrasound may be useful.

Imaging/Radiology

Plain film radiographs: PA and lateral views are helpful to reveal arthritic changes of osteoarthritis and rheumatoid arthritis prior to joint injection (Fig. 7.47). Calcium pyrophosphate deposition disease is suspected when there is chondrocalcinosis and radiocarpal joint indentation since calcium pyrophosphate deposition disease otherwise appears similar to osteoarthritis.

Ultrasound: This modality may be useful for bedside joint assessment as well as guidance for injection. It is useful for the evaluation of erosions and synovitis. It is also useful for evaluating the tendons and entheses (tendon insertions) of early osteoarthritis and rheumatoid arthritis (Østergaard et al. 2008).

Arthrography: Arthrography is useful for the assessment of carpal instability due to interosseous and triangular fibrocartilage complex ligament tears. It can be combined with CT or MRI to increase sensitivity for interosseous ligament and triangular fibrocartilage complex tears in the setting of joint instability.

CT: CT is not routinely used. It is slightly more sensitive than plain films for erosion, but less useful for

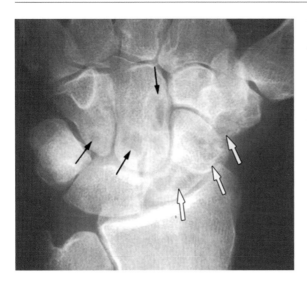

Fig. 7.47 A 42-year-old woman with rheumatoid arthritis. Posteroanterior radiograph reveals multiple erosions of carpal bones (*black and white arrows*) (Taouli et al. 2004)

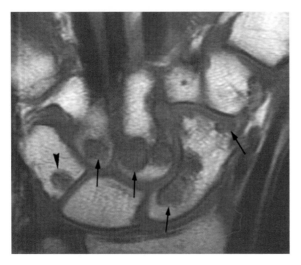

Fig. 7.48 A 42-year-old woman with rheumatoid arthritis. Unenhanced coronal T1-weighted spin-echo conventional high-field-strength MR image reveals multiple erosions of carpal bones (*arrows*). Triquetral erosion (*arrowhead*) is not visible on radiograph because of pisiform superposition (Taouli et al. 2004)

the evaluation of synovitis in assessing arthritis. It is however excellent for bone detail in occult fractures and avascular necrosis.

MRI: This imaging modality represents the gold standard for early rheumatoid arthritis. It is more sensitive than plain films for erosions, joint effusion, joint space narrowing, and synovitis (Fig. 7.48). It may be slightly superior or equivalent for the assessment of synovitis compared to ultrasound. MRI assesses

ligament tears or tendon abnormalities in the setting of joint instability. It is also able to detect occult fractures or avascular necrosis (Østergaard et al. 2008).

Bone scintigraphy: Bone scan is sensitive for inflammation by demonstrating increased uptake. However, it has low specificity. When combined with MRI, it can be helpful in the diagnosis of previously unclassified arthritis (Duer et al. 2008).

Indications

Common indications include arthritis,** mildly symptomatic scapholunate advanced collapse** (SLAC) (advanced degenerative arthritis initially localized to the scaphoid and radius that may progress to the capitate and lunate), and triscaphe arthritis** (degenerative arthritis localized to the trapezium, trapezoid, and distal scaphoid).

7.2.3.2 Aspiration and Injection for Ganglion Cyst of the Wrist (Fig. 7.49)

Anatomy

Ganglion cysts are the most frequent tumor of the wrist and hand. The content of a ganglion cyst is that of a thick liquid interior. It is formed by bulging of synovium secondary to chronic degeneration of the intercarpal ligaments, especially the scapholunate ligament. It originates from the dorsum of the wrist at the scapholunate joint (in 60–70% of cases), the volar wrist usually at the radioscaphoid or scaphotrapezial joint (in 20-25% of cases), and the flexor tendon sheath (in 10–15% of cases) at the A1 pulley or distal interphalangeal joint.

Function

Not applicable since this is not a normal structure.

Clinical Presentation

Ganglion cyst presents as a compressible mass, which are usually not (but may be) painful. There may be associated decreased range of motion. They can impinge on the median nerve if located within the carpal tunnel resulting in sensory or motor defects. An occult ganglion may be difficult to detect on physical

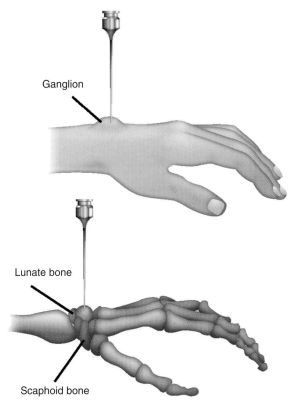

Ganglion

Lunate bone

Scaphoid bone

Fig. 7.49 Ganglion cyst of the wrist (Illustrated by Michael Dobryzcki)

exam if there is no swelling and may be manifested only by the presence of pain. However, in the setting of chronic dorsal wrist pain, it may be clinically difficult to distinguish an occult ganglion from synovitis.

Etiology

Etiologies include overuse/repetitive motion injury, trauma, or arthritis.**

Differential Diagnosis

Differential diagnoses include tumor,** infection,** inflammation including bursitis,** degenerative joint disease,** and trauma.** At the dorsal aspect of the wrist, differential diagnoses also include dorsal impaction syndrome,** extensor tenosynovitis,** avascular necrosis** of the lunate or scaphoid, inflammatory arthritis,** or neuropathy of the posterior interosseous nerve.** At the volar aspect of the wrist, differential diagnoses include tenosynovitis** of the flexor carpi

radialis in the setting of triscaphe degenerative joint disease,** accessory muscles (extensor digitorum brevis manus**), and pigmented villonodular synovitis** (giant cell tumor of the tendons sheath).

In the digits, differential diagnoses include a mucous cyst** at the distal interphalangeal joint or Dupuytren's disease (fixed flexion contracture of the hand where the fingers bend toward the palms and cannot be contracted).**

Injection Site

The needle is inserted directly into the cyst depending on its anatomic location. The cyst is aspirated first using a 20- to 30-mL syringe to create suction. Injection of steroid and local anesthetic may be performed while stabilizing the needle with a hemostat during and after aspiration.

Imaging/Radiology

Imaging is needed in the majority of cases to confirm the diagnosis. It is also necessary for preoperative evaluation.

Plain film radiographs: Plain films are helpful to rule out associated bony abnormalities such as degenerative joint disease of the scaphotrapeziotrapezoid joint. Ganglion cysts are usually difficult to detect with plain films if there is no associated soft tissue swelling.

Ultrasound: A high resolution 10- to 17-MHz transducer may allow optimal imaging. Combined with radiography, ultrasound allows definitive diagnosis in the preponderance of cases. It determines mass dimensions, contents, and relationships to nearby anatomy. Doppler assessment of vascularity may be performed to exclude other diagnoses. On ultrasound, a ganglion cyst is seen as a sonolucent structure, which may have septations or echogenic contents if it is more chronic (Fig. 7.50). At the dorsum of the wrist, the relationship to the scapholunate ligament may be assessed. At the volar aspect of the wrist, ultrasound may distinguish a ganglion from a pseudoaneurysm with color Doppler evaluation. It can also distinguish a ganglion from tenosynovitis of the flexor carpi radialis tendon. At the carpal tunnel, mass effect on the median nerve and tendon may be identified. In the digits, the anatomy with respect to the tendons and pulleys can

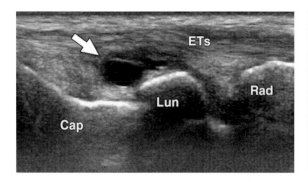

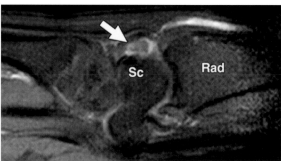

Fig. 7.50 A 24-year-old woman with a ganglion cyst of the dorsal aspect of the wrist. Sagittal sonogram obtained over the dorsal aspect of the wrist shows the ganglion cyst (*arrow*) located between the lunate (*Lun*) and extensor tendons (*ETs*). The ganglion cyst has a hypoechoic wall and thin internal septum. Internal viscid fluid appears anechoic. *Cap* capitate; *Rad* radius (Bianchi et al. 2008)

Fig. 7.51 A 24-year-old woman with a ganglion cyst of the dorsal aspect of the wrist (same patient as Fig. 7.50). Corresponding T1-weighted gadolinium-enhanced sagittal MR image obtained in slightly more lateral position than Fig. 7.51 shows that the ganglion cyst (*arrow*) has an isointense internal signal. Note contrast enhancement of wall. *Sc* scaphoid; *Rad* radius (Bianchi et al. 2008)

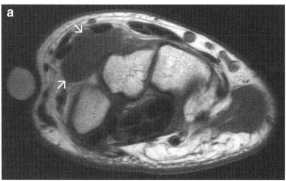

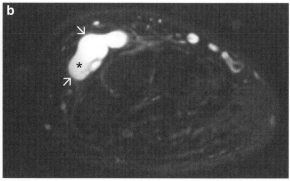

Fig. 7.52 A 23-year-old woman with MRI showing characteristic features of a ganglion cyst of the dorsal aspect of the wrist. (**a**) Focal, relatively large mass (*arrows*) is evident on the T1-weighted image. Placement of a vitamin capsule to demarcate

patient's pain site has slightly displaced soft tissues. Clinically, however, no soft-tissue swelling was evident. (**b**) Corresponding fast spin-echo T2-weighted axial image shows focal, fluid cystic mass (*arrows*) with internal septa (*asterisk*) (Anderson et al. 2006)

be seen. Ultrasound can be utilized for guidance of cyst aspiration and injection (Teefey et al. 2008).

MRI: A dedicated wrist coil is utilized. T1-weighted fat-saturated, T2, and STIR sequences are utilized with multiplanar imaging. MRI is helpful in the situation of chronic wrist pain without a palpable mass in identifying a ganglion cyst. It is comparable to ultrasound in diagnosing dorsal occult ganglion cyst. Similar to ultrasound, MRI can determine mass dimensions, contents, and relationship to nearby anatomy. A ganglion cyst is seen as a well-marginated round septated structure with enhancing walls (Figs. 7.51 and 7.52). MRI can distinguish a ganglion cyst from synovitis, which has indistinct margins, a concentric or flattened appearance, and enhances throughout its substance (Anderson et al. 2006).

Indications

The major indication for aspiration and injection is symptomatic ganglion cysts which cause pain and paresthesia.

7.2.3.3 Injection of the First Carpometacarpal Joint (Fig. 7.53)

Anatomy

The first carpometacarpal joint is a saddle type joint between the trapezium and the first metacarpal. It is the most commonly involved joint in arthritis of the hand. A thin capsule envelops the carpometacarpal

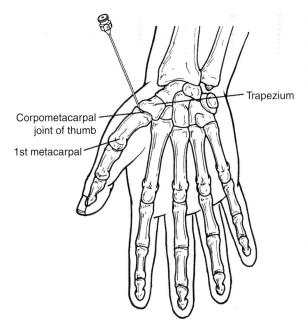

Fig. 7.53 First carpometacarpal joint injection (Weiss 2007m, Fig. 3-15)

joints. There are five ligaments at this joint including the anterior oblique, posterior oblique, dorsal radial ligament, intermetacarpal ligament, and ulnar collateral ligament.

Function

The first metacarpal joint permits apposition, flexion/extension, and abduction/adduction.

Clinical Presentation

The clinical presentation of first carpometacarpal joint arthritis is pain with motion and limitation of the range of motion. There is also tenderness over the volar aspect of the thumb.

Etiology

Etiologies include osteoarthritis,** rheumatoid arthritis,** calcium pyrophosphate deposition disease,** gout,** seronegative spondyloarthropathy** (ankylosing spondylitis** and psoriatic arthritis**), and infection.**

Differential Diagnosis

The differential diagnoses include de Quervain's tenosynovitis,** flexor carpi radialis tendinosis,** stenosing flexor tenosynovitis of the flexor pollicis longus,** chronic dislocation,** and fracture (Bennett's fracture**).

Injection Site

The site of injection involves the extensor surface of the first metacarpal joint just proximal to the first metacarpal. It is important to avoid the radial artery and the extensor pollicis tendon.

Imaging/Radiology

Plain film radiographs: AP, lateral, and oblique views are usually obtained. Radiographs may demonstrate findings of arthritis including joint space narrowing, subchondral sclerosis, osteophyte formation, cystic changes, bony fragmentation, and radial subluxation in advanced cases (Fig. 7.54).

Fluoroscopy: Fluoroscopy is useful for injection guidance, but may not be necessary even in advanced arthritis (Mandl et al. 2006).

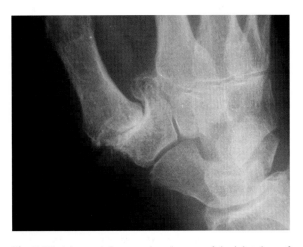

Fig. 7.54 Advanced degenerative changes of the joint: loss of joint space, subchondral sclerosis, large osteophyte, erosions, all with preservation of the adjacent joints (www.eatonhand. com/img/img00031.htm). (Reproduced with permission from Dr. Charles Eaton)

Ultrasound: This modality is useful for injection guidance and assessment of the joint. It is very sensitive for evaluation of erosions and synovitis. It is also sensitive for the evaluation of tendons and entheses in early osteoarthritis and rheumatoid arthritis. It is more sensitive than plain film radiographs.

MRI: High-resolution thin-slice images with a small surface coil are utilized. Coronal, axial, fast spin-echo, and STIR sequences are useful. MRI is useful for assessing the articular cartilage. It is very sensitive for effusions, erosions, and synovitis. It assesses the ligaments and tendons as well as cyst formation (Connell et al. 2004; Cardoso et al. 2009).

Indications

The two main indications for first carpometacarpal joint injection are: (1) arthritis and (2) overuse.

Complications

The principal complications encountered in first carpometacarpal joint injection are: (1) radial artery injection, and (2) extensor pollicis tendon injection.

7.2.3.4 Injection for de Quervain's Tenosynovitis (Fig. 7.55)

Anatomy

de Quervain's tenosynovitis is an entrapment tendinitis involving the abductor pollicis longus and extensor pollicis brevis, which are connected to the radial styloid by the extensor retinaculum. The tendons are coated in synovial sheath. Evaluation of histology shows no inflammation, but it shows thickening and mixed degeneration. Thus, chronic degeneration (tendinosis or tendinopathy) is a more accurate term.

Function

The extensor pollicis brevis and abductor pollicis longus move the thumb away from the hand in the plane of the hand (radial abduction).

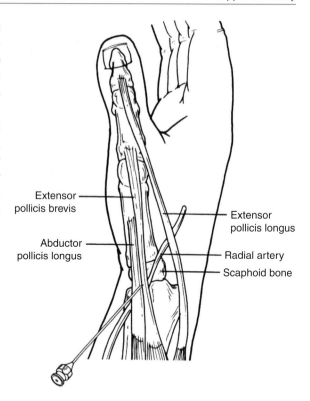

Fig. 7.55 de Quervain's injection (Weiss 2007n, Fig. 4-3)

Clinical Presentation

de Quervain's tenosynovitis is manifested clinically by pain and swelling involving the base of the thumb and radial styloid with tenderness, thickening, and firmness of the radial or first dorsal compartment of the wrist. The pain is worsened by movement of the thumb while there is simultaneous ulnar or radial deviation of the wrist. The Finkelstein maneuver is useful in the diagnosis. This test is performed by having the thumb positioned adjacent to the palm and the fingers folded over the thumb with simultaneous ulnar deviation of the wrist. de Quervain's tenosynovitis is seen in mothers of infants or childcare workers due to repetitive lifting. It can also be seen in trauma or rheumatoid arthritis.

Differential Diagnosis

Includes osteoarthritis of the first carpometacarpal joint,** intersection syndrome** (tenosynovitis of the radial wrist extensors), Wartenberg's syndrome/cheiralgia paresthetica** (radial superficial sensory nerve entrapment), Kienböck's disease (avascular necrosis

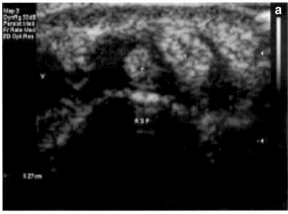

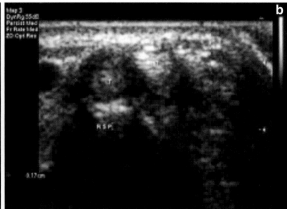

Fig. 7.56 (**a**) Ultrasonographic transverse image of the symptomatic tendons of the abductor pollicis longus and the extensor pollicis brevis, showing a diffuse circumferential hypoechoic thickening of the synovial sheath (0.27 cm), giving a characteristic double-target pattern, denoting de Quervain's tenosynovitis; (**b**) ultrasound transverse scans of the same patient. After 1 week of injection, note the decrease in thickening of the synovial sheath (0.17 cm). *T* tendon; *RSP* radial styloid process. 11 MHz (Kamel et al. 2002). (Reproduced from Annals of the Rheumatic Disease, Kamel et al, vol. 61, pp 1034-35, 2002 with permission from BMJ Publishing Group Ltd.)

of the lunate), carpal tunnel syndrome,** scaphoid fracture,** cervical radiculopathy,** lateral epicondylitis,** and pseudoaneurysm.**

Injection Site

The injection site is between the tendons of the abductor pollicis longus and extensor pollicis brevis at the tip of the radial styloid. The hand should be rested on a towel in a lateral position, ulnar aspect dependent to remove tension on the tendons.

Imaging/Radiology

Imaging may help in atypical or refractory cases.

Plain film radiographs: These are helpful to rule out fracture.

Ultrasound: Demonstrates a diffuse circumferential hypoechoic thickening of the synovial sheath (double-target pattern) (Fig. 7.56). Ultrasound is also useful in guidance for intrasynovial injection to avoid intratendon injection (Kamel et al. 2002; Jeyapalan and Choudhary 2009).

MRI: Axial images demonstrate a soft tissue mass corresponding to tendon sheath thickening with decreased signal intensity on T1- and T2-weighted images within and around the first extensor compartment of the wrist (peritendinous edema) (Fig. 7.57). There is increased signal intensity on STIR sequences

with enhancement. This is best seen on axial images (Anderson et al. 2004).

Bone scintigraphy: Bone scintigraphy demonstrates increased flow, blood pool, and skeletal phases. A three-phase bone scan may be useful to rule out a fracture of the scaphoid.

Indications

de Quervain's tenosynovitis is the main indication for this intervention.

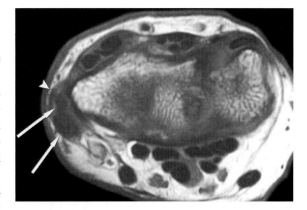

Fig. 7.57 de Quervain's tenosynovitis. Axial T1-weighted MR image shows increased thickness of the abductor pollicis longus and extensor pollicis brevis tendons (*arrows*) and increased intratendinous signal intensity. Also note the enlarged synovial sheath (*arrowhead*) (Clavero et al. 2003)

Complications

The three main complications encountered in injection for de Quervain's tenosynovitis include: (1) radial artery injection**; (2) extensor pollicis tendon injection**; (3) injury to the superficial branch of the radial nerve (sensory).

7.2.3.5 Injection for Trigger Finger (Stenosing Tenosynovitis) (Fig. 7.58)

Anatomy

The condition trigger finger occurs when there is thickening of the sheath surrounding the flexor tendon due to chronic inflammation. This is also known as stenosing tenosynovitis. Stenosing tenosynovitis results in an inability of the tendon to glide through the fibroosseous tunnel, usually at the A1 pulley overlying the metacarpophalangeal joint at its volar surface. (The pulley keeps the tendon sheath apposed to the finger during flexion.) The condition prevents extension or flexion of the finger depending on the site of tendon thickening with respect to the pulley.

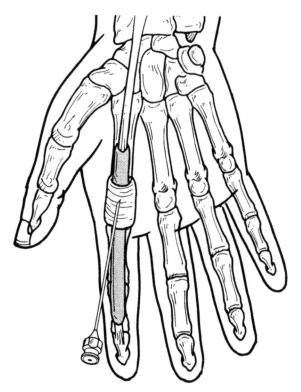

Fig. 7.58 Trigger finger injection (Weiss 2007o, Fig. 4-1)

Clinical Presentation

The patient clinically presents with finger and/or thumb that are painful to extend after flexion or vice versa. Difficulty with finger extension is more common than with flexion. There may be an associated clicking or snapping sound during flexion or extension. An external force may be required to extend or flex the finger. Stiffness and pain in the finger joints is common. A tender palpable nodule associated with the flexor tendon may be noted. The condition most commonly affects the forefinger (index finger) followed by the thumb (trigger thumb). Next, the middle finger and fourth finger may be affected.

Etiology

Etiologies include idiopathic, repetitive motion injury, rheumatoid arthritis,** gout,** diabetes, hypothyroidism, renal disease, amyloidosis,** and infection.** (Infectious etiologies include gonococcus, *Staphylococcus aureus*, streptococcus species, *Pasteurella multocida*, and *Eikenella corrodens*.)

Differential Diagnosis

Differential diagnoses include Dupuytren's contracture,** ganglion** of the tendon sheath, metacarpophalangeal osteoarthritis,** or joint injury**; flexor tendon/sheath tumor**; extensor tendon injury**; ulnar collateral ligament injury/gamekeeper's thumb** (for trigger thumb); de Quervain's tenosynovitis** (for trigger thumb).

Injection Site

The site of injection is the distal palmar crease over the flexor tendon sheath at the level of the A1 pulley. Intratendon injection should be avoided.

Imaging/Radiology

Imaging is usually not necessary as there is no history of injury or inflammatory arthritis (Makkouk et al. 2008).

Plain film radiographs: These can be useful to evaluate for foreign bodies or to exclude fracture as well as arthritis (Katzman et al. 1999).

Ultrasound: Ultrasound is useful in atypical presentations to confirm the diagnosis. Thickening and hypoechogenicity of the A1 pulley as well as hypervascularity of the A1 pulley with power Doppler imaging are pathognomonic (Fig. 7.59). Flexor tendinosis and tenosynovitis are frequently seen in approximately 50% of cases. Ultrasound is useful for guidance for injection and for percutaneous tendon release (Guerini et al. 2008; Bodorm et al. 2009).

MRI: MRI is useful to exclude other etiologies and atypical presentations. It is more sensitive than ultrasound in flexor and extensor tenosynovitis in early and untreated rheumatoid arthritis (Wakefield et al. 2007). MRI findings in stenosing tenosynovitis include thickening of the tendon or tendon sheath, increased fluid within the tendon sheath, and enhancement of the tendon sheath after intravenous gadolinium contrast. MRI is performed with high resolution imaging such as the use of a digit coil. Thin slices are utilized with T1- and T2-weighted fat-saturated imaging. Thickening of the tendon may be seen as well as increased signal intensity within the tendon. There may be a small amount of fluid within the tendon sheath as well as subcutaneous edema.

Indications

Trigger finger is the sole indication for intervention.

Complications

The two main complications encountered here are: (1) tendon rupture**; (2) acute bacterial tenosynovitis** (Fig. 7.60).

7.2.3.6 Injection for Interphalangeal Joint Arthritis (Fig. 7.61)

Anatomy

The interphalangeal joint is a hinged joint. Each joint has a volar ligament and two collateral ligaments. Extensor tendons stabilize the dorsal aspect. There is also a thin capsule which is lax dorsally spanning the joint. There are two interphalangeal joints (distal and

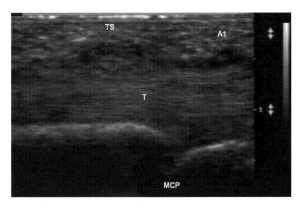

Fig. 7.59 Trigger finger. Longitudinal sonogram of trigger finger at the level of the metacarpophalangeal (*MCP*) joint shows focal tenosynovitis (*TS*) on the palmar aspect of flexor tendon (*T*) and thickened A1 pulley. There is hesitation of flexor tendon movement during extension as seen on dynamic imaging (Khoury et al. 2007)

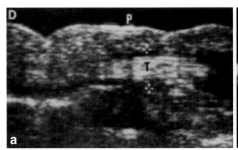
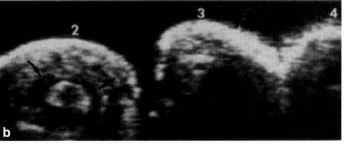

Fig. 7.60 Acute bacterial tenosynovitis after puncture wound to the hand. (**a**) Sagittal ultrasound scan of the flexor tendon of the right second digit at the level of the middle phalanx. Note diffuse enlargement of the flexor tendon (*T*). Cursors are on the outer margin of the hypoechoic tendon sheath. The *open arrow* denotes the middle phalanx. *P* palmar surface; *D* distal digit. (**b**) Transverse scan of the second, third, and fourth digits at the level of the proximal phalanx demonstrates a hypoechoic area (*arrows*) surrounding an enlarged, echogenic flexor tendon (*T*). The appearance is compatible with tendon sheath fluid, which was found to be pus at surgery (Jeffrey et al. 1987)

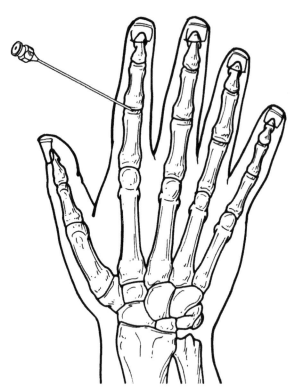

Fig. 7.61 Interphalangeal joint injection (Weiss 2007p, Fig. 3-17)

Etiology

Osteoarthritis** (includes degenerative change, which may be occupation related), rheumatoid arthritis,** gout,** calcium pyrophosphate deposition disease,** psoriatic arthritis,** and infection** (aspiration only). Rheumatoid arthritis usually involves the interphalangeal joints and metacarpophalangeal joints, whereas osteoarthritis involves the distal and proximal interphalangeal joints.

Differential Diagnosis

Differential diagnoses include ulnar neuropathy,** carpal tunnel syndrome,** Raynaud's syndrome, myositis,** fracture,** tendon/ligament injury,** cervical radiculopathy,** brachial plexus compression,** and peripheral arterial disease.**

Injection Site

The site of injection lies in the midline of the extensor aspect of the joint during flexion of the joint.

Imaging/Radiology

Plain film radiographs: PA, lateral, and oblique views are obtained. Osteoarthritis is manifested by joint space loss, osteophytes, subchondral sclerosis, and subluxation (Fig. 7.63). Osteophyte formation is the most sensitive and specific finding in osteoarthritis.

In rheumatoid arthritis, erosions, joint space loss, and periarticular osteopenia as well as soft tissue swelling is noted (Fig. 7.62).

Suspect calcium pyrophosphate deposition disease or hemochromatosis if there are osteoarthritis-like changes in the metacarpophalangeal joints.

Septic arthritis is manifest by joint space narrowing, osteopenia, with bone erosions. It represents a contraindication to injection, but is an indication for aspiration (Fig. 7.64).

Ultrasound: Ultrasound may be more sensitive than radiography in detecting osteophytes and joint space narrowing in osteoarthritis. Furthermore, ultrasound detects synovitis on gray-scale imaging as well as increased power Doppler signal in the setting of inflammation. It is also useful to evaluate pathology at the metacarpophalangeal and interphalangeal joints for detection of tenosynovitis. It is more sensitive than radiography and the

proximal interphalangeal joints) in the fingers, as well as a single interphalangeal joint in the thumb. The metacarpophalangeal joint is a condyloid joint. It is stabilized by palmar ligaments and collateral ligaments.

Function

The interphalangeal joint allows flexion and extension of the fingers and thumb. The metacarpophalangeal joint can perform flexion, extension, adduction, abduction, and circumduction.

Clinical Presentation

Interphalangeal joint arthritis presents with pain in the fingers especially with motion. There is usually stiffness and with progression of disease, there is limitation in the range of motion. There may be joint swelling/enlargement. In osteoarthritis, this may be manifested as Bouchard's nodes in the proximal interphalangeal joint and Heberden's nodes in the distal interphalangeal joint.

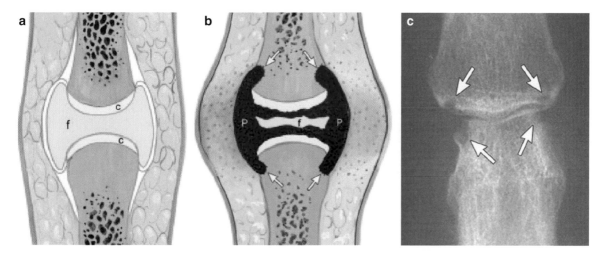

Fig. 7.62 (**a**) Illustration of synovial joint shows joint fluid (*f*) and articular cartilage (*c*). (**b**, **c**) Illustration (**b**) and radiograph (**c**) show inflammatory arthritis, synovitis, and pannus (*P*) caus-ing cartilage destruction. Marginal erosions (*arrows*) are seen where subchondral bone plate is exposed to intraarticular syno-vitis. *f* fluid (Jacobson et al. 2008)

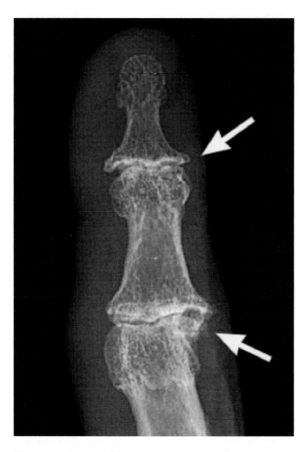

Fig. 7.63 Osteoarthritis. Posteroanterior radiograph shows interphalangeal joint space narrowing, subchondral sclerosis, and osteophyte formation (*arrows*) (Jacobson et al. 2008)

clinical exam in rheumatoid arthritis for erosions and inflammation (Keen et al. 2008; Szkudlarek et al. 2006).

CT: CT is slightly more sensitive than plain films for erosions. It is however less sensitive than ultra-sound or MRI for the detection of synovitis.

MRI: MRI represents the gold standard. It is more sensitive at visualization of early inflammatory change and destructive changes within the joints. This includes identification of erosions, synovitis, and bone marrow edema in the setting of arthritis. Furthermore, it is able to detect soft tissue pathology including tenosynovitis and abnormalities of the interphalangeal joints. Although it is superior to modalities including ultra-sound for the evaluation of changes associated with arthritis, it may be equivalent to ultrasound specifically for synovitis (Ostergaard et al. 2008).

Scintigraphy: Skeletal scintigraphy is highly sensi-tive for synovitis, but has low specificity.

7.3 Upper Extremity Nerves

7.3.1 Brachial Plexus Block (Axillary Approach) (Fig. 7.65)

7.3.1.1 Anatomy

The brachial plexus continues between the anterior and middle scalene muscle below the mid clavicle superior to the first rib into the axilla. In the axilla the brachial plexus forms the musculocutaneous, radial, median, and ulnar nerves as discrete entities as they

Fig. 7.64 (**a**, **b**) Septic arthritis. Posteroanterior (**a**) and oblique (**b**) radiographs show joint space narrowing (*arrows*), osteopenia, soft-tissue swelling, and bone erosion (*arrowhead*). *Note*: this is a contraindication to injection (Jacobson et al. 2008)

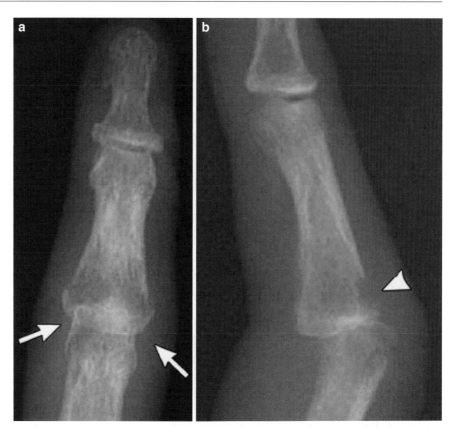

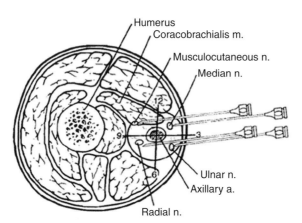

Fig. 7.65 Relative locations of the musculocutaneous, radial, median, and ulnar nerves of the brachial plexus in the axilla (Waldman 2001)

follow the axillary artery. The sheath that surrounds the axillary artery also tends to at least partially surround the median, radial, ulnar, and musculocutaneous nerves within the distal axillary region. In the axial view positioned around the axillary artery, the median nerve is found in the anterior medial quadrant, the ulnar nerve is found in the posterior medial quadrant, the radial nerve is found in the posterior lateral quadrant, and the musculocutaneous nerve is found in the anterior lateral quadrant.

7.3.1.2 Function

The function of these nerves is discussed in their respective sections.

7.3.1.3 Injection Site

The arm is abducted and the elbow flexed with the patient's fingertips adjacent to the ear. The axillary artery is identified by manual palpation. The needle is then advanced just posterior to the axillary artery. Bearing in mind that in the lower quadrants the ulnar and radial nerve are present, the operator identifies

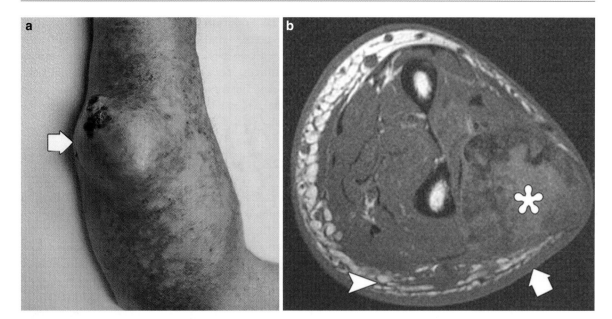

Fig. 7.66 Indication for upper extremity nerve injection. (**a, b**) High-grade undifferentiated pleomorphic sarcoma of the left forearm in an 85-year-old man who underwent preoperative radiation therapy (dose, 6,250 cGy). (**a**) Photograph obtained 3 months after the initiation of radiation therapy shows a large protruding mass (*arrow*) on the volar aspect of the forearm with overlying ulceration and extensive radiation dermatitis. (**b**) Axial T1-weighted MR image depicts the soft-tissue mass (*asterisk*), radiation-induced changes in the skin (*arrow*), and subcutaneous soft tissue (*arrowhead*) (Garner et al. 2009)

the type of paresthesia elicited with needle advancement. If aspiration test is negative and there is no continual paresthesia, injection is then performed at this site. If the initial paresthesia was radial in distribution, then the needle is withdrawn into the posterior medial quadrant in order to block the ulnar nerve. If the initial paresthesia was in the ulnar distribution, the needle is pulled back and repositioned for a slightly more anterior and lateral position into the posterior lateral quadrant containing the radial nerve. A similar procedure is then performed anterior to the axillary artery to block the median and musculocutaneous nerves.

7.3.1.4 Imaging/Radiology

Plain film radiographs: May be useful to identify bony anatomy in setting of trauma.

Ultrasound: This modality is useful for guidance. It can also directly image the nerves and can be used to identify soft tissue pathology for any of the indications.

CT: CT can identify fractures or dislocations in the setting of trauma, when plain films are inadequate.

MRI: MRI can better demonstrate soft tissue pathology in any of the indications. It can also directly image nerves (Fig. 7.66).

7.3.1.5 Indications

The following are the main indications for upper extremity nerve injections:

- Diagnosis and treatment of entrapment neuropathy (radial tunnel syndrome)**
- Traumatic or compressive neuropathic pain excluding spiral groove syndrome**
- Acute pain emergencies below the elbow in the setting of shingles, brachial plexus neuritis, Parsonage Turner syndrome,** trauma,** etc., until definitive treatment can be effective
- Contraindications to more proximal brachial plexus blockade (i.e., supraclavicular, infraclavicular, or interscalene) due to difficult access (altered anatomy,** clavicle fracture,** pacer**), or infection, etc.
- Refractory postoperative or post-traumatic pain
- Postamputation pain
- Traumatic nerve injury-related pain

- Cancer** (Fig. 7.66)
- Reflex sympathetic dystrophy**

7.3.1.6 Complications

Axillary artery hematoma,** pneumothorax,** and arterial injection (with resulting thrombosis**/emboli**/dissection**) are rare potential complications of a brachial plexus block via the axillary approach.

7.3.2 *Musculocutaneous Nerve* (Fig. 7.67)

7.3.2.1 Anatomy

The musculocutaneous nerve originates from the C5–C7 nerve roots. It originates from the upper and middle trunks, anterior division, and lateral cord of the brachial plexus (Fig. 7.68).

7.3.2.2 Function

The musculocutaneous nerve provides motor innervation for the coracobrachialis, biceps, and brachialis muscles. The nerve ends as the lateral cutaneous nerve of the forearm that provides sensory supply to the radial aspect of the forearm.

7.3.2.3 Injection Site

The axillary artery is palpated in the distal axilla. The injection is made inferior to the pectoralis muscle tendon. The needle is directed parallel to the arm in the direction of the coracoid process. Stimulation can be used to distinguish the median nerve from the musculocutaneous nerve.

7.3.2.4 Imaging/Radiology

Ultrasound: This modality is useful to provide guidance (Fig. 7.69).

7.3.2.5 Indications

The two main indications for musculocutaneous nerve injection are: (1) Tourniquet injury and (2) spasticity of the brachialis, coracobrachialis, and biceps muscles

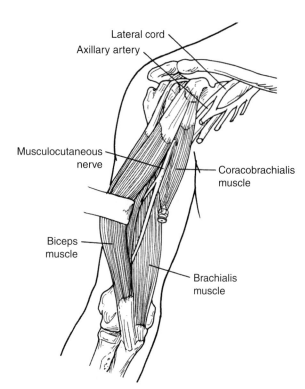

Fig. 7.67 Musculocutaneous nerve injection (Weiss 2007q, Fig. 6-3)

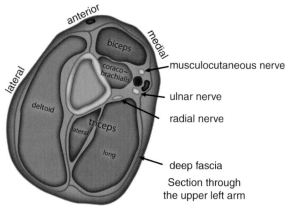

Fig. 7.68 Cross-sectional anatomy of the upper arm (Illustrated by Michael Dobryzcki)

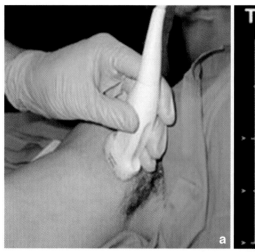

The Musculocutaneous Nerve

Fig. 7.69 (**a**) Ultrasound of the musculocutaneous nerve. (**b**) *Arrow* points to musculocutaneous nerve. *Arrowheads* point to the needle traversing the biceps muscle (Schafhalter-Zoppoth and Gray 2005)

7.3.2.6 Complications

A potential serious complication encountered in musculocutaneous nerve injection is axillary artery injection.

7.3.3 Radial Nerve

7.3.3.1 Injection for Radial Tunnel Syndrome/Posterior Interosseous Nerve Syndrome (Fig. 7.70)

Anatomy

This nerve travels adjacent to the humerus to the lateral intramuscular septum where it divides into a superficial sensory branch and the deep motor branch (the posterior interosseous nerve). The posterior interosseous nerve passes through the radial tunnel. The radial tunnel is formed by the radial humeral joint and the proximal portion of the supinator muscle. The arcade of Frohse is located at this site. This represents fibrous tissue linking the brachioradialis to the brachialis muscle. It is to be noted that the posterior interosseus nerve may be compressed at the level of the radial head by anomalous radial artery anatomy, the extensor carpi radialis brevis, and the arcade of Frohse (Fig. 7.71).

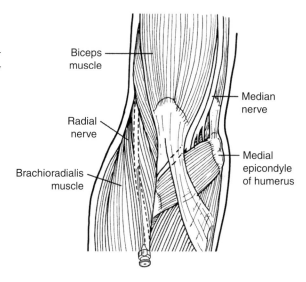

Fig. 7.70 Radial nerve injection (Weiss 2007r, Fig. 6-12)

Function

The posterior interosseous nerve provides innervation to all the muscles on the radial side and extensor surface of the forearm, with sparing of the brachioradialis, anconæus, and extensor carpi radialis longus. Therefore, the nerve supplies the muscles listed below:

- Extensor pollicis brevis
- Extensor carpi radialis brevis
- Extensor digitorum
- Extensor digiti minimi

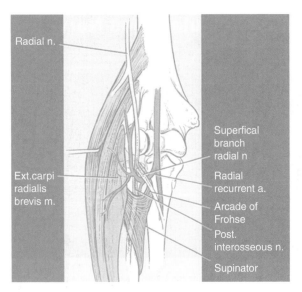

Fig. 7.71 Diagram of posterior interosseous nerve compression at the radial tunnel. The posterior interosseous nerve may be compressed at four typical sites: the fascial bands at the level of the radial head, the prominent recurrent radial vessels, the tendinous medial edge of the extensor carpi radialis brevis, and the arcade of Frohse, or proximal border of the supinator muscle. *a* artery; *Ext* extensor; *m* muscle; *n* nerve; *Post* posterior (Ferdinand et al. 2006)

- Supinator muscle
- Abductor pollicis longus
- Extensor pollicis longus
- Extensor carpi ulnaris
- Extensor indicis

Clinical Presentation

Radial tunnel syndrome presents as forearm pain at the extensor muscles without weakness. Posterior interosseous nerve syndrome presents as pain at the lateral elbow. There may be extensor weakness in the fingers and hand without sensory loss. Symptoms are worsened by wrist flexion and pronation of the forearm.

Etiology

Etiologies include overuse, external compression (ganglion cyst,** lipoma,** synovitis**), or trauma** (radial head fracture**/dislocation**), and soft tissue tumor**/swelling.**

Differential Diagnosis

Differential diagnoses include lateral epicondylitis,** chronic extensor compartment syndrome,** and cervical radiculopathy.**

Injection Site

The injection is at the antecubital region between the brachioradialis muscle and the biceps tendon with the needle directed in a cephalad, radial, and dorsal direction.

Imaging/Radiology

Plain film radiographs: Plain films exclude fracture, dislocation, and arthritis and can be helpful for identifying soft tissue masses and calcification.

Ultrasound: High resolution sonography can visualize entrapment of the posterior interosseus nerve inside the supinator muscle. The nerve may look edematous (enlarged and hypoechoic). Mass lesions may be identified compressing the nerve. Monteggia fractures (a dislocation of the proximal radioulnar joint that occurs with a forearm fracture) results in tandem areas of narrowing and swelling due to stretch injury amid the bellies of the supinator muscle.

MRI: MRI allows visualization of the posterior interosseous nerve being compressed as well. Usually, muscle edema associated with denervation can be seen. There may be abnormal signal intensity in the supinator, extensor carpi ulnaris, extensor digitorum, extensor digiti quinti, abductor pollicis longus, extensor indicis proprius, extensor pollicis longus, and extensor pollicis brevis (Figs. 7.72 and 7.73). There may or may not be involvement of the extensor carpi radialis depending on whether it is supplied by this nerve or not in any given patient. MRI can also evaluate pathology causing nerve compression such as lipomas, ganglion cysts, and rheumatoid synovitis.

Indications

The main indication for this block is radial tunnel syndrome.

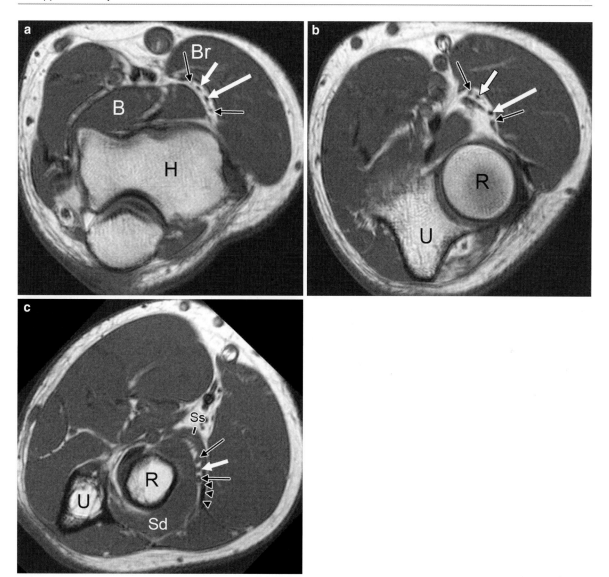

Fig. 7.72 (**a–c**) Normal MR imaging anatomy of the radial nerve and its branches. Transverse T2-weighted fast spin-echo MR images (3,350/60) at the level of (**a**) the distal humerus, (**b**) the proximal radioulnar joint, and (**c**) the proximal supinator muscle depict the posterior interosseous nerve (*long white arrow*) and the superficial radial nerve (*short white arrow*) as intermediate-signal-intensity structures within intermuscular fat. Note vessels that accompany nerves (*black arrows*). The posterior interosseous nerve enters the supinator muscle between the deep and superficial heads of the supinator muscle while superficial the radial nerve courses superficial to muscle. Note the tendinous origin of the superficial head of the supinator muscle, also known as the arcade of Frohse (*arrowheads* in **c**). *B* brachialis; *Br* brachioradialis; *H* humerus; *R* radius; *Sd* deep head of supinator muscle; *Ss* superficial head of supinator muscle; *U* ulna (Ferdinand et al. 2006)

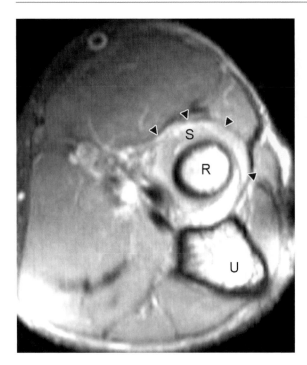

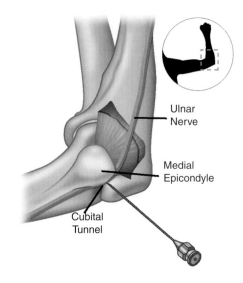

Fig. 7.74 Ulnar nerve anatomy at the elbow (Illustrated by Michael Dobrzycki)

Fig. 7.73 Supinator edema in a 74-year-old man clinically suspected of having radial tunnel syndrome. Transverse intermediate-weighted MR image (912/20) demonstrates edema within supinator muscle (*arrowheads*). The patient experienced relief of symptoms following injection of anesthetic in the region of the radial tunnel. *R* radius; *S* supinator; *U* ulna (Ferdinand et al. 2006 and Spinner et al. 1968)

7.3.4 Ulnar Nerve

7.3.4.1 Injection for Cubital Tunnel Syndrome (Ulnar Nerve at the Elbow) (Fig. 7.74)

Anatomy

Cubital tunnel syndrome is the second most frequent nerve entrapment in the upper extremity after carpal tunnel syndrome. This occurs due to pathological compression of the ulnar nerve inside the cubital tunnel. The cubital tunnel lies between the medial epicondyle (medial border) and the olecranon (lateral border), where the ulnar nerve passes under the cubital tunnel retinaculum (Osborn's band). The floor of the cubital tunnel is the ulnar collateral ligament. Sites of compression include the cubital tunnel itself or further distally between the two heads of the flexor carpi ulnaris.

Function

The ulnar nerve supplies motor function in the forearm to the flexor carpi ulnaris and flexor digitorum profundus (medial half). In the hand, the ulnar nerve supplies (through the deep branch of the ulnar nerve): the hypothenar muscles (including the opponens digiti minimi, abductor digiti minimi, and flexor digiti minimi brevis), adductor pollicis, flexor pollicis brevis (deep head), the third and fourth lumbrical muscles, dorsal interossei, and palmar interossei. In the hand, the ulnar nerve supplies (through the superficial branch of ulnar nerve) the palmaris brevis. The ulnar nerve also supplies sensation to the dorsal and palmar surface of the hand (ulnar portion) and the ulnar half of the fourth finger and entire fifth digit.

Clinical Presentation

Cubital tunnel syndrome is manifested with achy pain in the elbow region worsened by pressure on the medial elbow. There is numbness and tingling in the fourth and fifth fingers. Handgrip weakness may be seen due to supply of this nerve to the intrinsic muscles of the hand. In advanced stages, an ulnar claw deformity of the fourth and fifth fingers may develop. This may be due to the chronic repetitive injury vs. an acute form due to trauma. Guyon's canal syndrome is distinguished from cubital tunnel syndrome by numbness in the ulnar extensor aspect of the hand in cubital tunnel syndrome. The elbow flexion test is useful in the diagnosis. It consists of full elbow flexion with full extension of the wrists for 3 min causing a reproduction of symptoms.

Etiology

Etiologies include overuse, subluxation of the ulnar nerve, fracture of the humerus,** osteochondral fractures,** degenerative joint disease** with enthesophyte formation, extrinsic compression due to a soft tissue mass including ganglion** or a bony mass** such as osteochondroma.** Other etiologies include synovitis** due to rheumatoid arthritis** as well as infection** and external compression.

Differential Diagnosis

Differential diagnoses include medial epicondylitis,** cervical disk disease,** brachial plexopathy,** thoracic outlet syndrome,** Pancoast tumor,** arthritis of the elbow joint,** medial elbow joint instability,** and snapping triceps syndrome** (dislocation of the medial head of the triceps muscle or tendon over the medial epicondyle during elbow flexion or extension resulting in snapping at the elbow that may be associated with medial elbow discomfort).

Injection Site

A posterior medial approach with the elbow flexed just medial to the medial epicondyle overlying the ulnar groove is used. The needle is advanced at a 45° angle to the skin surface for a relatively superficial injection.

Imaging/Radiology

Plain film radiographs: The cubital tunnel view can be helpful for evaluation. Plain films can be useful in identifying osteophytes and degenerative joint disease. It can also be helpful in identifying valgus deformity or osteochondral bodies as well as an osteochondroma. Tumor and infection can also be identified.

CT: CT easily can visualize the osseous portion of the cubital tunnel with axial slices.

Ultrasound: Ultrasound demonstrates hypoechoic enlargement of the ulnar nerve with loss of its fascicular pattern (>7.5 mm^2). Dynamic imaging during elbow flexion can reveal nerve impingement due to flattening within the cubital tunnel (Martinoli et al. 2004). Etiologies can be detected including muscle anomalies and mass lesions.

MRI: Cubital tunnel syndrome may be demonstrated as enlargement of the nerve or increased signal intensity on T2-weighted or STIR sequences within the nerve (Fig. 7.75). Ulnar dislocation may be seen during elbow flexion. There may also be ulnar muscle denervation manifested by edema or atrophy of the flexor digitorum profundus or flexor carpi ulnaris. MRI may also visualize secondary causes such as synovitis, degenerative joint disease, or tumor (Andreisek et al. 2006).

7.3.4.2 Injection for Guyon's Canal Syndrome (Ulnar Nerve at the Wrist) (Fig. 7.76)

Anatomy

Guyon's canal syndrome is caused by entrapment of the ulnar nerve as it courses through Guyon's canal. This is the second most frequent cause of ulnar nerve entrapment. Guyon's canal is a fibro-osseous tunnel formed by the space between the hook of the hamate and pisiform bone (Fig. 7.77). The tunnel is covered by the volar carpal ligament and pisohamate ligament. The ulnar nerve bifurcates into superficial and deep branches within the tunnel.

Proximal to Guyon's canal, the dorsal cutaneous branch in the distal forearm provides sensation to the dorsal ulnar half of the hand and fingers (Hence it is spared in Guyon's canal syndrome but not in cubital tunnel syndrome.).

Function

The ulnar nerve within Guyon's canal via the deep motor branch supplies the hypothenar muscles including two ulnar and lumbrical muscles, as well as the interossei muscle to the hand (see Sect. 7.3.4.1). This

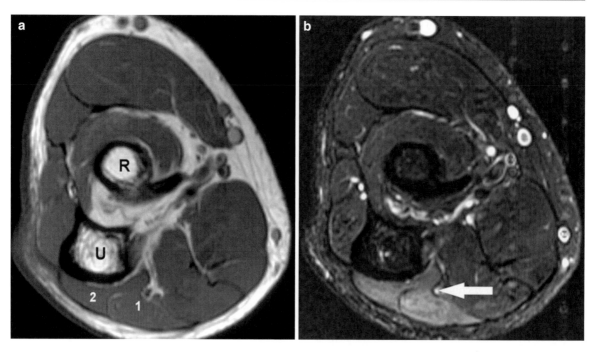

Fig. 7.75 (**a**, **b**) Cubital tunnel syndrome in a 44-year-old man with pain in the forearm while playing the transverse flute. Axial T1-weighted SE MR image (500/16) (**a**) and corresponding axial T2-weighted fat-suppressed SE MR image (5,340/58) (**b**) depict normal muscle volume but high signal intensity in the flexor carpi ulnaris (*1* in **a**) and flexor digitorum profundus (*2* in **a**) muscles, respectively. Increased signal intensity in the ulnar nerve in (**b**) is indicative of focal neuritis (*arrow*). *R* radius; *U* ulna (Andreisek et al. 2006)

nerve also provides innervation to the deep head of the flexor pollicis brevi. This portion of the ulnar nerve is responsible for 50–80% of pinch strength, 50% of grip strength, and lateral deviation of the fingers as well as the ability to perform proximal interphalangeal and metacarpophalangeal joint flexion. The superficial cutaneous branch provides sensation to the ulnar aspect of the palm and the flexor surfaces of the entire fifth finger and the ulnar half of the fourth finger. The superficial branch also provides motor innervation to the palmaris brevis.

Clinical Presentation

Guyon's canal syndrome results in numbness and paresthesia of the fourth and fifth fingers along with burning pain in the wrist. There is associated clumsiness of the hand. It is hard to spread the fingers and pinch with them. Guyon's canal syndrome is distinguished from cubital tunnel syndrome by numbness in the ulnar extensor aspect of the hand in cubital tunnel syndrome.

There are four subtypes of Guyon's canal syndrome. Type I is due to compression of the ulnar nerve in the proximal portion of Guyon's canal (proximal to the bifurcation of the ulnar nerve). It is the most common form of Guyon's canal syndrome. This may be associated with a fracture of the hook of the hamate or ganglion cyst. This manifests as motor weakness of the intrinsic muscle of the hand and sensory loss to the ulnar portion of the palm and flexor surface of the ulnar one and a half fingers. (The dorsal ulnar sensation to the hand and last two fingers is spared.)

Type II is manifested by compression of the ulnar nerve within the distal wrist (motor branch of the ulnar nerve after its bifurcation). There is sparing of the superficial cutaneous branch. It involves the muscles of the hand supplied by the ulnar nerve at this site. This may result in a clawing deformity of the hand.

Type III involves an impingement of the deep motor branch peripherally, which allows sparing of the hypothenar muscles, but weakness in the interosseus and lumbrical musculature.

Type IV involves a lesion of the superficial branch that results in pure sensory loss without weakness.

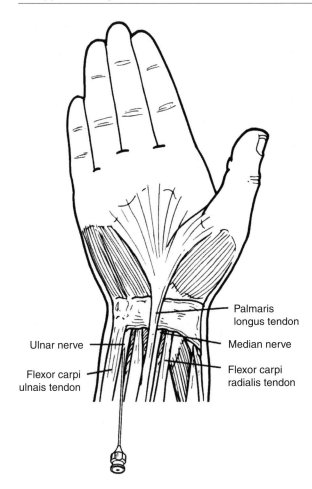

Fig. 7.76 Ulnar nerve injection in the wrist (Weiss 2007s, Fig. 6-14)

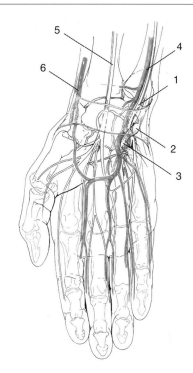

Fig. 7.77 A palmar view of the course of the ulnar nerve (*1*) as it passes through Guyon's canal, which is located between the pisiform bone (*2*) and the hook of the hamate (*3*). In addition to the ulnar nerve, Guyon's canal contains the ulnar artery (*4*), fat, and, occasionally, veins, (*5*) median nerve; (*6*) radial artery (Andreisek et al. 2006)

Etiology

Guyon's canal syndrome is caused by repetitive motion injury of the wrist and hand as a result of wrist flexion and abduction, gripping, or twisting. It may be seen in cyclists, weightlifters, jackhammer operators, or people with crutches. It may also be seen in golfers and batters. In addition, it may be secondary to trauma including fracture of the hamate bone,** ganglion cyst,** anomalous musculature,** ulnar artery aneurysm,** or osteoarthritis of the pisotriquetral joint.**

Differential Diagnosis

Differential diagnoses include cervical radiculopathy,** brachial plexus injury,** thoracic outlet syndrome,** Pancoast tumor,** epicondylitis,** rheumatoid arthritis,** wrist fracture,** ulnar artery aneurysm/thrombosis,** or rupture of the deep transverse ligament.**

Injection Site

The injection is performed at the volar aspect of the wrist with the wrist in flexion and the hand clenched. The injection is made at the radial aspect of the flexor carpi ulnaris tendon between this tendon and the ulnar artery.

Imaging/Radiology (Hochman and Zilberfarb 2004)

Plain film radiographs: The radially deviated with thumb abducted lateral view is useful for identifying a fracture of the hook of the hamate, carpal bone dislocation, or soft tissue mass. It may also identify calcific tendinitis at the insertion of the flexor carpi ulnaris.

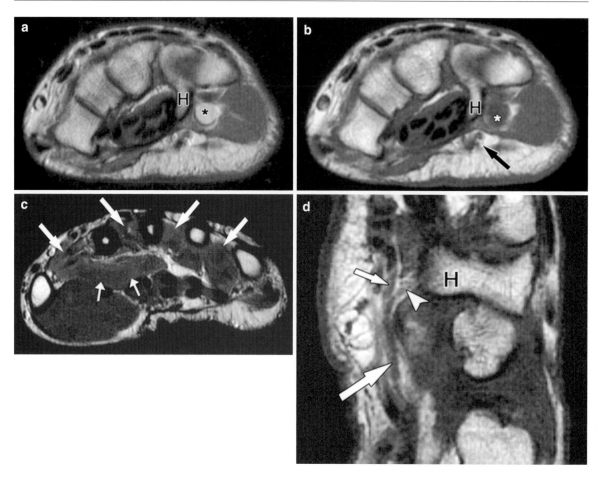

Fig. 7.78 (**a–d**) Ulnar nerve compression due to a ganglion cyst in the hand of a 57-year-old man. (**a**) Axial intermediate-weighted MR image (3,500/40) at the level of the hook of the hamate (*H*) shows a hyperintense ganglion cyst (*asterisk*). (**b**) Corresponding axial T1-weighted SE MR image (420/11) demonstrates the location of the ganglion cyst (*asterisk*) next to the hook of the hamate (*H*) and near the ulnar nerve (*arrow*). (**c**) Axial intermediate-weighted MR image (3,500/40) at the level of the metacarpal bones shows increased signal intensity in the adductor pollicis (*small arrows*) and in all the interosseous muscles (*large arrows*). (**d**) Sagittal T1-weighted SE MR image (540/12) at the level of the hook of the hamate (*H*) depicts the ulnar nerve (*large arrow*) and its bifurcation into a superficial sensory branch (*small arrow*) and a deep motor branch (*arrowhead*) (Andreisek et al. 2006)

The semi-supinated oblique views may identify a dislocation of the pisiform or fracture of the pisiform.

Ultrasound: The nerve is seen overlying the pisiform as a narrow filament at the ulnar aspect of the ulnar artery. Anomalous muscles as well as cysts and other mass lesions may be visualized.

CT: CT may identify bony abnormalities such as fractures of the pisiform hamate or triquetrum. It has the highest accuracy for fracture. It can also identify dislocations, which can simulate Guyon's canal syndrome.

MRI: MRI is usually not necessary. However, it is excellent at visualizing the ulnar nerve inside Guyon's canal as well as its two branches throughout their peripheral extent. The signal intensity within the nerve and its size can be studied. Anomalous musculature, cysts, or other mass lesions may be demonstrated causing compression of the nerve (Fig. 7.78). Denervation edema within the intrinsic hand musculature can be ascertained with a high degree of sensitivity (Andreisek et al. 2006).

Indications

The main indication for this injection is Guyon's canal syndrome**:

Complications

The two main complications associated with ulnar nerve injection are: (1) Flexor carpi ulnaris tendon rupture,** (2) ulnar artery injection.**

7.3.5 *Median Nerve*

7.3.5.1 Injection for Pronator Teres Syndrome (Median Nerve at the Elbow) (Fig. 7.79)

Anatomy

The median nerve originates from the C6–T1 nerve roots specifically from the medial and lateral cords of the brachial plexus. The nerve courses in the arm adjacent to the axillary artery and continues past the elbow along the volar lateral aspect of the distal humeral epicondyle at the trochlea. It continues into the forearm between the humeral and ulnar heads of the pronator teres muscle (Fig. 7.80). Pronator teres syndrome usually results from compression of the median nerve between the two heads of the pronator teres. Other anastomotic sites of entrapment include the lacertus fibrosis or bicipital aponeurosis, as well as the arch of the origin of the flexor digitorum superficialis. A rare source of compression is an anatomic variant, the supracondylar process of the distal humerus shaft. This forms a fibro-osseous tunnel to the medial humeral epicondyle via the ligament of Struthers.

The median nerve travels adjacent to the brachial artery within the medial arm amid the biceps brachii and brachialis muscles. It is lateral to the artery in the arm, but then courses in front to lie medial to the artery within the peripheral portion of the arm and antecubital fossa. The median nerve then gives off the anterior interosseus branch in the proximal forearm.

Function

The unbranched median nerve in the antecubital fossa innervates the following muscles:

- Pronator teres
- Palmaris longus
- Flexor carpi radialis
- Flexor digitorum superficialis muscle

This includes supply to the anterior interosseus branch of the median nerve that includes the:

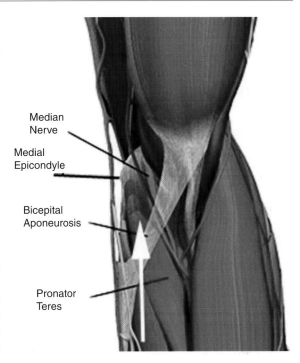

Median Nerve

Medial Epicondyle

Bicepital Aponeurosis

Pronator Teres

Fig. 7.79 Median nerve injection for pronator teres syndrome. *White arrow* denotes injection site (www.primalpictures.com)

- Lateral portion of the flexor digitorum profundus
- Pronator quadratus
- Flexor pollicis longus

Within the hand the median nerve supplies the first and second lumbricals and the muscles of the thenar eminence (see Sect. 7.3.5.2).

The median nerve's sensory supply includes the volar aspect of the first, second, third and, half of the fourth digit, the extensor aspect of the distal phalanges of these digits. The radial portion of the palm is innervated by the palmar cutaneous branch of the median nerve that branches off the median nerve central to the flexor retinaculum.

Clinical Presentation

The clinical presentation of pronator syndrome is that of pain, paresthesias, and numbness in the flexor aspect of the elbow and forearm including also the distribution of the distal median nerve. Weakness may or may not be associated. There may be weakness of abduction of the thumb, flexion of the thumb and index finger, as well as numbness in the first three fingers and palm.

Etiology

Typical etiologies can include anatomical or congenital abnormalities of the muscles** (pronator teres** or biceps brachii**) or bone** (ulna**). Other etiologies include: trauma** (hematoma**/fracture of the elbow**), prolonged external compression, mass lesions,** ulnar head abnormalities,** and repetitive actions (professional cleaners, weight lifters, professional vehicle drivers).

Differential Diagnosis

Cervical radiculopathy,** brachial plexus injury,** carpal tunnel syndrome,** medial epicondylitis,** fracture,** dislocation,** myositis,** and elbow arthritis.**

Injection Site

At the elbow crease midway between the medial epicondyle and the biceps tendon, an injection is made directly into the pronator teres muscle.

Imaging/Radiology

Plain film radiographs: Plain film radiographs are useful to exclude the supracondylar process on plain films and also to evaluate for elbow joint abnormalities.

Ultrasound: There is very limited experience with ultrasound.

MRI: Axial MRI demonstrates a small round thread-like structure between the brachialis and pronator teres. It is difficult to see the normal nerve, but swelling of the nerve with increased signal intensity may be seen. It is best diagnosed by denervation edema in the muscle supplied including the pronator teres. This is manifested by increased signal intensity on T2-weighted fat-suppressed and STIR images (Fig. 7.81).

Indications

The three main indications for median nerve injection at the antecubital fossa are: (1) Pronator syndrome, (2) anterior interosseus nerve syndrome, and (3) carpal tunnel syndrome.

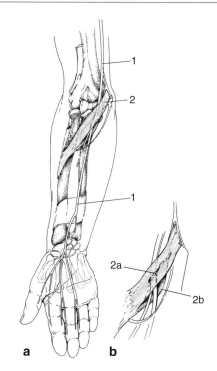

Fig. 7.80 (**a**) An anterior view of the course of the median nerve (*1*) along the elbow, through the two heads of the pronator teres muscle (*2*), and into the forearm. (**b**) A close-up detail of the most common site of pronator syndrome, where the nerve courses between the humeral head (*2a*) and the ulnar head (*2b*) of the muscle (Andreisek et al. 2006)

Complications

A potential serious complication encountered in median nerve injection at the antecubital fossa is brachial artery injection, with resultant thrombosis,** emboli,** and dissection,** all of which could result is ischemia.

7.3.5.2 Injection for Carpal Tunnel Syndrome (Fig. 7.82)

Anatomy

Carpal tunnel syndrome is the most common nerve entrapment of the upper extremity. It occurs due to pathological compression of the median nerve (C6–T1). This nerve is located superficially within the carpal tunnel between the flexor digitorum superficialis and the flexor pollicis longus tendon. It lays on top of the second flexor digitorum superficialis just deep to the flexor retinaculum.

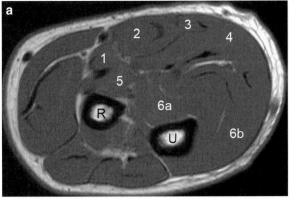
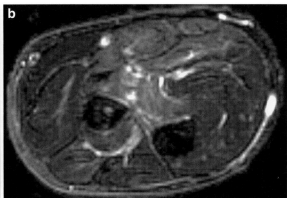

Fig. 7.81 Pronator syndrome in a 58-year-old man after repeated pronation-supination stress from snow shoveling. (**a**) Axial T1-weighted SE MR image (repetition time ms/echo time ms, 560/9) at a middle level in the forearm shows normal volume and normal signal intensity of the proximal forearm muscles (*1* pronator teres; *2* flexor carpi radialis; *3* palmaris longus; *4* flexor digitorum superficialis; *5* flexor pollicis longus; *6a* radial part of the flexor digitorum profundus; *6b* ulnar part of

the flexor digitorum profundus) and normal signal intensity of the radius (*R*) and ulna (*U*). (**b**) Corresponding T2-weighted fat-suppressed fast SE MR image (4,340/106; echo train length, 8) demonstrates increased signal intensity indicative of edema in all of the muscles that are innervated by the median nerve. The ulnar part of the flexor digitorum profundus muscle, which is innervated by the ulnar nerve, is unaffected (Andreisek et al. 2006)

Function

The median nerve at the level of the carpal tunnel and within the hand innervates the first and second lumbricals and the muscles of the thenar eminence.

The median nerve's sensory supply includes the volar aspect of the first, second, third and radial half the fourth digit, as well as the extensor aspect of the distal phalanges of these digits. The radial portion of the palm is innervated by the palmar cutaneous branch of the median nerve that branches off the median nerve central to the flexor retinaculum.

Clinical Presentation

Carpal tunnel syndrome presents with wrist pain and gradually worsening numbness and tingling. It involves the thumb and first three fingers as well as the radial portion of the fourth finger. Symptoms are worsened by repetition, wrist extension and flexion, and are most bothersome at night. Clumsiness of the hand may develop in advanced stages.

Etiology

Chronic repetition injury, trauma,** masses** (ganglion cyst,** lipoma,** etc.), systemic disease, carpal bone fracture** (capitate,** hamate,** etc.).

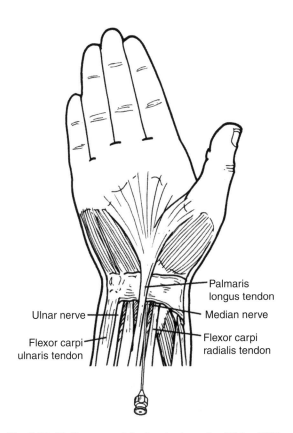

Fig. 7.82 Median nerve injection in the wrist (Weiss 2007s, Fig. 6-13)

Ulnar nerve

Flexor carpi ulnaris tendon

Palmaris longus tendon

Median nerve

Flexor carpi radialis tendon

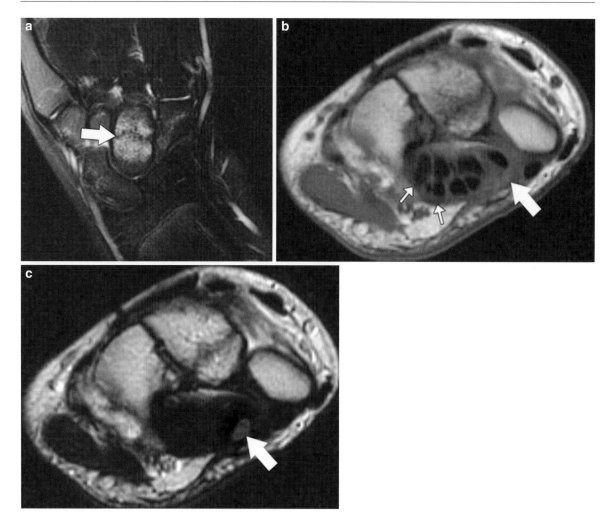

Fig. 7.83 Carpal tunnel syndrome in a 14-year-old female patient with a wrist trauma-related fracture of the capitate bone. Electrodiagnostic testing revealed a complete conduction block of the median nerve at the level of the carpal tunnel. (**a**) Coronal T2-weighted fat-suppressed fast SE MR image (3,500/100; echo train length, 12) of the wrist shows a fracture of the capitate bone (*arrow*) without dislocation. (**b**) Axial T1-weighted SE MR image (540/10) at the level of the carpal tunnel depicts moderate bowing of the flexor retinaculum (*small arrows*) and normal size of the median nerve (*large arrow*). (**c**) Axial T2-weighted fast SE MR image (4,200/100; echo train length, 12) at the same level as (**b**) depicts increased signal intensity of the median nerve (*arrow*), a finding consistent with carpal tunnel syndrome (Andreisek et al. 2006)

Differential Diagnosis

Differential diagnoses include cervical radiculopathy,** thoracic outlet syndrome,** brachial plexus pathology,** ulnar neuropathy,** pronator teres syndrome,** and de Quervain's tenosynovitis.**

Injection Site

The usual injection site lies at the volar aspect of the wrist at the ulnar edge of the flexor carpi radialis tendon adjacent to the level of the wrist crease. If the palmaris longus is present, the injection is made between the tendons of the flexor carpi radialis and palmaris longus. The median nerve is just deep to these tendons.

Imaging/Radiology

Carpal tunnel syndrome is usually diagnosed via clinical exam and/or electromyogram/nerve conduction velocity study. Imaging may be necessary in indeterminate cases and after recurrent or failed relief of symptoms following carpal tunnel release.

Plain film radiographs: These are not usually helpful. A carpal tunnel view to demonstrate osteophytes, fracture, and carpal instability may be performed.

CT: CT is useful for carpal bone anatomy, especially with 3D reconstruction.

Ultrasound: The median nerve is well seen with ultrasound including the nerve fascicles. These are easily distinguished from flexor tendons with dynamic imaging (during flexion and extension of the fingers). The nerve is also well distinguished from the ulnar artery. The median nerve may be swollen at the level of the pisiform (proximally) such that it is greater than 15 mm². This has a sensitivity of 88% and a specificity of 96% with a negative predictive value of 86%. The nerve may be flattened at the level of the hamate. Palmar bowing of the flexor retinaculum may also be seen (Lee et al. 1999; Buchberger 1997).

MRI: The normal nerve is well detected on MRI using axial high resolution images including demonstration of its vesicles. It is flattened normally at the site of the pisiform bone. MRI imaging is usually not necessary since carpal tunnel syndrome is generally a clinical diagnosis. However, for carpal tunnel syndrome, MRI has sensitivity between 37–96% and specificity between 23–87%. Since the specificity is low, MRI does not have a role in the clinical evaluation of carpal tunnel syndrome.

However, Axial images will demonstrate a swollen median nerve at the level of the pisiform and flattening of the median nerve at the level of the hamate. There is increased signal intensity of the nerve on T2-weighted fat suppressed images and STIR images (Fig. 7.83). In addition, palmar bowing of the flexor retinaculum at the hook of the hamate is seen. A caveat is to be noted that MRI findings are nonspecific with similar findings seen in asymptomatic people. There is no significant difference between ultrasound and MRI in cross-sectional area determination and flattening of the nerve. MRI, however, is superior at revealing ganglion cyst, flexor retinaculum bowing, mild nerve compression, and tendon sheath hypertrophy. MRI is useful in excluding other etiologies such as rheumatoid arthritis or gout. It is also useful in the postoperative setting following carpal tunnel release. Furthermore, it is useful in the detection of mass lesions and congenital anomalies including the bifid median nerve. It is also useful in detecting tenosynovitis (Andreisek et al. 2006; Hochman and Zilberfarb 2004; Buchberger 1997).

Indications

Carpal tunnel syndrome is the main indication for this procedure prior to considering surgery. This procedure can be predictive of pain relief following surgery.

References

Weiss LD. Easy injections. Philadelphia: Elsevier, 2007a, p. 16

Weiss LD. Easy injections. Philadelphia: Elsevier, 2007b, p. 17

Jacobson JA, Lin J, Jamadar DA, Hayes CW. Aids to successful shoulder arthrography performed with a fluoroscopically guided anterior approach. Radiographics. 2003;23(2):373-8; discussion 379

Sommer OJ, Kladosek A, Weiler V, Czembirek H, Boeck M, Stiskal M. Rheumatoid arthritis: a practical guide to state-of-the-art imaging, image interpretation, and clinical implications. Radiographics. 2005;25(2):381-98

Papatheodorou A et al. Ultrasound of the shoulder, rotator cuff, and non-rotator cuff disorders. Radiographics. 2006a; 26:E23

Mengiardi B, Pfirrmann CW, Gerber C, Hodler J, Zanetti M. Frozen shoulder: MR arthrographic findings. Radiology. 2004;233(2):486-92. Epub 2004 Sep 9

Weiss LD. Easy injections. Philadelphia: Elsevier, 2007c, p. 20

Alasaarela E, Tervonen O, Takalo R, Lahde S, Suramo I. Ultrasound evaluation of the acromioclavicular joint. J Rheumatol. 1997;24(10):1959-63

Fialka C, Krestan CR, Stampfl P, Trieb K, Aharinejad S, Vécsei V. Visualization of intraarticular structures of the acromioclavicular joint in an ex vivo model using a dedicated MRI protocol. AJR Am J Roentgenol. 2005;185(5):1126-31

Strobel K, Pfirrmann CW, Zanetti M, Nagy L, Hodler J. MRI features of the acromioclavicular joint that predict pain relief from intraarticular injection. AJR Am J Roentgenol. 2003; 181(3):755-60

Weiss LD. Easy injections. Philadelphia: Elsevier, 2007d, p. 86

Hambly N, Fitzpatrick P, MacMahon P, Eustace S. Rotator cuff impingement: correlation between findings on MRI and outcome after fluoroscopically guided subacromial bursography and steroid injection. AJR Am J Roentgenol. 2007;189(5): 1179-84

Tallia AF, Cardone DA. Diagnostic and therapeutic injection of the shoulder region. Am Fam Physician. 2003;67(6):1271-8

Fongemie AE, Buss DD, Rolnick SJ. Management of shoulder impingement syndrome and rotator cuff tears. Am Fam Physician. 1998;57(4):667-74, 680-2

Weiss LD. Easy injections. Philadelphia: Elsevier, 2007e, p. 73

Saupe N, Pfirrmann CW, Schmid MR, Jost B, Werner CM, Zanetti M. Association between rotator cuff abnormalities and reduced acromiohumeral distance. AJR Am J Roentgenol. 2006;187(2):376-82

del Cura JL, Torre I, Zabala R, Legórburu A. Sonographically guided percutaneous needle lavage in calcific tendinitis of the shoulder: short- and long-term results. AJR Am J Roentgenol. 2007;189(3):W128-34

Mulligan ME. CT-guided shoulder arthrography at the rotator cuff interval. AJR Am J Roentgenol. 2008;191(2):W58-61

Papatheodorou A, Ellinas P, Takis F, Tsanis A, Maris I, Batakis N. US of the shoulder: rotator cuff and non-rotator cuff disorders. Radiographics. 2006b;26(1):e23

Serafini G, Sconfienza LM, Lacelli F, Silvestri E, Aliprandi A, Sardanelli F. Rotator cuff calcific tendonitis: short-term and 10-year outcomes after two-needle us-guided percutaneous treatment – nonrandomized controlled trial. Radiology. 2009;252(1):157-64

Kijowski R, Farber JM, Medina J, Morrison W, Ying J, Buckwalter K. Comparison of fat-suppressed T2-weighted fast spin-echo sequence and modified STIR sequence in the evaluation of the rotator cuff tendon. AJR Am J Roentgenol. 2005;185(2):371-8

de Jesus JO, Parker L, Frangos AJ, Nazarian LN. Accuracy of MRI, MR arthrography and ultrasound in the diagnosis of rotator cuff tears: a meta-analysis. AJR Am J Roentgenol. 2009;192(6):1701-7

Weiss LD. Easy injections. Philadelphia: Elsevier, 2007f, p. 65

Robinson P. Sonography of common tendon injuries. AJR Am J Roentgenol. 2009;193(3):607-18

Krief OP. MRI of the rotator interval capsule. AJR Am J Roentgenol. 2005;184(5):1490-4

Tung GA, Entzian D, Green A, Brody JM. High-field and low-field MR imaging of superior glenoid labral tears and associated tendon injuries. AJR Am J Roentgenol. 2000;174(4): 1107-14

Hodler J, Gilula LA, Ditsios KT, Yamaguchi K. Fluoroscopically guided scapulothoracic injections. AJR Am J Roentgenol. 2003;181(5):1232-4

Huang CC, Ko SF, Ng SH, Lin CC, Huang HY, Yu PC, Lee TY. Scapulothoracic bursitis of the chest wall: sonographic features with pathologic correlation. J Ultrasound Med. 2005; 24(10):1437-40

Fujikawa A, Oshika Y, Tamura T, Naoi Y. Chronic scapulothoracic bursitis associated with thoracoplasty. AJR Am J Roentgenol. 2004;183(5):1487-8

Weiss LD. Easy injections. Philadelphia: Elsevier, 2007g, p. 25

Martinoli C, Bianchi S, Giovagnorio F, Pugliese F. Ultrasound of the elbow. Skeletal Radiol. 2001;30(11):605-14. Epub 2001 Aug 30

Bhutani N, Chhabra A, Batra K, Elbow MRI. http://emedicine. medscape.com/article/401161-overview

Steinbach LS, Palmer WE, Schweitzer ME. Special focus session. MR arthrography. Radiographics. 2002;22(5): 1223-46

Cotten A, Jacobson J, Brossmann J, Pedowitz R, Haghighi P, Trudell D, Resnick D. Collateral ligaments of the elbow: conventional MR imaging and MR arthrography with coronal oblique plane and elbow flexion. Radiology. 1997;204(3): 806-12

Sonin AH, Tutton SM, Fitzgerald SW, Peduto AJ. MR imaging of the adult elbow. Radiographics. 1996;16(6):1323-36

Weiss LD. Easy injections. Philadelphia: Elsevier, 2007h, p. 67

Levin D, Nazarian LN, Miller TT, O'Kane PL, Feld RI, Parker L, McShane JM. Lateral epicondylitis of the elbow: US findings. Radiology. 2005a;237(1):230-4

Levin D, Nazarian LN, Miller TT, O'Kane PL, Feld RI, Parker L, McShane JM. Lateral epicondylitis of the elbow: US findings. Radiology. 2005b;237(1):230-4. Epub 2005 Aug 18

Miller TT, Shapiro MA, Schultz E, Kalish PE. Comparison of sonography and MRI for diagnosing epicondylitis. J Clin Ultrasound. 2002;30(4):193-202

Bredella MA, Tirman PF, Fritz RC, Feller JF, Wischer TK, Genant HK. MR imaging findings of lateral ulnar collateral ligament abnormalities in patients with lateral epicondylitis. AJR Am J Roentgenol. 1999;173(5):1379-82

Weiss LD. Easy injections. Philadelphia: Elsevier, 2007i, p. 70

Park GY et al. Diagnostic value of ultrasound for clinical medical epicondylitis. Arch Phys Med Rehabil. 2008;89(4):738-42

Kijowski R et al. Magnetic resonance imaging findings in patients with medial epicondylitis Skeletal Radiol. 2005; 34(4):196-202

Genovese MC. Joint and soft-tissue injection. A useful adjuvant to systemic and local treatment. Postgrad Med. 1998;103(2): 125-34

Weiss LD. Easy injections. Philadelphia: Elsevier, 2007j, p. 89

Blankstein A et al. Ultrasonographic findings in patients with olecranon bursitis. Ultraschall Med. 2006;27(6):568-71

Floemer F, Morrison WB, Bongartz G, Ledermann HP. MRI characteristics of olecranon bursitis. AJR Am J Roentgenol. 2004;183(1):29-34

Weiss LD. Easy injections. Philadelphia: Elsevier, 2007k, p. 28

Weiss LD. Easy injections. Philadelphia: Elsevier, 2007l, p. 30

Taouli B, Zaim S, Peterfy CG, Lynch JA, Stork A, Guermazi A, Fan B, Fye KH, Genant HK. Rheumatoid arthritis of the hand and wrist: comparison of three imaging techniques. AJR Am J Roentgenol. 2004;182(4):937-43

Østergaard M, Pedersen SJ, Døhn UM. Imaging in rheumatoid arthritis – status and recent advances for magnetic resonance imaging, ultrasonography, computed tomography and conventional radiography. Best Pract Res Clin Rheumatol. 2008;22(6):1019-44

Duer A, Østergaard M, Hørslev-Petersen K, Vallø J. Magnetic resonance imaging and bone scintigraphy in the differential diagnosis of unclassified arthritis. Ann Rheum Dis. 2008; 67(1):48-51. Epub 2007 Feb 8

Teefey SA, Dahiya N, Middleton WD, Gelberman RH, Boyer MI. Ganglia of the hand and wrist: a sonographic analysis. AJR Am J Roentgenol. 2008;191(3):716-20

Bianchi S, Della Santa D, Glauser T, Beaulieu JY, van Aaken J. Sonography of masses of the wrist and hand. AJR Am J Roentgenol. 2008;191(6):1767-75

Anderson SE, Steinbach LS, Stauffer E, Voegelin E. MRI for differentiating ganglion and synovitis in the chronic painful wrist. AJR Am J Roentgenol. 2006;186(3):812-8

Weiss LD. Easy injections. Philadelphia: Elsevier, 2007m, p. 33

Mandl LA, Hotchkiss RN, Adler RS, Ariola LA, Katz JN. Can the carpometacarpal joint be injected accurately in the office setting? Implications for therapy. J Rheumatol. 2006;33(6): 1137-9

Connell DA, Pike J, Koulouris G, van Wettering N, Hoy G. MR imaging of thumb carpometacarpal joint ligament injuries. J Hand Surg Br. 2004;29(1):46-54

Cardoso FN, Kim HJ, Albertotti F, Botte MJ, Resnick D, Chung CB. Imaging the ligaments of the trapeziometacarpal joint: MRI compared with MR arthrography in cadaveric specimens. AJR Am J Roentgenol. 2009;192(1):W13-9

Weiss LD. Easy injections. Philadelphia: Elsevier, 2007n, p. 63

Kamel M, Moghazy K, Eid H, Mansour R. Ultrasonographic diagnosis of de Quervain's tenosynovitis. Ann Rheum Dis. 2002;61(11):1034-5

Jeyapalan K, Choudhary S. Ultrasound-guided injection of triamcinolone and bupivacaine in the management of de

Quervain's disease. Skeletal Radiol. 2009;38(11):1099-103. Epub 2009 Jun

Anderson SE, Steinbach LS, De Monaco D, Bonel HM, Hurtienne Y, Voegelin E. "Baby wrist": MRI of an overuse syndrome in mothers. AJR Am J Roentgenol. 2004;182(3): 719-24

Clavero JA, Golanó P, Fariñas O, Alomar X, Monill JM, Esplugas M. Extensor mechanism of the fingers: MR imaging-anatomic correlation. Radiographics. 2003;23(3):593-611

Weiss LD. Easy injections. Philadelphia: Elsevier, 2007o, p. 59

Makkouk AH et al. Trigger finger: etiology, evaluation, and treatment. Curr Rev Musculoskelet Med. 2008;1(2):92-96

Katzman BM et al. Utility of obtaining radiographs in patients with trigger finger. Am J Orthop. 1999;28(12):703-5

Guerini H et al. Sonographic appearance of trigger fingers J. Ultrasound Med. 2008;27(10):1407-13

Bodorm M et al. Ultrasound-guided first annular pulley injection for trigger finger. J Ultrasound Med. 2009;28(6):737-43

Khoury V, Cardinal E, Bureau NJ. Musculoskeletal sonography: a dynamic tool for usual and unusual disorders. AJR Am J Roentgenol. 2007;188(1):W63-73

Wakefield RJ et al. Finger tendon disease and untreated early rheumatoid arthritis comparison of ultrasound and magnetic resonance imaging. Arthritis Rheum 2007;57(7):1158-64

Jeffrey RB Jr, Laing FC, Schechter WP, Markison RE, Barton RM. Acute suppurative tenosynovitis of the hand: diagnosis with US. Radiology. 1987;162(3):741-2

Weiss LD. Easy injections. Philadelphia: Elsevier, 2007p, p. 35

Jacobson JA, Girish G, Jiang Y, Resnick D. Radiographic evaluation of arthritis: inflammatory conditions. Radiology. 2008;248(2):378-89

Keen HI et al. Can ultrasonography improve on radiographic assessment in osteoarthritis of the hands? A comparison between radiographic and ultrasonographic detected pathology. Ann Rheum Dis. 2008;67(8):1116-20

Szkudlarek M et al. Ultrasonography of the metacarpophalangeal and proximal interphalangeal joints in rheumatoid arthritis: a comparison with MRI, conventional radiography, and clinical examination. Arthritis Res Ther. 2006;8(2):R52

Ostergaard M et al. Imaging in rheumatoid arthritis – status and recent advances for MRI, ultrasound, CT, and computed radiography. Best Pract Res Clin Rheumatol. 2008;22(6): 1019-44

Waldman SD. Interventional pain management, 2nd ed. Philadelphia: Saunders, 2001

Garner HW, Kransdorf MJ, Bancroft LW, Peterson JJ, Berquist TH, Murphey MD. Benign and malignant soft-tissue tumors: posttreatment MR imaging. Radiographics. 2009;29(1): 119-34

Weiss LD. Easy injections. Philadelphia: Elsevier, 2007q, p. 109

Schafhalter-Zoppoth I, Gray AT. The musculocutaneous nerve: ultrasound appearance for peripheral nerve block. Reg Anesth Pain Med. 2005;30(4):385-90

Weiss LD. Easy injections. Philadelphia: Elsevier, 2007r, p. 120

Ferdinand BD, Rosenberg ZS, Schweitzer ME, Stuchin SA, Jazrawi LM, Lenzo SR, Meislin RJ, Kiprovski K. MR imaging features of radial tunnel syndrome: initial experience. Radiology. 2006;240(1):161-8

Spinner M. The arcade of Frohse and its relationship to posterior interosseous nerve paralysis. J Bone Joint Surg Br. 1968; 50:809-812

Martinoli C, Bianchi S, Pugliese F, Bacigalupo L, Gauglio C, Valle M, Derchi LE. Sonography of entrapment neuropathies in the upper limb (wrist excluded). J Clin Ultrasound. 2004;32(9):438-50

Andreisek G, Crook DW, Burg D, Marincek B, Weishaupt D. Peripheral neuropathies of the median, radial, and ulnar nerves: MR imaging features. Radiographics. 2006;26(5): 1267-87

Weiss LD. Easy injections. Philadelphia: Elsevier, 2007s, p. 123

Hochman MG, Zilberfarb JL. Nerves in a pinch: imaging of nerve compression syndromes. Radiol Clin North Am. 2004; 42(1):221-45

Lee D et al. Diagnosis of carpal tunnel syndrome: ultrasound versus electromyography. Radiol Clin North Am. 1999; 37(4):859-72

Buchberger W. Radiologic imaging of the carpal tunnel. Eur J Radiol. 1997;25(2):112-7

Lower Extremity

8

8.1 Introduction

The main strengths and weaknesses of imaging modalities for diagnosis in the lower extremity are discussed below.

8.1.1 Plain Film Radiographs

This is the first-line modality in imaging for lower extremity pathology. This technique enables one to image the bone, effusions, and any calcified pathology, as well as radiodense foreign bodies. It is also able to evaluate fracture/dislocations, arthritis, infection, and tumor.

8.1.2 Bone Scan

This technique is performed using nuclear medicine scintigraphy. It is sensitive for pathology, but very non-specific and vague in localizing the exact anatomic site. However, it can be useful in the evaluation of radiographically occult fractures (stress fractures), osteomyelitis/septic arthritis, and reflex sympathetic dystrophy (complex regional pain syndrome).

8.1.3 Ultrasound

This method is used more commonly outside the US. It is useful for evaluating soft tissue pathology such as joints, tendons, and ligaments. It can also be used complementary to MRI for assessing tendon and ligament pathology. Although it has real-time imaging capability, one disadvantage is its operator dependency.

8.1.4 CT

This technique enables cross-sectional imaging for the evaluation of bone and joint pathology. It is less useful for soft tissue pathology compared to MRI. It is available in acute or emergency settings in the hospital 24/7.

8.1.5 MRI

MRI is the modality of choice for musculoskeletal imaging for nearly all pathology due to its superior soft tissue contrast and its ability to image in any plane. However, it is poor in imaging cortical bone due to lack of signal in the cortical bone, although this is considered a relatively minor weakness. CT is superior to MRI in evaluating cortical bone. MRI is able to directly image the musculature, cartilage of joints, joint spaces, tendons, ligaments, bursae, and nerves. In addition, MR arthrography is useful in increasing the sensitivity of articular pathology. However, its limitations include metal artifacts and calcified pathology.

M.I. Syed and A. Shaikh, *Radiology of Non-Spinal Pain Procedures*,
DOI: 10.1007/978-3-642-00481-0_8, © Springer-Verlag Berlin Heidelberg 2011

8.1.6 Major Clinical Scenarios to Exclude

- Joint infection (septic arthritis)
  - Cortical indistinctness
  - Periosteal reaction
  - Joint space loss
  - Periarticular osteopenia
  - Joint fluid or effusion
      Joint aspiration may be necessary to diagnose prior to any steroid injection
  - MRI and CT are more sensitive in diagnosis compared to plain films
- Fracture
  - Would appear as cortical discontinuity
  - Periosteal reaction if subacute
  - Malalignment if fracture is complete
  - MRI and CT are more sensitive than plain film radiograph
- Diabetic foot (Chatha et al. 2005)
  - Charcot foot (diabetic neuroarthropathy) can mimic osteomyelitis clinically and radiologically
      Presenting symptoms are an erythematous and edematous foot in both scenarios
      MRI: both entities demonstrate, subchondral bone marrow signal abnormality, joint fluid, periosteal reactions, and soft tissue inflammation
      Distinguish based on distribution of disease on MRI
        Osteomyelitis tends to occur at pressure points and ulcers at bony prominences (metatarsal heads, interphalangeal joints, plantar aspect of the posterior calcaneus or distal fibula)
        Neuropathic changes are usually localized to the midfoot
      Nuclear medicine indium-labeled WBC scanning may be helpful
- Bleeding diathesis
- Avascular necrosis
- Acute traumatic soft tissue injury (ACL, PCL, MCL, meniscus tear, and osteochondral fracture for knee joint injection)
- Maximum limit of steroid dose attained
- Joint prosthesis for joint injections only
- Impending joint surgery (within days)

8.1.7 Complications of Injections in the Lower Extremity

The principal complications encountered in the upper extremity are:

- Hematoma/bleeding
- Infection
- Transient synovitis (post-injection steroid flare)
- Transient lower extremity weakness and paresthesias (can be seen in hip, popliteal cyst, ischiogluteal bursa, iliopsoas bursa, and nerve injections)
- Artery or vein injury for hip and popliteal injection

8.2 Lower Extremity Joints, Bursae, and Tendons

8.2.1 Hip and Surrounding Structures

8.2.1.1 Hip Joint Injection (Figs. 8.1 and 8.2)

Anatomy (Fig. 8.3)

The hip joint is a synovial ball-and-socket joint formed by the femoral head and pelvic acetabulum, which are

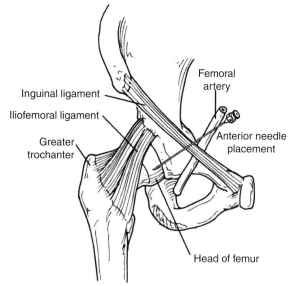

Hip joint injection—anterior approach

Fig. 8.1 Hip joint injection, anterior approach (Weiss 2007a, Fig. 3-21)

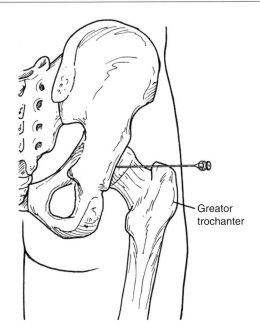

Fig. 8.2 Hip joint injection, lateral approach (Weiss 2007b, Fig. 3-23)

lined by hyaline cartilage. The joint contains synovial fluid. The hip joint capsule is attached between the base of the femoral neck and base of the acetabular lip such that its rim projects into the capsule. The joint capsule consists of both longitudinal and circular fibers. The circular fibers are also known as the zona orbicularis and surround the femoral neck. The acetabulum is surrounded by a ring of fibrocartilage, the acetabular labrum, which hugs the head of the femur to further stabilize the joint. The hip joint is strengthened by four extracapsular ligaments (iliofemoral, ischiofemoral, and pubofemoral ligaments). The ligamentum teres is an intracapsular ligament, which attaches the fovea of the femoral head to the acetabular notch. It contains an arterial branch to supply the femoral head. The transverse ligament spans the inferior aspect of the acetabulum. It also attaches to the ligamentum teres.

Function

The hip supports the body in both active and stationary positions. It provides external/internal rotation, flexion/extension, and abduction/adduction.

Clinical Presentation

Hip joint pain presents as pain and stiffness in the hip, buttock, groin, and thigh. There can even be associated low back pain. Pain emanating from the hip joint is exacerbated by motion. There is also a decreased ability to ambulate due to pain. In addition, there is loss of range of motion.

Etiology

Etiologies include osteoarthritis** (** Signifies that the entity may be imaged. It is understood that an entity may represent a clinical syndrome but that its underlying pathology may actually be imaged (cervical radiculopathy** may be imaged via imaging of cervical spondylosis or disc herniation [HNP]).), rheumatoid arthritis**, gout**, CPPD**, psoriatic arthritis**, ankylosing spondylitis**, and infection**.

Differential Diagnosis

Differential diagnoses include lumbar radiculopathy**, avascular necrosis of the hip**, intraarticular osteochondral fragments**, sacroiliac joint pain**, pelvic pathology**, bursitis**, tendonitis**, hernia**, fracture**, kidney stone**, aneurysm**, neoplasm**, myositis**, and herpes zoster.

Injection Site

The anterior approach originates 4 cm lateral to the common femoral artery inferior to the inguinal ligament over the femoral head. The lateral approach originates 2 cm superior to the greater trochanter. The oblique vertical approach is an anterolateral approach, which avoids the common femoral neurovascular bundle (Fig. 8.4).

Imaging/Radiology

Plain film radiographs: Plain films demonstrate joint space loss (superolateral), osteophyte formation, subchondral sclerosis, and cyst formation in

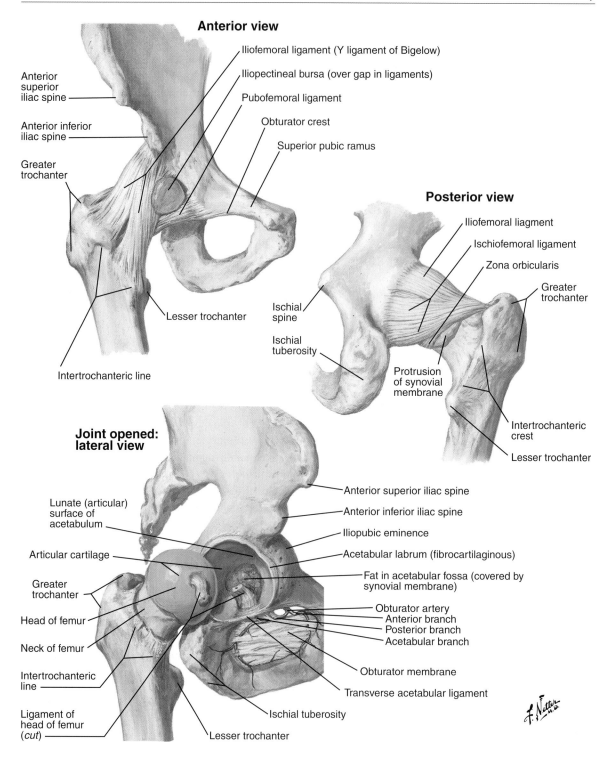

Anterior view

Iliofemoral ligament (Y ligament of Bigelow)

Iliopectineal bursa (over gap in ligaments)

Pubofemoral ligament

Obturator crest

Superior pubic ramus

Anterior superior iliac spine

Anterior inferior iliac spine

Greater trochanter

Lesser trochanter

Intertrochanteric line

Posterior view

Iliofemoral liagment

Ischiofemoral ligament

Zona orbicularis

Greater trochanter

Ischial spine

Ischial tuberosity

Protrusion of synovial membrane

Intertrochanteric crest

Lesser trochanter

Joint opened: lateral view

Lunate (articular) surface of acetabulum

Articular cartilage

Greater trochanter

Head of femur

Neck of femur

Intertrochanteric line

Ligament of head of femur (*cut*)

Lesser trochanter

Ischial tuberosity

Anterior superior iliac spine

Anterior inferior iliac spine

Iliopubic eminence

Acetabular labrum (fibrocartilaginous)

Fat in acetabular fossa (covered by synovial membrane)

Obturator artery
Anterior branch
Posterior branch
Acetabular branch

Obturator membrane

Transverse acetabular ligament

Fig. 8.3 Anterior, posterior, and lateral view of the hip (http://www.netterimages.com/)

osteoarthritis (Fig. 8.5). Rheumatoid arthritis is characterized by joint space loss (central and uniform), erosions, and osteopenia with a much higher

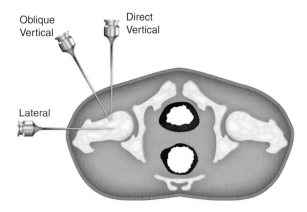

Fig. 8.4 Various approaches for access to the hip joint: direct vertical, oblique vertical, and lateral (Peterson et al. 2008)

frequency of acetabular protrusio (medial migration of the hip). Large joint effusion may be seen in both forms of arthritis and are detected through lateral displacement of the femoral head. Avascular necrosis as an alternative diagnosis in the setting of hip pain can be seen but at a later stage than that with MRI. Plain films can also demonstrate fractures and dislocations in the setting of trauma.

Soft tissue calcifications can also be seen that can lead to the alternate diagnosis of calcific tendonitis or bursitis.

Fluoroscopy: Fluoroscopy is useful for guidance of hip joint aspiration and injection, as well as arthrography.

Ultrasound: This modality is useful for detecting moderate hip joint effusions and for guidance (Pourbagher et al. 2005). It is helpful in visualizing the surrounding soft tissues.

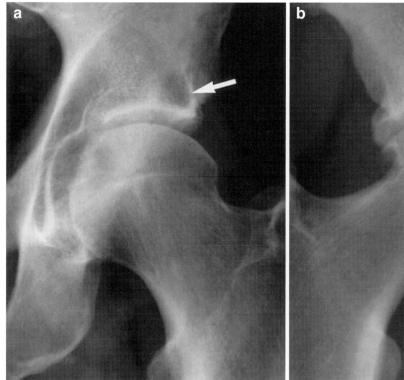
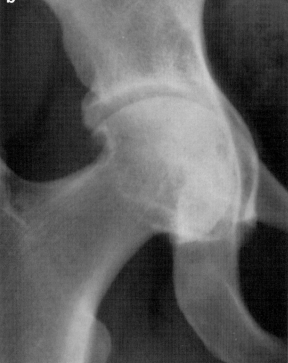

Fig. 8.5 (**a**, **b**) Osteoarthritis. (**a**) AP radiograph of the *left* hip shows early osteoarthritis with no significant cartilage loss; the disease is heralded by a small subchondral cyst (*arrow*) in the acetabulum. A minimal osteophyte is seen at the lateral margin of the femoral head. (**b**) AP radiograph of the *right* hip in another patient shows a more unusual pattern of osteoarthritis. In this case, the direction of migration is medial, with protrusio. This appearance is often mistaken for that of rheumatoid arthritis. However, note the normal bone density and the osteophyte formation. The patient represents one of the 20% of those with osteoarthritis who have a pattern of medial migration of the hip (Manaster 2000)

CT: CT is useful for detecting bone tumors including osteoid osteoma (localizes the nidus better than MRI). It is sensitive for evaluation after trauma to detect radiographically occult fracture, especially of the pelvis and intraarticular osteochondral fragments, as well as hematomas. CT can also characterize soft tissue calcifications. It can provide guidance for radiofrequency ablation or injection by avoiding the neurovascular bundle (Fig. 8.6).

MRI: MRI is sensitive for labral tears, effusions, erosions, subchondral cysts, intraarticular loose bodies, and bone marrow edema, as well as surrounding soft tissue pathology. It is the most sensitive modality for evaluating the bone marrow and for detecting avascular necrosis as well as stress fractures. It is very useful in characterizing neoplasms.

MR arthrography: This modality increases sensitivity for acetabular labral tears and cartilage loss in early forms of arthritis (Figs. 8.7 and 8.8).

Nuclear medicine: Sensitive for pathology, but nonspecific. This modality can be helpful in detecting metastases, avascular necrosis, stress fractures, arthritis, and Paget's disease.

Indications (Mauffrey and Pobbathy 2006)

Interventions in the hip are generally made on the basis of the following:

- Primarily used for patients who are not surgical candidates
- Hip pain
- Osteoarthritis (Reference: Flouroscopically guided steroid injection effective in hip osteoarthritis) **
- Rheumatoid arthritis**
- Crystal-induced arthritis**
- Femoroacetabularimpingementsyndrome(Wisniewski and Grogg 2006; Crawford and Villar 2005) **
- Painful hip arthroplasty**
- Diagnostically to determine the likelihood of achieving pain relief after primary or revision hip arthroplasty

Contraindications

Avascular necrosis** would be a contraindication for steroid injection, but the use of viscosupplementation

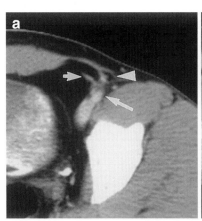
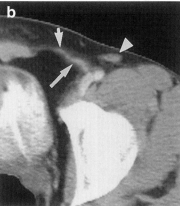
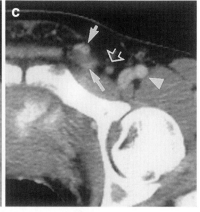

Fig. 8.6 (**a–c**) CT anatomy is depicted to demonstrate normal cross-sectional anatomy, especially the neurovascular bundle. Normal anatomic characteristics of the groin on contrast-enhanced computed tomographic (CT) scans obtained at the level of the hip joint, from superior (**a**) to inferior (**c**). (**a**) The inferior epigastric artery (*short arrow*) arises from the external iliac artery (*long arrow*). Fat surrounds the spermatic cord (*arrowhead*) where it enters the deep inguinal ring. (**b**) The inguinal ligament (*short arrow*), spermatic cord in the inguinal canal (*long arrow*), and normal superficial lymph node (*arrowhead*) are shown. (**c**) The spermatic cord is at the superficial inguinal ring (*short solid arrow*). The inguinal ligament (*long arrow*) is shown. The femoral canal lies laterally and contains the common femoral vessels/neurovascular bundle (*arrowhead*) and node of Cloquet (*open arrow*) (Shadbolt et al. 2001)

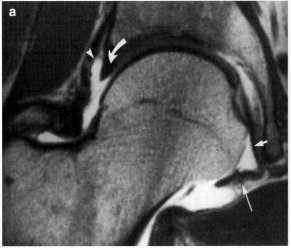 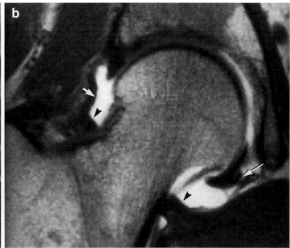

Fig. 8.7 (**a**, **b**) Normal anatomy in a 43-year-old-man with chronic hip pain is depicted on T1-weighted (repetition time ms/echo time ms = 600/17) MR images obtained with intra-articular contrast material. (**a**) Midline coronal MR image shows the long axis of the ligamentum teres (*short arrow*) and its insertion onto the transverse ligament (*long arrow*). A normal superior labrum (*curved arrow*) and the larger superior perilabral recess (*arrowhead*) are seen. (**b**) On a more posterior coronal MR image, the circular fibers of the zona orbicularis (*arrowheads*) are evident, as are the longitudinal fibers of the iliofemoral ligament (*short arrow*). A cleft is seen where the transverse ligament and labrum start to merge (*long arrow*) (Petersilge 2000)

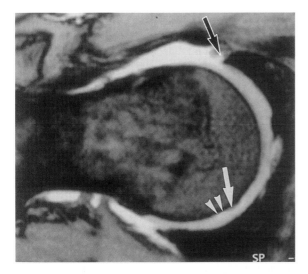

Fig. 8.8 Oblique-transverse FLASH MR image (400/11, 60° flip angle) shows a small contrast material-filled femoral cartilage defect (*arrowheads*) in a 42-year-old-woman with early osteoarthritis of the *right* hip joint. Adjacent cartilage (*white arrow*) has a hypointense signal. Partial detachment of the anteroinferior acetabular labrum (*black arrow*) without an adjacent cartilage defect also is seen (Schmid et al. 2003)

(hylan G-F 20) has been reported (Liang and Ma). Infection is also a contraindication for injection (not aspiration).

Complications (Peterson et al. 2008)

The three main complications (Peterson et al. 2008) encountered in hip interventions are: (1) Transient lower extremity weakness; (2) transient lower extremity paresthesia; (3) femoral artery or vein injury**.

8.2.1.2 Injection for Greater Trochanteric Pain Syndrome (Fig. 8.9)

Anatomy

The greater trochanteric bursa lies adjacent to the greater trochanter between the insertions of the gluteus minimus and the gluteus medius muscle. There is in fact a complex of bursae (subgluteus maximus, medius,

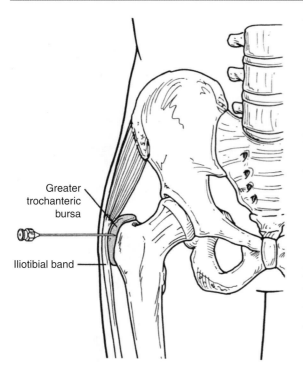

Greater trochanteric bursa

Iliotibial band

Fig. 8.9 Trochanteric bursa injection (Weiss 2007c, Fig. 5-5)

and minimus). Greater trochanteric pain syndrome is a new classification of a regional pain syndrome that includes both greater trochanteric bursitis and gluteus medius tendon abnormalities. Most cases of greater trochanteric pain syndrome may in fact be due to gluteal tendon injury rather than to an actual bursitis (which, if present, may be secondary to the gluteal tendon injury).

Function

The bursa decreases the friction between the muscles next to it. It also absorbs the impact of blunt forces. The gluteus medius muscle is responsible for hip abduction.

Clinical Presentation (Greater Trochanteric Pain Syndrome)

The patient typically presents with pain in the anterior and lateral hip region, tenderness in the lateral hip region, and/or inability to lie in the decubitus positions on the site of pain. This pain is often worse at night. There may

be pain or weakness with hip abduction. Trendelenburg's sign (resisted hip abduction) may be helpful in confirming greater trochanteric pain syndrome.

Etiology

Etiologies for greater trochanteric pain syndrome include: Gluteal medius tendon pathology**, greater trochanteric bursitis**, rheumatoid arthritis**, uneven leg length/pelvic tilt**, and iliotibial band syndrome**.

Differential Diagnosis

Differential diagnoses includes lumbar radiculopathy**, meralgia paresthetica, snapping hip syndrome**, hernia**, hip joint pathology**, avascular necrosis**, fracture**, tumor** (osseous or soft tissue) in the pelvis or thigh.

Injection Site

A lateral approach is utilized over the site of the greater trochanter. The needle traverses the gluteus medius tendon/iliotibial tract into the greater trochanteric bursa.

Imaging/Radiology

Plain film radiographs: Plain films are usually not helpful, but calcific deposits may be seen in the vicinity of the greater trochanteric bursa. Leg length discrepancy can be identified as a cause of pelvic tilt. It can also exclude other sources of hip pain.

Ultrasound: Ultrasound depicts fluid-filled sacs adjacent to the greater trochanter between tendons of gluteus medius and maximus. The gluteus medius and minimus insertions can be evaluated for tendinopathy (Kong et al. 2007). Ultrasound can be useful in guidance of injection.

CT: CT may demonstrate a fluid collection within the bursa, but may be less sensitive than ultrasound or MRI.

MRI: MRI is less operator-dependent than ultrasound. It is able to demonstrate bone marrow edema in the greater trochanter. Bursal fluid collection is easily seen. Tendinopathy (tendinosis, peritendinitis, partial and complete tear) in the adjacent gluteal tendon can be seen and other causes of lateral hip pain may be excluded (Kong et al. 2007) (Figs. 8.10–8.12).

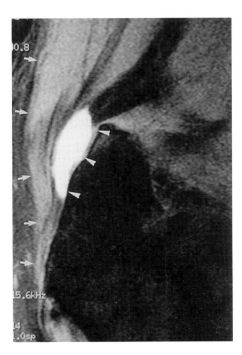

Fig. 8.10 Cadaveric study. Coronal T1-weighted fat-saturated MR image (500/22) through the lateral facet of the greater trochanter after bursography shows the subgluteus medius bursa (*arrowheads*) deep to the lateral part of the gluteus medius tendon and muscle (*arrows*) (Pfirrmann et al. 2001)

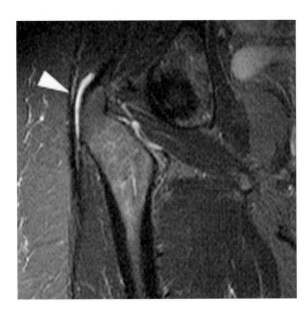

Fig. 8.11 Coronal short tau inversion recovery (STIR) image demonstrating high signal adjacent to the greater trochanter indicating trochanteric bursitis (*arrowhead*) (Fang and Teh 2003)

Indications

The main indication for intervention is greater trochanteric bursitis** or gluteus medius tendinopathy.

Contraindications

It is important to exclude fracture of the hip including greater trochanter prior to injection** (Feldman and Staron 2004; Jones and Erhard 1997).

8.2.1.3 Iliopsoas Bursa Injection (Fig. 8.13)

Anatomy

The iliopsoas bursa is the largest bursal sac in the body. It is located anterior to the hip between the iliopsoas muscle and iliopectineal eminence of the superior pubic ramus. (The iliopectineal eminence is a subtly raised structure over the superior pubic ramus and demarcates the medial aspect of the groove over which the iliacus and psoas muscle pass together). The iliopsoas bursa communicates with the hip joint in 15% of people. Some authors distinguish between iliopectineal and iliopsoas bursae. These authors describe the true iliopsoas bursa as being located medially in the femoral triangle near the insertion of the iliopsoas muscle at the lesser trochanter. These authors describe the previously mentioned bursa anterior to the hip joint as the iliopectineal bursa.

Function

The iliopsoas bursa cushions the musculotendinous junction of the iliopsoas muscle from the pelvic brim or superior pubic ramus.

Clinical Presentation

Iliopsoas bursitis presents as anterior hip pain, which may radiate to the anterior thigh all the way to the knee joint. This radiation of pain may occur if the adjacent femoral nerve is irritated. The pain is worsened with hip extension and rotation especially with ambulation. There is associated groin tenderness. The syndrome may also be associated with a mass. There may be

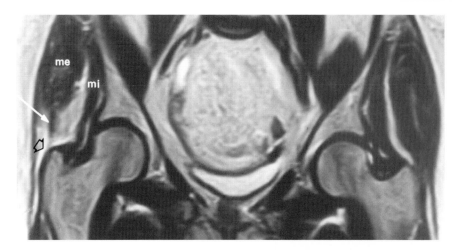

Fig. 8.12 A 74-year-old-woman with surgically confirmed focal full-thickness tear in right abductor tendon cuff with trochanteric (subgluteus maximus) bursitis. Coronal T2-weighted fast spin-echo image (TR/TE, 3,879/102) of hips (obtained at 0.2 T with postprocessing) reveals gluteus medius (*me*) and gluteus minimus (*mi*) muscles, elongated and distally discontinuous right gluteus medius tendon (*solid arrow*), and a sheet of high signal intensity outlining lateral and superior margins of the greater trochanter (pattern 2) (*open arrow*). In general, visualization of pattern 2 T2 hyperintensity superior to greater trochanter alone is sufficient to diagnose a tear (Cvitanic et al. 2004)

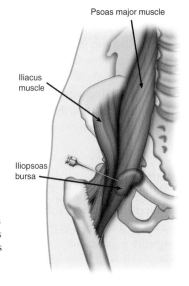

Fig. 8.13 Iliopsoas bursa injection: anatomy of the psoas major muscle, iliacus muscle, and iliopsoas bursa (Illustrated by Michael Dobryzcki)

associated numbness and tingling. Iliopsoas bursitis may also be associated with internal snapping hip syndrome (medial extraarticular snapping hip syndrome). This is a sensation of snapping with hip flexion/extension that is associated with an audible noise and pain. It is caused by the iliopsoas tendon rubbing on the anterior superior iliac spine and lesser trochanteric or iliopectineal ridge during hip extension.

Etiology

It can be a post total hip arthroplasty** status. Additionally, etiologies include overuse of the hip during running, soccer, ballet, hurdling or jumping, trauma, arthritis** (osteoarthritis** or rheumatoid arthritis**), synovial chondromatosis**, and avascular necrosis**.

Differential Diagnosis

Differential diagnoses include inguinal hernia**, hip joint pathology**, neoplasm**, lumbar radiculopathy**, and meralgia paresthetica.

Injection Site

A lateral approach is utilized with ultrasound, CT or fluoroscopic guidance at the level of the joint line at the iliopectineal eminence. The distended iliopsoas bursa is targeted at this site if present. Otherwise, injection is performed between the iliopsoas tendon and the hip capsule.

Imaging/Radiology

Ultrasound: This can demonstrate the iliopsoas tendon snapping over the iliopectineal eminence in internal snapping hip syndrome. However, it is highly operator dependent. A fluid-filled enlarged iliopsoas bursa may also be identified. Sonography can be useful for injection of the iliopsoas bursa and injection of the iliopsoas tendon (Adler et al. 2005) (Fig. 8.14).

CT: CT may demonstrate a fluid collection. This is usually located anterior to the hip between the iliopsoas muscle and iliopectineal eminence of the superior pubic ramus (Fig. 8.15). CT may also show a thickened iliopsoas tendon. Associated hip joint disease may be identified. CT may be helpful in combination with hip arthrography to identify a communication of the bursa with the hip joint in order to confirm the diagnosis.

MRI: MRI is the modality of choice for evaluating the iliopsoas bursa. Iliopsoas bursitis is characterized by an enlarged fluid-filled bursa which may communicate with the hip joint (Fig. 8.15). There may be associated findings of iliopsoas tendonitis/tendinosis manifested by increased signal intensity on T2-weighted sequences.

Indications

The main indications for intervention in the iliopsoas bursa are: (1) Iliopsoas bursitis**, and (2) snapping

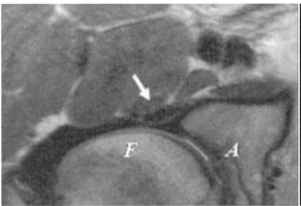
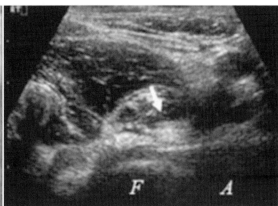

Fig. 8.14 Axial image of the iliopsoas tendon at the level of the joint line in a 19-year-old-man. Fast spin-echo proton density image (*left*) and corresponding sonogram (*right*) show the anatomic relationship of the iliopsoas tendon (*arrow*), femoral head (*F*), and iliopectineal eminence of acetabulum (*A*). The tendon (*arrow*) is seen as an elliptic structure situated medial and superficial to the joint capsule and along the lateral margin of the iliopectineal eminence (Adler et al. 2005)

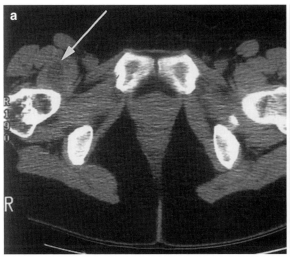
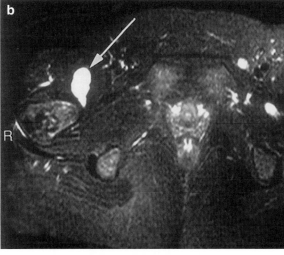

Fig. 8.15 (**a**, **b**) Groin pain and limitation of hip flexion in a 41-year-old-woman. (**a**) Unenhanced CT scan shows a low-attenuation region (*arrow*) within the iliopsoas muscle. (**b**) T2-weighted MR image obtained with fat saturation helps confirm the region as a fluid collection (*arrow*). This is the classic location of the iliopectineal bursa, which in this case is inflamed. MR imaging allowed better depiction of the fluid nature of the bursa and greater diagnostic confidence (Shadbolt et al. 2001)

iliopsoas tendon syndrome (which can be imaged with ultrasound)**.

Complications

The principal complications encountered in intervention in the iliopsoas bursa are: (1) Weakness (transient due to femoral nerve involvement), and (2) paresthesia (transient due to femoral nerve involvement).

8.2.1.4 Ischiogluteal Bursa Injection (Fig. 8.16)

Anatomy

The ischiogluteal bursa lies between the ischial tuberosity and the gluteus maximus muscle. It is medial to the sciatic nerve and adjacent to the origin of the semitendinosus and biceps femoris muscles (hamstrings).

Function

It cushions the musculotendinous junction of the hamstring muscles from the ischial tuberosity.

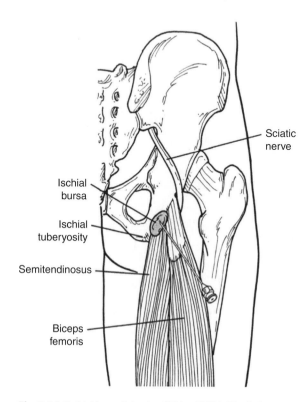

Fig. 8.16 Ischial bursa injection (Weiss 2007d, Fig. 5-7)

Clinical Presentation

Ischiogluteal bursitis presents as pain in the buttock region, which can be excruciating. The pain is worsened with sitting, climbing stairs, or running. The pain may extend to the posterior thigh if there is sciatic nerve irritation or compression. The site over the ischiogluteal bursa is tender to palpation. Ischiogluteal bursitis needs to be distinguished from piriformis syndrome because the presentation is similar. The condition is seen in professional automobile/truck drivers as well as sewing machine operators, who are subject to prolonged periods of sitting. It is also seen in athletes, who are prone to falls or who perform prolonged sitting (rowing). It can also be seen in debilitated patients where weight-bearing has shifted onto the ischial tuberosity.

Etiology

Etiologies include overuse syndromes (prolonged sitting), athletics, repetitive falls (trauma**), weight loss, and debilitation.

Differential Diagnosis

Differential diagnoses include hematoma**, solid tumors**, and abscess**. Pigmented villonodular synovitis** as well as synovial chondromatosis**, synovial hemangioma**, lipoma**, and synovial sarcoma** can mimic ischiogluteal bursitis. Piriformis syndrome** can also mimic ischiogluteal bursitis.

Injection Site

The needles should be advanced to the ischial tuberosity while avoiding the sciatic nerve, which is at the lateral aspect of the ischial tuberosity.

Imaging/Radiology

Plain film radiographs: There may be cortical irregularity of the involved ischial tuberosity in a chronic condition. There may also be associated adjacent calcification.

Ultrasound: Ultrasound may demonstrate a fluid-filled sac adjacent to the lower posterior medial aspect of the ischial tuberosity. This may have echogenic contents.

CT: CT may demonstrate a fluid collection adjacent to the ischial tuberosity at the inferior posterior medial aspect.

MRI: This is the imaging modality of choice. It excludes pathology involving the hip and pelvis as well as surrounding soft tissues. It can also excludes pathology originating from the spine. The findings on MRI include a cystic-appearing enlarged bursa, which has a characteristic location at the lower posterior medial aspect of the ischial tuberosity (Fig. 8.17). There is a propensity for blood fluid levels within the structure. The appearance on T1-weighted images is variable. It is hyperintense on T2-weighted images, however. There is enhancement of the bursal lining as well as peribursal soft tissues. Ischiogluteal bursitis can mimic soft tissue or bone metaphysis in the cancer patient. Biopsy is therefore required in this situation. It is also necessary to exclude infection in the appropriate clinical setting by aspiration (i.e., tuberculosis). If the bursa is ruptured, the diagnosis is difficult due to the spread of bursa contents into the posterior thigh or towards the sciatic nerve. This can be associated with referred pain to the posterior thigh.

Indications

The principal indication for intervention is ischiogluteal bursitis**.

Complications

The main complication encountered is transient lower extremity weakness and paresthesia due to sciatic nerve involvement.

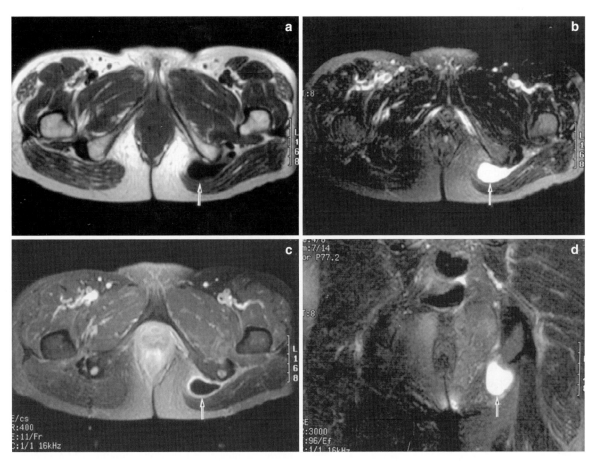

Fig. 8.17 Ischiogluteal bursitis in 68-year-old-woman. (**a**) T1-weighted image: a hypo-intense mass (*arrow*) in comparison with that of the adjacent muscle is seen at the soft tissue just posterior to the ischial tuberosity. (**b**) T2-weighted image: a hyper-intense mass (*arrow*) at the ischial tuberosity. (**c**) Contrast-enhanced T1-weighted image: the bursal wall is enhanced hyper-intensely at the ischial tuberosity (*arrow*). The bursa extends medially to the ischial tuberosity. (**d**) T2-weighted image on the coronal section shows a homogeneously hyper-intense mass (*arrow*) at the ischial tuberosity. The enlarged bursa extends inferiorly and medially to the inferior surface of the ischial tuberosity (Cho et al. 2004)

8.2.1.5 Pubic Symphysis Joint injection for Osteitis Pubis (Fig. 8.18)

Anatomy

The pubic symphysis is a joint (non-synovial), which contains a cartilaginous disk in the midst of the joint space. The joint is lined by hyaline cartilage lining the inner margins of the pubic bones, strengthened by the superior and inferior ligaments as well as the anterior and posterior ligaments. The adductor group muscles and anterior abdominal wall musculature (rectus abdominis, external oblique, internal oblique, and transversus abdominis) attach to the pubic symphysis and stabilize the anterior pelvis.

Function

This joint performs slight cephalocaudal translation as well as slight widening/narrowing to absorb the impact of ambulation. It allows childbirth by widening in women.

Clinical Presentation (Osteitis Pubis)

The presentation of osteitis pubis is that of a dull aching groin pain and pain overlying the pubic symphysis. There can also be sharp pain associated with shifting direction, running, or kicking, as well as loss of range of motion within the groin. The pain may radiate from the pubic symphysis to the groin and pelvis. There is also tenderness over the pubic bone and there may be a limping gait.

Etiology

Repetitive motion injury in athletes is related to running and jumping. Other causes include: Exercise on hard surfaces or uneven ground, increasing the intensity or duration of exercise too rapidly, poorly fitting shoes, gait disturbance or leg length discrepancy**, pregnancy**, and prior pelvic surgery**.

Differential Diagnosis

Differential diagnoses include adductor muscle injury**, pubic stress fracture**, prostatitis**, urinary tract infection, pelvic inflammatory disease**, hernia**, and osteomyelitis.

Injection Site

The needle is directed under fluoroscopic guidance toward the pubic symphysis at the midline into the joint space. CT or ultrasound may also be used for guidance.

Imaging/Radiology

Plain film radiographs: Plain films can be negative in early stages of osteitis pubis. Plain films can demonstrate symmetric marginal sclerosis of the inner aspect of the pubic bone, marginal erosions, and marginal osteophytes. Significant widening of the joint space and indistinct cortical margins (as a result of marginal erosions) can be visualized less frequently. In advanced cases, there is evidence of joint disruption with malalignment of the pubic bones (Fig. 8.20).

Fluoroscopy/pubic symphyseal cleft injection: In most patients with osteitis pubis, contrast injection results in extrusion above or below the symphyseal margins or penetration of bone defects at the lateral and inferior joint margins. However, in mild cases extrusion may be absent (Fig. 8.19). Extension of contrast beyond the lateral and inferior joint margins is associated with chronic avulsion

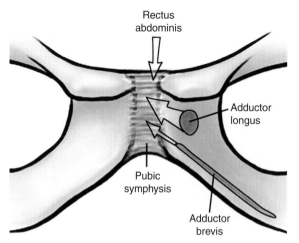

Fig. 8.18 Male cadaver dissection, normal anatomy. The line diagram shows the relative position of tendinous attachments with the direction (*arrows*) of involvement over symphyseal capsular tissues (Robinson et al. 2007)

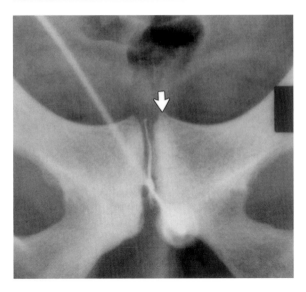

Fig. 8.19 A 19-year-old-male athlete with osteitis pubis. Anteroposterior radiograph shows normal findings after symphyseal cleft injection. Contrast material is confined to the central cleft of the fibrocartilaginous disk with no evidence of extrusion. Sclerosis and marginal osteophyte (*arrow*) are seen on the medial margins of pubic bones (O'Connell et al. 2002)

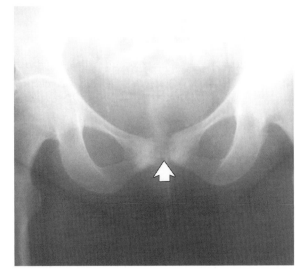

Fig. 8.20 A 29-year-old-male soccer player. Anteroposterior radiograph shows extensive erosive changes of osteitis pubis and widening of joint space (*arrow*) (O'Connell et al. 2002)

of the adductor longus or gracilis muscles. In cases of severe inflammation, venous or lymphatic intravasation may be seen.

MRI: MRI findings include marrow edema at the pubic symphysis that may be symmetric or asymmetric, dorsal or cephalad symphyseal disk extrusion, and adductor avulsion that may be unilateral

or bilateral (Figs. 8.21 and 8.22). The symphysis may become widened and develop irregularity of its margins as well as erosions. Intra-articular fluid may also be identified. Signal intensity within the pubis may become low on both T1- and T2-weighted sequences as the disease progresses (Omar et al. 2008).

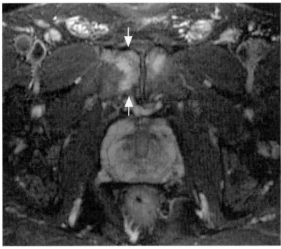

Fig. 8.21 Mild osteitis pubis in a male ultra-marathoner. (**a**) Axial T2-weighted image of the pubic symphysis shows marrow edema (*arrows*) that extends the full anteroposterior thickness of both pubic bodies (Omar et al. 2008)

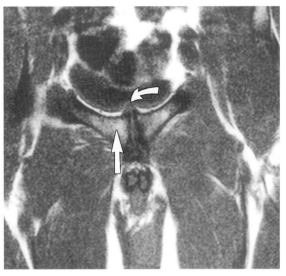

Fig. 8.22 A 22-year-old-male athlete with osteitis pubis. Coronal T1-weighted MR image (TR/TE, 620/20) shows irregularity in joint surface and fatty replacement of para-articular marrow (*straight arrow*). Note superior extrusion of fibrocartilaginous disk indenting bladder (*curved arrow*) (O'Connell et al. 2002)

Bone scintigraphy: Moderate to marked uptake may be seen at the pubic symphysis even in early stage of the disease. SPECT (single photon emission computed tomography) imaging is useful in the pelvis. Uptake is usually bilateral, but can be unilateral. Findings of uptake representing adjacent adductor avulsion injury may be identified.

Indications

Osteitis pubis** is the main indication for pubic symphysis injection.

Contraindications

The principal contraindication to pubic symphysis injection is infection (Ross and Hu 2003) **, usually established on clinical grounds, although biopsy and microbiologic examination are often required to distinguish infection more accurately. Bone destruction is more prominent than in osteitis. Osteomyelitis is progressive whereas osteitis is self-limited.

8.2.2 *Knee and Surrounding Structures*

8.2.2.1 Knee Joint Injection for Arthritis
(Figs. 8.23 and 8.24)

Anatomy

The knee joint is a pivotal hinge joint with femorotibial and patellofemoral components. It is the largest and most complicated joint in the body. The joint capsule is lined with synovial membrane and contains synovial fluid. The lateral and medial condyles of the femur articulate with the tibial condyles. The intercondylar eminence between the tibial condyles has both a medial and a lateral tubercle.

The patella has a lateral and medial surface. It is attached to the anterior aspect of the joint capsule and articulates with the anterior aspect of the femoral condyles.

The lateral and medial menisci are large cartilage discs that supplement the articular cartilage of the femur and tibia. They provide additional support and absorb impact.

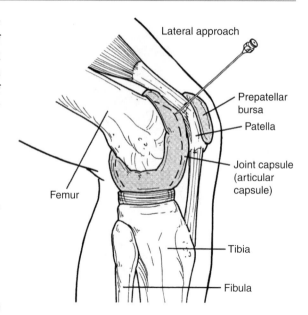

Fig. 8.23 Knee joint injection, lateral approach (Weiss 2007e, Fig. 3-25)

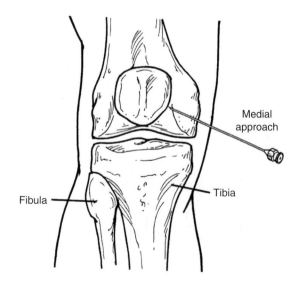

Fig. 8.24 Knee joint injection, medial approach (Weiss 2007f, Fig. 3-27)

There are multiple ligaments associated with the knee that are both intracapsular and extracapsular. These include the anterior cruciate ligament, posterior cruciate ligament, and transverse ligaments. There is also the patellar ligament, patellar retinaculum, as well as the medial and lateral collateral ligaments. In addition, there is an oblique popliteal ligament and arcuate popliteal ligament. Discussion of these ligaments is beyond the scope of this section (Figs. 8.25–8.27).

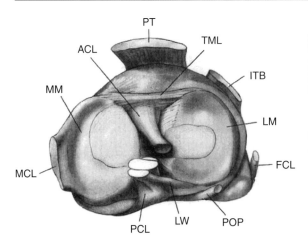

Fig. 8.25 Knee joint anatomy. *MM* medial meniscus; *ACL* anterior cruciate ligament; *PT* patellar tendon; *TML* transverse meniscal ligament; *ITB* iliotibial band; *LM* lateral meniscus; *FCL* fibulocollateral ligament; *POP* popliteus tendon; *LW* ligament of Wrisberg; *PCL* posterior cruciate ligament; *MCL* medial collateral ligament (Peterson et al. 2008)

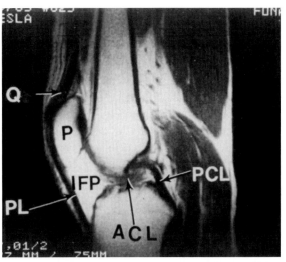

Fig. 8.27 Sagittal section through the intercondylar fossa shows the posterior cruciate ligament (*PCL*), quadriceps femoris (*Q*), patella (*P*), patellar ligament (*PL*), infrapatellar fat pad (*IFP*), and a vague image of the anterior cruciate ligament (*ACL*). Note the posterior bowing of the posterior cruciate ligament (Mesgarzadeh et al. 1988)

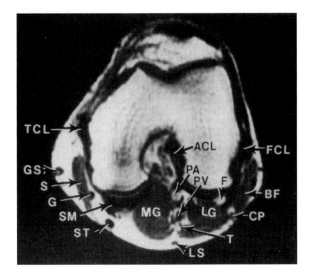

Fig. 8.26 Transaxial MRI and anatomic sections at the level at which the tibial collateral ligament (*TCL*) and fibular collateral ligament (*FCL*) attach to the femoral epicondyles. At this level, the anterior cruciate ligament (*ACL*) is attaching to the lateral condyle. The interval between the semimembranosus (*SM*) and the medial head of gastrocnemius (*MG*) marks the location of the semimembranosus-gastrocnemius bursa. The common peroneal nerve (*CP*) descends behind the biceps femoris (*BF*). The fabella (*F*) is seen within the lateral head of gastrocnemius (*LG*). The sartorius (*S*), gracilis (*G*), and semitendinosus (*ST*) will fuse at a lower level to form the pes anserinus. Also visualized are the patella, greater (*GS*) and lesser (*LS*), saphenous veins, popliteal artery (*PA*) and vein (*PV*), and tibial nerve (*T*) (Mesgarzadeh et al. 1988)

Function

The knee supports bodyweight for flexion and extension. It also performs slight medial and lateral rotation.

Clinical Presentation (Arthritis)

Arthritis generally presents with knee pain and stiffness, which worsen with activity, as well as decreased range of motion.

Etiology

Etiologies include osteoarthritis**/degenerative joint disease**, rheumatoid arthritis**, CPPD**, gout**, and infection**.

Differential Diagnosis

Differential diagnoses include fracture**, bursitis**, tendonitis**, tear of the ligament** or meniscus**, osteonecrosis of the tibia** or femur**, hip**, ankle disorders**, tumor**, and pigmented villonodular synovitis**.

Injection Site

Anterolateral and anteromedial approaches are common. The anterolateral approach is performed at the lateral aspect of the patella at its upper half. The needle is directed between the patella and lateral femoral condyle. The anteromedial approach is performed at the medial aspect of the patella by directing the needle between the patella and medial femoral condyle.

Imaging/Radiology

Plain film radiographs: Plain films are usually the initial and most important study for evaluation. They usually include AP, lateral, and tangential views (to evaluate the patellofemoral joint). Weightbearing views may be performed in the setting of arthritis to evaluate for joint space loss.

In osteoarthritis findings include non-uniform or focal joint space narrowing as well as osteophyte formation. There is subchondral sclerosis and cyst formation also present.

In rheumatoid arthritis, there is uniform joint space narrowing with effusion. There are also findings of soft tissue swelling, osteopenia, and erosions. Joint space subluxation, synovial cyst, and periostitis are also demonstrated on plain film radiographs. In juvenile rheumatoid arthritis, growth disturbances may be seen such as epiphyseal overgrowth.

In CPPD (calcium pyrophosphate deposition disease), there is involvement of the medial femoral tibial joint. Isolated patellofemoral degenerative joint disease is suggestive. Chondrocalcinosis is commonly seen. There may be surrounding calcifications of the ligaments and tendons (Fig. 8.28).

Fluoroscopy: Fluoroscopy is useful for guidance in knee joint injection or aspiration. This can be useful for both the medial and lateral approaches especially in obese patients or patients with patellofemoral osteoarthritis. An anteromedial or anterolateral approach may be utilized just medial or lateral to the patellar tendon via an approach inferior to the patella where the needle may contact the medial or lateral femoral condyle.

Ultrasound: This modality can be very useful for guidance in the postoperative patients or in the setting of extreme soft tissue edema. An approach through the quadriceps tendon a few centimeters superior to the superior margin of the patella may be used. Alternatively, superomedial or superolateral approach may be utilized to access the suprapatellar recess, which has the

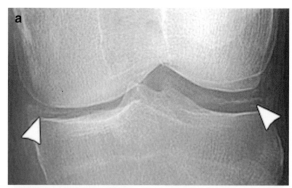

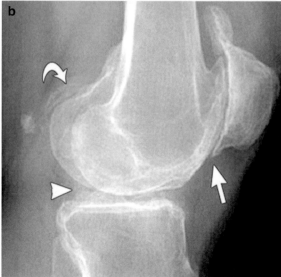

Fig. 8.28 (**a**, **b**) CPPD crystal deposition disease in the knee. Anteroposterior (**a**) and lateral (**b**) radiographs show chondrocalcinosis involving the menisci (*arrowhead*) and hyaline cartilage, predominant patellofemoral joint osteoarthritis (*straight arrow*), and calcification of the gastrocnemius tendon origin (*curved arrow*) (Jacobson et al. 2008)

advantage of avoiding neurovascular structures. Ultrasound is well suited to evaluating the soft tissue structures around the knee joint, but less sensitive to evaluating the knee joint itself. The soft tissue structures could include the tendons, muscles, ligaments, and bursae. Ultrasound can assess joint effusion, synovial thickening, articular cartilage abnormality, and even the bony cortex as well as loose bodies in the setting of arthritis, but is operator dependent. Furthermore, it may not be possible to visualize weightbearing areas. It is thus less sensitive than MRI for the assessment of synovial thickness, bone erosions, and cartilage abnormality.

CT: CT is not as useful for imaging unless concurrent fracture is suspected.

MRI: MRI is the most sensitive radiological modality in the setting of both osteoarthritis and rheumatoid arthritis, as well as other arthropathies. In osteoarthritis as well as rheumatoid arthritis, it is very sensitive at detecting synovial thickening, effusions, cartilage abnormality, popliteal cyst, and intracapsular ligament tears (intracapsular ligament tears such as in the anterior cruciate ligament may not be visualized with ultrasound). It can also demonstrate bone marrow edema at areas of remodeling, which may not be visible with ultrasound. In the setting of rheumatoid arthritis, synovial hypertrophy and joint effusions have been found to correlate with active synovitis. However, gadolinium enhancement may be needed in order to distinguish joint effusion from synovial hypertrophy since they are both bright on T2-weighted and STIR sequences.

MR arthrography has an increased sensitivity for meniscal tears and osteochondritis dissecans compared to standard MRI or arthrography.

Scintigraphy: Nuclear medicine bone scintigraphy is sensitive, but not specific.

Indications for Arthrocentesis

Indications include unexplained monarthritis**, crystal-induced arthropathy**, hemarthrosis**, unexplained joint effusion**, limiting joint damage from an infectious** process, and symptomatic relief of a large effusion**.

Indications for Injection of the Knee Joint

The following represent the main indications (Calmbach and Hutchens 2003a; Zuber 2002) for injection of the knee joint:

- Osteoarthritis**
- Inflammatory arthropathy (rheumatoid arthritis)**
- Crystal-induced arthritis (gout and CPPD)**
- Overuse syndromes**
  - Patellofemoral syndrome (chondromalacia patellae)**
  - Medial plica syndrome [remnant fetal tissue that forms synovial folds in the knee which is prone to inflammation/injury] (Calmbach and Hutchens 2003b) **

Contraindications

The four principle contraindications to intervention in the knee include: (1) Acute injury (ACL, PCL, MCL, LCL, medial meniscus, lateral meniscus, and osteochondral fracture)**; (2) hemarthrosis**; (3) impending joint surgery (scheduled within days); (4) joint prosthesis**.

8.2.2.2 Injection for Iliotibial Band Syndrome (Fig. 8.29)

Anatomy

The iliotibial band or tract is a laterally reinforced tendon-like portion of the tensor fasciae latae muscle. The iliotibial band has its origin at the anterior iliac crest. It proceeds inferiorly overlying the lateral thigh including the greater trochanter (specifically the trochanteric bursa). It continues inferiorly and attaches to the lateral femoral epicondyle and lateral tibial condyle at Gerdy's tubercle. At its inferior aspect, the iliopatellar band splits off of the iliotibial tract and merges within the lateral retinaculum to connect with the lateral patella. The gluteus maximus and gluteus medius insert into the iliotibial tract at its proximal portion.

Function

The iliotibial tract provides lateral stability for the knee joint by its connections to the distal femur and proximal tibia.

Clinical Presentation

Iliotibial band syndrome occurs when the tensor fasciae latae and iliotibial band become tense. The band creates friction over the lateral knee and lateral femoral epicondyle. There is pain at these sites as well as the

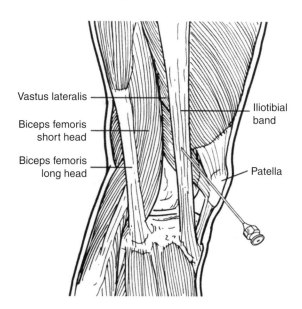

Fig. 8.29 Iliotibial band injection (Weiss 2007g, Fig. 4-17)

greater trochanter, occasionally where there also may be friction. There can be associated tenderness overlying the iliotibial tract especially over Gerdy's tubercle. Symptoms can be worsened with climbing stairs, squatting, and running. The syndrome is seen in long-distance runners, cyclists, tennis players, and military recruits. The syndrome can be associated with snapping syndrome of the hip (external). This is also known as lateral extraarticular snapping syndrome of the hip.

Injection Site

Injection is made at the point of maximum tenderness at the iliotibial band. This is usually at the lateral femoral condyle.

Etiology

Etiologies may include running long distances, prolonged squatting, or stair-climbing.

Differential Diagnosis

Differential diagnoses include hamstring strain**, degenerative joint disease**, myofascial pain, overuse injury, medial collateral** and lateral collateral ligament injury**, patellofemoral syndrome**, meniscal injury**, trochanteric bursitis**, biceps femoris tendonitis**, and popliteus tendonitis**.

Imaging/Radiology

Imaging is usually not necessary, but may be helpful if the clinical findings are ambiguous or the patient is not responding to therapy/injection.

Plain film radiographs: Plain films are useful to exclude other causes such as fracture or arthritis.

Ultrasound: Sudden motion of the iliotibial band over Gerdy's tubercle can be visualized with real-time scanning. However, this is highly operator dependent.

MRI: MRI of T2-weighted fat-suppressed images may demonstrate edema between the iliotibial band and the lateral femoral condyle. There is also thickening of the iliotibial band and enhancement of fat deep to the iliotibial band. Complete disruption or tear of the iliotibial band would be seen as absence of this structure at its expected location (Figs. 8.30 and 8.31).

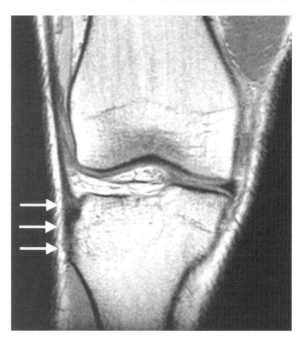

Fig. 8.30 Normal appearance of the iliotibial band. Coronal fast spin-echo proton density-weighted MR image of a 24-year-old-woman shows insertion of superficial fibers of the iliotibial band (*arrows*) on Gerdy's tubercle of the anterior tibia. This tendinous insertion is the main one for iliotibial band (Haims et al. 2003)

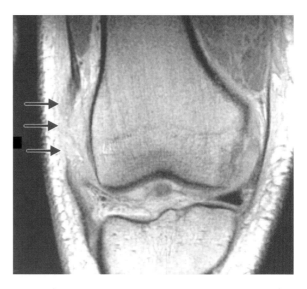

Fig. 8.31 Injuries to the iliotibial band. Coronal fast spin-echo proton density-weighted MR image illustrates disruption of fibers of the iliotibial band (*arrows*) in a 34-year-old-man with multiple ligamentous knee injuries (Haims et al. 2003). (A complete tear of the iliotibial band as seen above would be less likely to respond to injection)

Indications

The principal indication for intervention here is iliotibial band syndrome (Khaund and Flynn 2005)**.

8.2.2.3 Injection for Prepatellar Bursitis (Housemaid's Knee) (Fig. 8.32)

Anatomy

The prepatellar bursa is a superficial structure, which overlies the patellar just below the skin.

Function

The function of the prepatellar bursa is to separate the patella from the skin, thereby decreasing the friction between the skin and patella.

Clinical Presentation

Prepatellar bursitis presents with anterior knee pain localized to the patella with associated swelling.

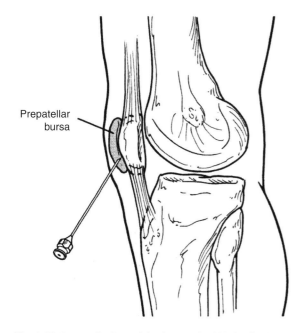

Fig. 8.32 Prepatellar bursa injection (Weiss 2007h, Fig. 5-11)

Etiology

Etiologies include trauma or chronic kneeling. There can be associated infection** due to superficial trauma. It is seen in professions such as carpet laying, coal mining, roofing, gardening, and plumbing. It may also be seen in rheumatoid arthritis** or gout**.

Differential Diagnosis

The differential diagnosis includes Morel-Lavallee effusions**. This is a degloving injury involving separation of skin and subcutaneous fat from the adjacent deeper fascia. It is seen in wrestlers and football players.

The following entities are also included in the differential diagnosis: patellofemoral syndrome**, other forms of patellar pathology**, femoral neuropathy**, knee ligament**, cartilage** or joint pathology**, and quadriceps tendonitis**.

Injection Site

Injection is generally made using an anterior approach with the needle angle parallel to the plane of the patella.

Imaging/Radiology

Plain film radiographs: Soft tissue swelling may be seen in the plain films. There may be associated calcification if there has been a history of associated bleeding into the bursa. Plain films are usually not needed unless one is excluding other clinically relevant pathology such as fracture or dislocation.

CT and *MRI*: These modalities are usually needed only in difficult clinical scenarios such as failed treatment or injection. The findings consist of a fluid pocket anterior to the patella with an associated thickened bursal lining (Fig. 8.33).

Indications

The major indication for prepatellar bursa treatment (injection) is prepatellar bursitis (housemaid's knee, wrestler's knee)**.

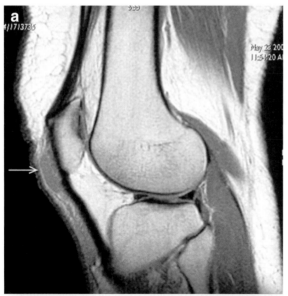

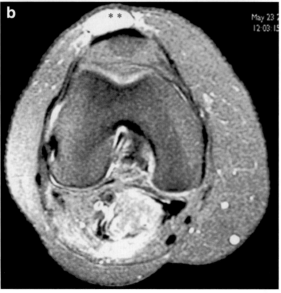

Fig. 8.33 (**a, b**) Housemaid's knee. (**a**) Sagittal T1-weighted magnetic resonance (MR) image of the knee shows fluid (*arrow*) in the prepatellar bursa. (**b**) Axial fat-saturated intermediate-weighted MR image also shows the fluid (*asterisk*) in the prepatellar bursa (Lee et al. 2004)

8.2.2.4 Injection for Infrapatellar Bursitis (Clergyman's Knee) (Fig. 8.34)

Anatomy

There are two infrapatellar bursae. The superficial bursa is just deep to the skin inferior to the patellar

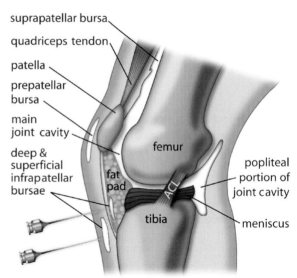

Fig. 8.34 Anatomy demonstrating the infrapatellar bursa (http://www.kneeguru.co.uk/KNEEnotes/infrapatellar-bursitis)

tendon at its inferior aspect. The deep bursa is located deep to the patellar tendon, but superficial to the anterior superior aspect of the tibia near the attachment of the patellar tendon.

Function

Both bursae decreased friction between the patellar tendon and adjacent structures.

Clinical Presentation

Infrapatellar bursitis presents with anterior knee pain and associated swelling of the bursa. The presentation is similar to infrapatellar tendinitis/tendinopathy.

Etiology

Etiologies of infrapatellar bursitis include overuse (repetitive kneeling) and trauma**.

Differential Diagnosis

Differential diagnoses include knee ligament injury**, infrapatellar tendinitis**, meniscal tear**, chondromalacia of the patella**, arthritis**, tendon injury**, and Osgood-Schlatter disease**.

Injection Site

The approach for injection is similar to that of infrapatellar tendon injection.

Imaging/Radiology

Plain film radiographs: Plain films are usually not revealing or helpful.

Ultrasound: Sonography demonstrates an anechoic fluid collection in the superficial infrapatellar bursa. There may be hypertrophy of the anterior wall of the superficial infrapatellar bursa.

MRI: This modality demonstrates soft tissue swelling with a fluid collection involving the infrapatellar bursa. MRI is frequently necessary for diagnosis and to exclude other pathology (Figs. 8.35 and 8.36).

Indications

The main indication for infrapatellar injection is infrapatellar bursitis.

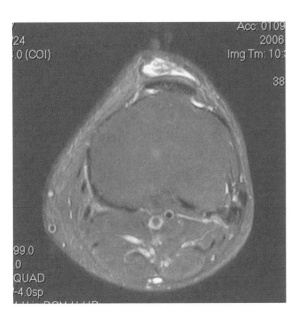

Fig. 8.35 Axial proton density fat-saturated MRI shows a fluid collection involving the infrapatellar bursa (http://www.mskcases.com/index.php?module=article&view=40) [Courtesy of Elvedin Kulenovic, MD, Ph.D.]

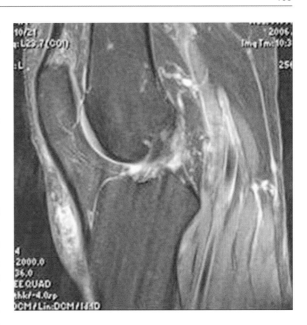

Fig. 8.36 Sagittal T2 fat-saturated MRI shows a fluid collection involving the infrapatellar bursa (http://www.mskcases.com/index.php?module=article&view=40 [Courtesy of Elvedin Kulenovic])

8.2.2.5 Injection for Infrapatellar Tendinitis/Tendinopathy (Jumper's Knee) (Fig. 8.37)

Anatomy

The infrapatellar tendon attaches the inferior aspect of the patella to the tibial tubercle. It is surrounded by a paratenon of loose connective tissue instead of a synovial sheath. Thus, para-tendinitis occurs rather than tenosynovitis.

Function

This tendon is involved in knee extension.

Clinical Presentation

Infrapatellar tendinitis presents as anterior knee pain localized inferior to the patella with associated tenderness of the site. It is related to jumping or running (chronic overload).

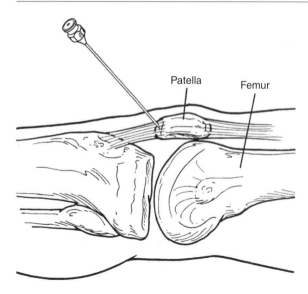

Patella   Femur

Fig. 8.37 Infrapatellar tendon injection (Weiss 2007i, Fig. 4-19)

Etiology

The etiology of infrapatellar tendinitis is overuse usually related to jumping, running, or trauma.

Differential Diagnosis

Differential diagnoses include:

- Avulsion fractures** related to the infrapatellar tendon (patellar sleeve fracture**).
- Sinding-Larsen-Johansson syndrome** which is a chronic overuse syndrome involving the patellar insertion site.
- Osgood-Schlatter disease** that is a chronic overuse syndrome involving the tibial insertion site.
- Infrapatellar plica injury**, which is pathological thickening of the infrapatellar plicae.
- Patellar tendon – lateral femoral condyle friction syndrome**. This involves lateral subluxation of the patella with inflammation of the lateral portion of the infrapatellar tendon, which is adjacent to the lateral femoral condyle.
- Hoffa's syndrome**. This represents trauma-related pathology in the infrapatellar fat pad.

Injection Site

Injection is performed using an anterior approach to the inferior aspect of the patella at the site of point tenderness.

Imaging/Radiology

Plain film radiographs: Plain films can detect calcifications within the tendon.

Ultrasound: Some authors rank this modality as the study of choice. It allows fast dynamic imaging with superior spatial resolution to MRI. However, it is operator-determined and most radiologists in the US may not be experienced with evaluation of the infrapatellar tendon. Tendinopathy manifests as thickening with areas of decreased echogenicity. Calcification is seen as foci of increased echogenicity. Paratenonitis or inflammation of the paratenon may manifest as an interrupted sonolucent margin surrounding the tendon. Partial tears of the tendon can mimic tendinopathy on ultrasound. It is therefore differentiated on a clinical basis. A full thickness tear can be seen as a gap within the tendon.

MRI: MRI is useful when ultrasound is normal and to exclude the differential diagnosis. It is also useful for surgical planning in the situation of suspected tears. Tendinopathy will manifest as localized regions of intermediate signal intensity on T1-weighted imaging and bright signal on T2-weighted images (Figs. 8.38 and 8.39). It usually involves the posterior aspect of the tendon adjacent to the patella. Marrow edema may be seen within the lower tip of the patella. Calcification may manifest as decreased foci of low signal intensity. Partial tears can mimic tendinopathy as with ultrasound. It is again differentiated based on the patient's clinical presentation. Full thickness tears are seen as gaps in the tendon.

Indications

The main indication for infrapatellar tendon injection is infrapatellar tendinitis. Injection of the tendon is controversial however due to the risk of rupture.

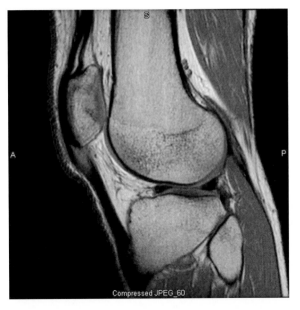

Fig. 8.38 Sagittal proton density MRI on jumper's knee or infrapatellar tendonitis. Note signal abnormality at the inferior aspect of the patella within the patellar tendon (http://www.mskcases.com/index.php?module=article&view=news&PAGER_limit=34&PAGER_start=102&PAGER_section=4) [Courtesy of Elvedin Kulenovic, MD, Ph.D.]

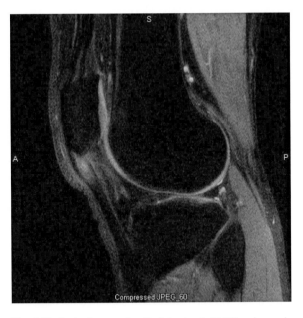

Fig. 8.39 Sagittal proton density fat-saturated MRI on jumper's knee or infrapatellar tendonitis. Note signal abnormality at the inferior aspect of the patella within the patellar tendon (http://www.mskcases.com/index.php?module=article&view=news&PAGER_limit=34&PAGER_start=102&PAGER_section=4) [Courtesy of Elvedin Kulenovic, MD, Ph.D.]

Complications

The main complication of infrapatellar tendon injection is infrapatellar tendon rupture**.

8.2.2.6 Popliteal Cyst Injection and/or Aspiration (Fig. 8.40)

Anatomy

The popliteal cyst is a synovial lined fluid-filled structure, which has a narrow neck that connects it to the knee joint at the posteromedial aspect between the semimembranosus and gastrocnemius tendon.

Function

The popliteal cyst is thought to provide decompression for the joint space in the setting of effusion via a valve-like mechanism. This may prevent joint destruction by reducing pressure inside the joint.

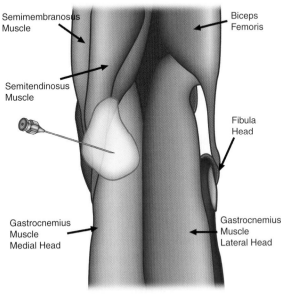

Popliteal Cyst

Fig. 8.40 Popliteal cyst (Illustrated by Michael Dobryzcki)

Clinical Presentation

Popliteal cysts may present as a popliteal mass with dull aching pain. There may be associated knee effusion. The presentation may also be similar to that of thrombophlebitis since the popliteal cyst may compress the popliteal vein and result in venous obstruction.

Etiology

The origin of popliteal cyst can lie in arthritis of various etiologies including osteoarthritis**, rheumatoid arthritis**, gout**, Reiter's disease**, psoriatic arthritis**, and systemic lupus erythematosus**. Trauma including fracture** or ligament injury**, end-stage renal disease**, pigmented villonodular synovitis**, and sarcoidosis** may also be implicated.

Differential Diagnosis

Differential diagnoses can include aneurysm**, cystic adventitial disease**, tumor**, meniscal cyst**, ganglion cyst**, gastrocnemius tear**, deep vein thrombosis**, and hematoma**.

Injection Site

A posterior approach using ultrasound guidance may be very helpful. The cyst is generally first aspirated and may be injected with a steroid.

Imaging/Radiology

Plain film radiographs: Plain films may demonstrate internal calcification, bone erosion, and mass effect on a calcified popliteal artery (Fig. 8.41). Findings of arthritis may also be identified.

Ultrasound: Sonography is extremely useful and is the modality of choice for diagnosis. It demonstrates fluid in a typical location between the semimembranosus and medial gastrocnemius tendons in communication with the posterior knee joint (Fig. 8.42). It excludes aneurysm or deep vein thrombosis. The link to the

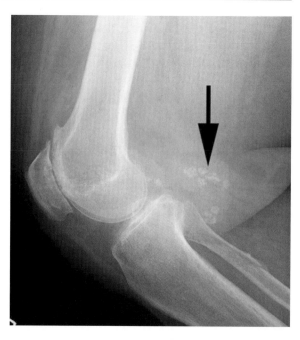

Fig. 8.41 Popliteal cyst with ossified loose bodies in a 64-year-old-woman. Lateral radiograph shows ossified loose bodies (*arrow*) that correspond to the round low-signal-intensity foci seen on MR images. This case emphasizes the importance of knowing the bursal anatomy and correlating MR images with radiographs (Stacy and Dixon 2007)

joint may be difficult to visualize on ultrasound, however, when the cyst is large. Ultrasound also provides guidance for aspiration.

CT: CT demonstrates a fluid-filled structure at the posteromedial aspect of the knee joint between the semimembranosus and gastrocnemius tendons.

MRI: MRI demonstrates a cystic mass. It is extremely useful in establishing definitive diagnosis on axial images by identifying the neck of the cyst that links to the knee joint. The neck usually lies between the tendons of the medial head of the gastrocnemius and semimembranosus muscle (Fig. 8.43). MRI is useful in excluding other cystic masses. Furthermore, it detects and assesses arthritis, such as rheumatoid arthritis, at very early stages. Fat-saturated T2-weighted images are usually part of the imaging protocol in the axial plane. Enhancement may be useful to assess synovitis. MRI is considered the gold standard in diagnosing popliteal cysts, but ultrasound may be very comparable (Ward et al. 2001).

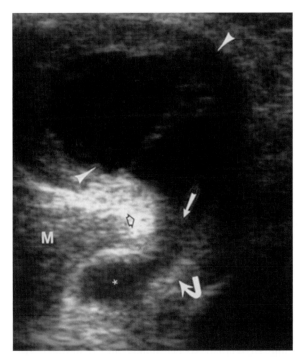

Fig. 8.42 A 60-year-old-woman with a Baker's cyst. Axial sonogram of the posterior knee shows the Baker's cyst (*arrowheads*) with fluid (*solid straight arrow*) between semimembranosus tendon (*curved arrow*) and medial gastrocnemius tendon (*open arrow*). Note the subgastrocnemius component (*asterisk*) of the Baker's cyst. Note that *top* of image is posterior; *right side* of image is medial. *M* medial gastrocnemius muscle (Ward et al. 2001)

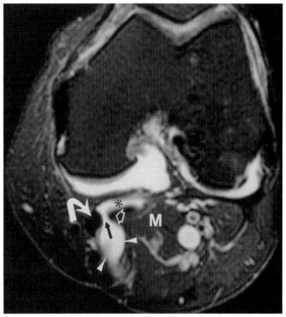

Fig. 8.43 A 60-year-old-woman with a Baker's cyst. Axial proton density-weighted MR image with fat saturation reveals the Baker's cyst (*arrowheads*) with fluid (*black arrow*) between the semimembranosus tendon (*curved white arrow*) and medial gastrocnemius tendon (*open arrow*). Note subgastrocnemius component (*asterisk*) of the Baker's cyst. *M* medial gastrocnemius muscle (Ward et al. 2001)

Indications

The main indication for intervention here is popliteal cyst or Baker's cyst**.

Contraindications

A popliteal artery aneurysm can appear similar to a popliteal cyst. Therefore, aneurysm of the popliteal artery must be excluded by duplex sonography prior to intervention**.

Complications

The two principal complications encountered are: (1) Lower extremity weakness and paresthesia due to tibial nerve injury in the popliteal fossa, and (2) popliteal artery or vein injury**.

8.2.2.7 Injection for Pes Anserine Bursitis
(Fig. 8.44)

Anatomy

The pes anserine bursa is located in the medial knee between the insertions of the sartorius, gracilis, and semitendinosus tendons as it separates these tendons from the tibial plateau. The anserine origin is based on the "goose's foot" appearance of the three-pronged inflamed bursa as it is confined by the three tendons. It lies adjacent to the medial collateral ligament of the knees (Fig. 8.45).

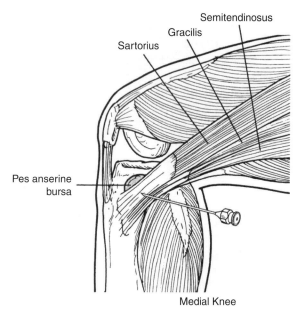

Fig. 8.44 Pes anserine bursa injection (Weiss 2007j, Fig. 5-9)

Function

The pes anserine bursa separates the fused tendons of the gracilis, sartorius, and semitendinosus muscles from the medial tibial plateau.

Clinical Presentation

Pes anserine bursitis is associated with medial knee pain upon standing up from a sitting or climbing position especially when going downstairs. There is swelling and tenderness along the medial aspect of the knee.

Etiology

Pes anserine bursitis is seen in chronic overuse such as in sports requiring rapid lateral shifts and body positions (basketball, soccer, tennis, and swimming "frog kicks"). It may also be seen in running. It is associated with pes planus**, obesity, degenerative joint disease**, valgus knee**, and trauma**.

Differential Diagnosis

Differential diagnoses include:

- Synovial cyst** and meniscal tear** with parameniscal cyst** (in pes anserine bursitis, there is no tear of the medial meniscus or medial collateral ligament and no communication with the joint).
- Periosteal tibial ganglion**.
- Tibial collateral ligament bursitis** (fluid collection is deep to the collateral ligament medially).
- Semimembranosus-tibial collateral ligament bursitis**.
- Semimembranosus, tendinosis**, or partial thickness tears** with tenosynovitis**.

Injection Site

A puncture site is selected for a medial approach about 3–4 cm inferior to the superior edge of the medial tibial plateau where the pes anserine conjoint tendon inserts on the tibia. The needle penetrates the conjoint tendon into the underlying bursa.

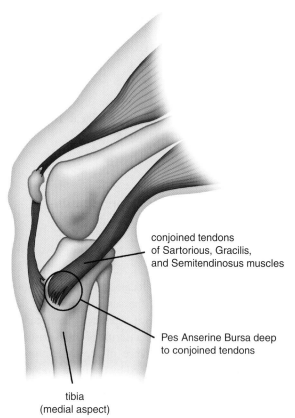

Fig. 8.45 Pes anserine bursitis (Illustrated by Michael Dobryzcki)

Fig. 8.46 (**a**, **b**) Pes Anserine bursitis. Axial (**a**) and coronal (**b**) T2-weighted gradient-echo MR images show a distended anserine bursa (*asterisk*) at medial aspect of the proximal part of the tibia, superficial to the tibial collateral ligament (*arrow*) (courtesy of Richard Eddy, Victoria, B.C.) (Janzen et al. 1994)

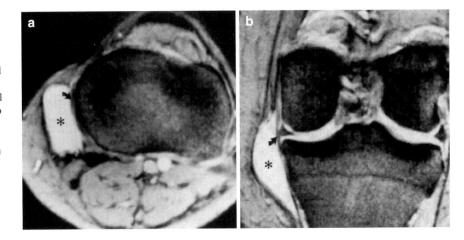

Imaging/Radiology

Plain film radiographs: Cortical scalloping due to remodeling may be seen at the proximal medial tibial cortex.

Ultrasound: Ultrasound may be useful for guidance; however, in small studies it appears to have low sensitivity in diagnostic evaluation (Unlu et al. 2003).

MRI: MRI usually demonstrates a cystic (fluid-filled) structure adjacent to the medial proximal tibial plateau, which is hypointense on T1- and bright T2-weighted images and does not communicate with the joint (Fig. 8.46). There is no associated tear of the medial malleolus or medial collateral ligament. MRI may also be helpful in distinguishing medial meniscal tear and other pathology from pes anserine bursitis (Beaman and Peterson 2007).

Indications

Pes anserine bursitis** is the major indication for treatment (injection).

8.2.3 Ankle and Foot

8.2.3.1 Ankle Joint Injection (Fig. 8.47)

Anatomy

The ankle is also known as the talocrural joint. It is a synovial hinge joint, which is lined with cartilage. The ankle articulates the tibia and fibula with the talus.

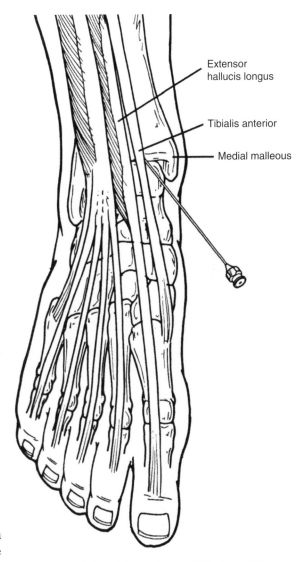

Extensor hallucis longus

Tibialis anterior

Medial malleous

Fig. 8.47 Ankle joint injection (Weiss 2007k, Fig. 3-29)

Medially, the deltoid ligament attaches the medial malleolus to the sustentaculum tali, calcaneonavicular ligament, and medial aspect of the navicular and talus. Laterally, the anterior and posterior talofibular ligaments attach the lateral malleolus to the anterior and posterior aspect of the talus. The calcaneofibular ligament connects the lateral aspect of the calcaneus to the lateral malleolus (Fig. 8.48).

Function

The ankle permits dorsiflexion and plantarflexion.

Clinical Presentation for Ankle Arthritis

Clinical presentation includes ankle pain and stiffness, which worsen with activity, and decreased range of motion.

Etiology

Etiologies include osteoarthritis**, rheumatoid arthritis**, CPPD**, traumatic arthritis**, Reiter's disease**, gout**, mixed connective tissue disease**, pigmented villonodular synovitis**, infectious arthritis**.

Differential Diagnosis

Differential diagnoses include:

- Charcot's joint (neuropathic joint)**
- Pigmented villonodular synovitis**
- Os trigonum syndrome**
- Anterolateral impingement syndrome**
- Sinus tarsi syndrome**
- Tuberculosis, sarcoidosis, and fungal infections**
- Fracture**

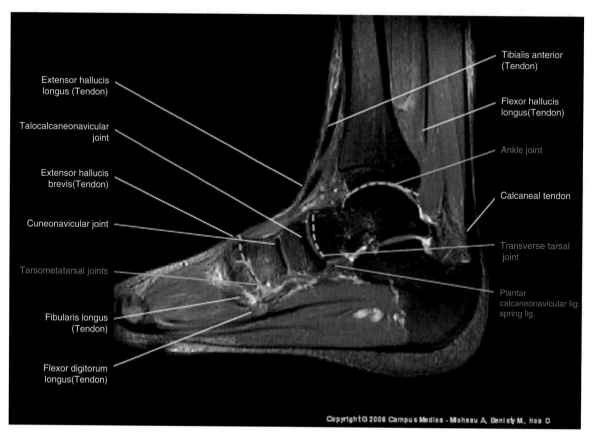

Fig. 8.48 Anatomy: sagittal view of the ankle – PD-SPIR weighted (http://www.e-anatomy.org/anatomy/human-body/limbs-skeletal/ankle-foot.html) (courtesy of e-Anatomy - Micheau A, Hoa D, www.imaios.com) www.imaios.com)

- Bursitis**
- Tendonitis**
- Ligament injury**

Injection Site

An anteromedial approach is used. The needle approach is just medial to the tibialis anterior tendon over the ankle joint.

Imaging/Radiology

Plain film radiographs: Plain films are insensitive for early bone erosion and soft tissue inflammatory change. They can be helpful for the detection of intraarticular joint body and fracture as well as arthritis. Infection (septic arthritis) may also be suggested on plain films.

Ultrasound: Ultrasound is helpful if the plain film radiographs are negative, as well as for direct visualization of early arthritic change in the joint and soft tissues. This includes synovitis of the joint and tenosynovitis of the tendons.

CT: CT is useful to exclude fracture and to evaluate the intraarticular joint bodies (osteochondral segment).

MRI: MRI is helpful to detect arthritis if the plain films are negative (Fig. 8.49). It is sensitive for synovitis and tenosynovitis. It may be useful in complex clinical situations even if ultrasound is positive.

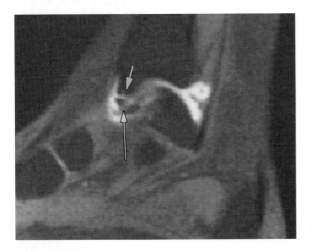

Fig. 8.49 Arthritis in the tibiotalar joint: clinical anteromedial impingement in a female hockey player. Sagittal T1-weighted fat-suppressed MR image shows anteromedial tibiotalar osteophytes (*arrows*) (Robinson and White 2002)

Indications

The three main indications for ankle joint injection are: (1) Arthritis (osteoarthritis, rheumatoid arthritis, crystal-induced arthropathy, and traumatic)**, (2) mixed connective tissue disease**, (3) synovitis**.

8.2.3.2 Injection for Achilles Tendinitis (Fig. 8.50)

Anatomy

The Achilles tendon connects the gastrocnemius and soleus muscles to the posterior aspect of the calcaneus. This tendon does not have a direct blood supply, but rather is nourished via the tendon sheath or paratendon. In the setting of Achilles tendon pathology, some

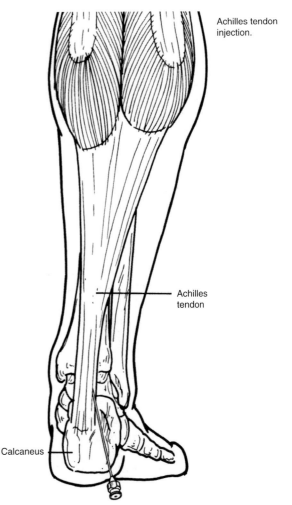

Achilles tendon injection.

Achilles tendon

Calcaneus

Fig. 8.50 Achilles tendon injection (Weiss 2007l, Fig. 4-15)

authors believe that the term Achilles tendinosis is preferable to tendinitis since there may only be intra-tendon degeneration without significant inflammation.

Function

The Achilles tendon permits plantarflexion during walking, running, or jumping. It is susceptible to injury due to the large stress placed on it by the gastrocne-mius and soleus muscles.

Clinical Presentation

Achilles tendinitis presents with pain at the back of the ankle with activity. The pain may be improved with the use of thick-heeled shoes compared to thin-heeled shoes.

Etiology

Etiologies of Achilles tendon pathology include over-use, overpronation, systemic disease such as diabetes, gout**, or other forms of arthritis**.

Differential Diagnosis

Differential diagnoses include symptomatic entheso-phyte**, ruptured plantaris tendon**, Haglund's dis-ease** (enlargement of the calcaneal tuberosity in response to chronic irritation due to compression of the retro-Achilles bursa against the posterolateral calcaneal prominence. This normally manifests as excessive fluid in the retrocalcaneal bursa, fluid in the retro-Achilles bursa, and with enlarged calcaneal tuberosity. It is also known as "pump bump."), and peroneal tendon dislocation**.

Injection Site

The injection is made several centimeters proximal to the insertion site of the Achilles tendon on the calcaneus.

Imaging/Radiology

Plain film radiographs: These are usually negative for any findings. There may be nonspecific findings for

Achilles tendinitis. These include tendon calcification associated with tendinosis or enthesophyte at the inser-tion of the Achilles tendon on the calcaneus.

Ultrasound: Real-time scanning allows dynamic evaluation of the tendon as well as assessment of pathologic thickening. The tendon appears hypoechoic compared to the adjacent soleus muscle. The study has the advantage of being performed quickly and is rela-tively inexpensive compared to MRI or CT. However, it is limited by operator dependency and the inability to distinguish a partial tear from tendinosis on MRI.

In the setting of tenosynovitis (inflammation of the tendon sheath) or peritendinitis (inflammation adjacent to the tendon), there may be an echogenic tendon sur-rounded by fluid in the tendon sheath. In the setting of tendinosis/tendinitis vs. partial rupture, the appearance may be similar on ultrasound. There are foci of decreased echogenicity with increase in the size of the tendon as well as indistinctness of the tendon margins. In the setting of complete tendon rupture, there may be a gap in the tendon with contraction of the disrupted segments. Ultrasound is useful for injections.

CT: CT is inferior to MRI in the detection of most pathology including tenosynovitis, peritendinitis, ten-dinitis, tendon rupture, and tendon dislocation or sub-luxation. It is also less sensitive than MRI in the detection of tendon degeneration as well as inflamma-tory fluid. Additionally, it is less sensitive in distin-guishing scar from edema. It is however superior to MRI in demonstrating calcifications, bone fragments, or spurs, which may complicate tendon dislocation or rupture. It is also superior to MRI in detecting the con-genital abnormality of convex retromalleolar groove. (The retromalleolar groove of the distal fibula stabi-lizes the peroneal tendons when concave. There is a predisposition to peroneal tendon dislocation and injury when the retromalleolar groove is convex in the axial plane). See differential diagnosis section.

MRI: MRI is useful for presurgical evaluation and in the evaluation of recalcitrant situations when there is suspected partial or complete tendon rupture. It is superior overall compared to all other radiological modalities. In the setting of tenosynovitis or peritendi-nitis, there is fluid in and around the tendon, which may in turn be surrounded by the low signal intensity tendon sheath. Pannus and scar can be shown by inter-mediate signal intensity around the tendon. In the set-ting of tendinosis/tendinitis, there is increased signal within the tendon itself on both T1-weighted and pro-ton density weighted images. In chronic tendinitis or peritendinitis, there is a hypertrophied tendon with decreased signal intensity on both T1- and T2-weighted images (this is not usually detectable on CT) (Fig. 8.51). In the clinical scenario of tendon rupture, the early or type I rupture is manifested by an enlarged tendon with heterogeneously increased signal intensity (Fig. 8.52). In type II tendon rupture, there is focal decrease in the size of the tendon at the site of the rupture. In complete tendon rupture (type III), there is a gap in the substance of the tendon with contraction of the disrupted segments (Schweitzer and Karasick 2000; Cheung et al. 1992).

Indication

The main indication for injection is Achilles tendinopathy** (Ryan et al. 2010). This is a controversial procedure however due to the risk of tendon rupture.

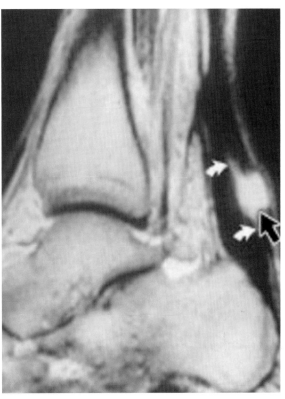

Fig. 8.52 A 58-year-old-woman with partial Achilles tendon tear. Sagittal T2-weighted MR image (TR/TE, 6,000/80) shows partial posterior Achilles tendon tear (*black arrow*). Longitudinal interstitial tear (*white arrows*) and evidence of underlying hypoxic degeneration with thickened tendon can also be seen (Schweitzer and Karasick 2000)

Complications

Tendon rupture** is the chief complication of Achilles tendon injection.

8.2.3.3 Subtalar Joint Injection for Sinus Tarsi Syndrome (Subtalar Impingement Syndrome) (Figs. 8.53 and 8.54)

Anatomy

The sinus tarsi is a space between the neck of the talus and the anterosuperior calcaneus, talocalcaneonavicular joint, and the posterior facet of the subtalar joint. The sinus tarsi contain fat arteries, joint capsules, and nerves. The five ligaments within the space include the cervical ligament, the interosseous talocalcaneal ligament, as well as the medial, intermediate, and lateral root of the

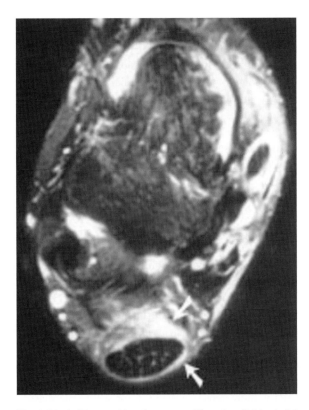

Fig. 8.51 A 47-year-old-male runner with peritendinitis. Axial T2-weighted fat-suppressed MR image (TR/TE, 4,000/78) shows thin rim of partially circumferential high signal (*arrows*), which represents mild peritendinitis. Background mucoid degeneration within tendon and intratendon signal can be seen (Schweitzer and Karasick 2000)

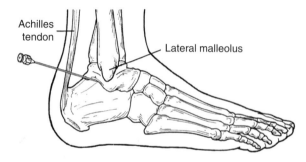

Fig. 8.53 Subtalar joint injection, lateral approach (Weiss 2007m, Fig. 3-33)

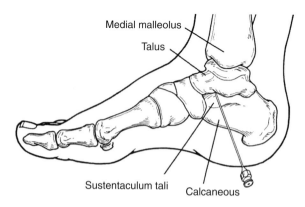

Fig. 8.54 Subtalar joint injection, medial approach. (Weiss 2007n, Fig. 3-31)

inferior extensor retinaculum. All of these ligaments are involved in stabilizing the hindfoot. Sinus tarsi syndrome is caused by repeated impingement of the sinus tarsi space when the foot has more pronation than normal.

Clinical Presentation

Pain in the lateral and anterior ankle region worsened with prolonged weightbearing associated with swelling and tenderness of the lateral ankle joint. Subtalar arthroscopy is the diagnostic study of choice.

Injection Site

A lateral approach may be utilized between the lateral malleolus and the Achilles tendon. A medial approach may also be utilized between the sustentaculum tali and the medial malleolus.

Etiology

Etiologies include trauma**, interosseous talocalcaneal ligament tear**, subtalar instability**, fibrous tarsal coalition**, chronic inflammation**, osteochondral injuries** of the subtalar joint, ankylosing spondylitis**, rheumatoid arthritis**, gout**, ganglion cyst**, foot deformities (pes cavus** and pes planus**), and pigmented villonodular synovitis** (Frey et al. 1999).

Differential Diagnosis

Differential diagnoses include arthritis**, anterolateral ankle impingement**, chronic ankle sprain**.

Imaging/Radiology

Plain film radiographs: Plain films are usually normal, but degenerative joint disease of the subtalar joint may be seen.

Fluoroscopy and ultrasound: Most injections can be performed safely and accurately using palpation of anatomic landmarks by experienced operators. Fluoroscopy or ultrasound may be helpful in challenging situations. Ultrasound can avoid the overlying neurovascular bundle or tendons. There is limited peer reviewed literature on the diagnostic utility of ultrasound in evaluating the sinus tarsi or subtalar joint.

CT: Rupture of the interosseus ligaments may be seen on CT when soft tissue or fluid is occupying the sinus tarsi, which normally contains fat. Thin-slice coronal CT may demonstrate the ligaments in normal patients however; they may not be seen when torn.

MRI: Multiplanar thin section (1- to 3-mm slice thickness) including 3D coronal gradient-echo imaging is performed. Inflammatory and fibrotic change of the tarsal sinus fat may be seen (Fig. 8.55). The interosseous talocalcaneal ligament may be torn. There may also be tears of the cervical ligament. In addition, synovial thickening may be identified. It is noted, however, that MRI is inadequate compared to arthroscopy for detecting interosseous talocalcaneal ligament tear. MRI is more sensitive than CT for soft tissue masses and ligament tears (Lee et al. 2008) MR arthrography in conjunction with 3D MRI may further improve the sensitivity of detection of sinus tarsi interosseus ligament tears (Lektrakul et al. 2001).

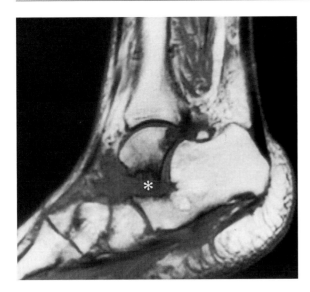

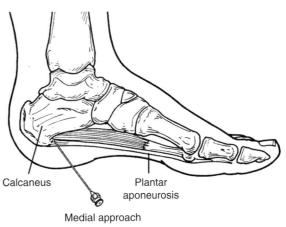

Fig. 8.56 Plantar fascia injection (Weiss 2007o, Fig. 4-13)

Fig. 8.55 Sinus tarsi syndrome in a patient with rheumatoid arthritis. Sagittal T1-weighted MR image shows obliteration of fat by an area of fluid-like signal intensity in the subtalar joint (*asterisk*) (Rosenberg et al. 2000)

Indications

The four main indications in Sinus tarsi syndrome** include: (1) Inversion injury**, (2) lateral collateral ligament tear**, (3) biomechanical strain (secondary to posterior tibial tendon tear in flat foot deformity)**, and (4) rheumatoid arthritis**.

8.2.3.4 Plantar Fasciitis Injection (Fig. 8.56)

Anatomy

The plantar fascia is a fibrous structure often called an aponeurosis that attaches between the proximal phalanges and the base of the calcaneus at the medial calcaneal tuberosity. In plantar fasciitis, there is really no significant inflammation present. It is more accurately classified as a tendinosis. The pathologic changes consist of increased fibroblast activity and lack of organization of the collagen fibers.

Function

The plantar fascia supports the arch of the foot. It is somewhat longer than normal in pes planus (flatfeet deformity) and somewhat shorter than normal in pes cavus.

Clinical Presentation

Plantar fasciitis is most common cause of heel pain in adults. The heel pain is characterized as being worst in the initial steps upon weightbearing in the morning. The pain is improved with continued ambulation, but worsened with further prolonged weightbearing. There is associated tenderness at the medial calcaneal tuberosity.

Etiology

Etiologies include overuse (running), obesity, and repetitive trauma.

Differential Diagnosis

Differential diagnoses include:

- Symptomatic heel spur**
- Plantar fascia rupture**
- Lateral plantar nerve entrapment/tarsal tunnel syndrome**
- Injury or pathology of the medial calcaneal branch of the posterior tibial nerve**
- Abductor digiti quinti nerve entrapment**
- Neuropathy
- Heel contusion**
- Posterior tibial tendonitis**
- Calcaneal enthesitis**
- Calcaneal stress fracture**
- Paget's disease**
- Calcaneal tumor**

Injection Site

The injection site is at the medial aspect of the foot along the medial calcaneus.

Imaging/Radiology

Plain film radiographs: There is limited usefulness for plain film radiographs. Calcification can be seen in the soft tissues along with enthesophyte formation (heel spurs). Enthesophytes at the insertion of the plantar fascia tendon are not specific and can be seen in asymptomatic patients. Plain films can be useful in evaluating for other etiologies of heel pain such as osteomyelitis, foreign bodies, or fracture.

Ultrasonography: Chronic plantar fasciitis may demonstrate thickening of the heel aponeurosis at 6–10 mm in thickness vs. the normal thickness of 2–4 mm. A complete tear may be seen as an area of discontinuity of the aponeurosis.

MRI: MRI is usually not necessary for the evaluation of plantar fasciitis. It may be useful however in patients refractory to conservative therapy by excluding the differential diagnosis. In situations of chronic plantar fasciitis, there is thickening of the plantar fascia greater than 5 mm with surrounding edema (Fig. 8.57). There may be increased signal intensity on T1-weighted images involving the plantar fascia as well as adjacent calcaneal marrow edema. A plantar enthesophyte may also be visualized on MRI. A plantar fascia tear will be visualized as discontinuity of the plantar fascia. There may be linear intrafascial increased signal intensity on the STIR sequence.

Scintigraphy: Nuclear medicine bone scintigraphy has excellent sensitivity for plantar fasciitis, but has decreased specificity. Plantar fasciitis is manifested as increased focal activity at the plantar fascia insertion on the calcaneal tuberosity.

Indications

The main indication for injection is plantar fasciitis**.

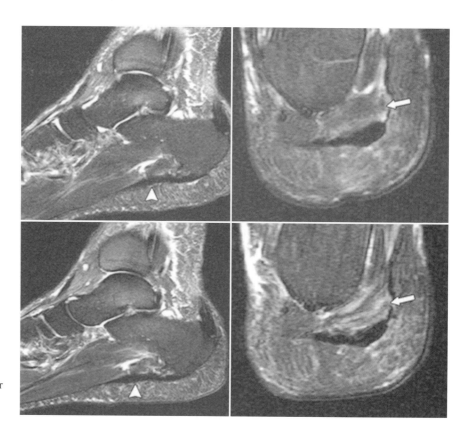

Fig. 8.57 Plantar fasciitis. Sagittal (4,000/108) (*left*) and coronal (4,000/108) (*right*) T2-weighted fat-saturated fast SE images of the hind foot before (*top*) and after (*bottom*) ESWT. Mild soft-tissue and perifascial edema (*arrow*) and thickened plantar fascia (*arrowhead*) are clearly depicted on the pre-ESWT images; the perifascial and surrounding soft-tissue edema increased after ESWT. Thickness of the fascia was little affected (9.0 mm before and 9.2 mm after ESWT on sagittal and 9.1 mm both before and after ESWT on coronal images) (Zhu et al. 2005)

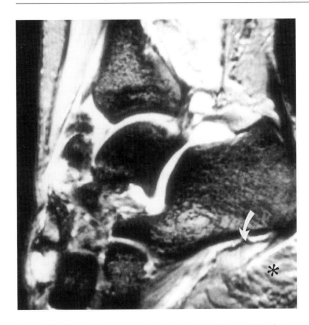

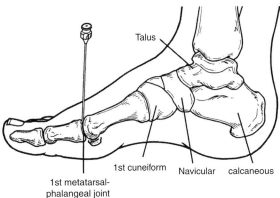

Fig. 8.59 First metatarsal-phalangeal joint injection (Weiss 2007p, Fig. 3-37)

Fig. 8.58 Tear of the plantar fascia. Sagittal T2*-weighted gradient-echo MR image demonstrates discontinuity and intrasubstance tearing at the calcaneal insertion site of the plantar fascia (*arrow*). Note also the edematous subcutaneous tissue (*asterisk*) (Rosenberg et al. 2000)

with the distal first metatarsal (metatarsosesamoid joint). The sesamoid also lies within a reinforced portion of the joint capsule called the plantar plate.

Function

The first metatarsophalangeal joint performs flexion and extension as well as minimal medial and lateral excursion or circumduction.

Complications

The main complication encountered in plantar fascia injection is plantar fascia tendon rupture** (Fig. 8.58).

Clinical Presentation

Metatarsophalangeal joint arthritis presents with pain and stiffness of the first metatarsophalangeal joint especially with motion. There may also be associated decreased range of motion.

8.2.3.5 Injection for First Metatarsophalangeal Joint Arthritis (Fig. 8.59)

Etiology

Etiologies include osteoarthritis**, gout**, inflammatory arthritis** (rheumatoid arthritis**, psoriatic arthritis**, and Reiter's disease**), and infection**.

Anatomy

The first metatarsophalangeal joint is a condyloid type synovial joint where the distal first metatarsal is convex and the base of the first proximal phalanx is slightly concave. The joint is surrounded by a joint capsule between the base of the first proximal phalanx and the neck of the distal metatarsal. The joint is stabilized by ligaments, the sesamoid complex, as well as the plantar plate and surrounding tendons. There is a collateral ligament medially and laterally spanning the joint. The extensor tendon expands at the joint to stabilize it at the dorsal surface of the joint. There are adjacent sesamoid bones within each of the heads of the flexor hallucis tendon. The superior aspect of the sesamoid forms a joint

Differential Diagnosis

Differential diagnoses include turf toe** (tear or sprain of the first metatarsophalangeal joint capsule and ligaments at the plantar surface), nerve impingement involving the medial branch of the plantar digital nerve, Freiberg's infraction (avascular necrosis of the distal first metatarsal), and absent sesamoid bone**.

Injection Site

Injection is made at the extensor aspect of the first metatarsophalangeal joint.

Imaging/Radiology

Plain film radiographs: Osteoarthritis is manifested by joint space loss, subchondral sclerosis, osteophytes, and cystic changes.

Gout is manifested by erosions at the medial dorsal surface of the distal first metatarsal with overhanging margins being characteristic. There is preservation of normal bone density. Joint space loss, however, is seen late and may be non-uniform. There is paraarticular soft tissue swelling, which has a cloud-like appearance (tophi) with associated amorphous calcification. There may be punctate sclerosis within the bone representing intraosseous tophi.

Rheumatoid arthritis is manifested by marginal erosion joint space loss, cyst, and periarticular osteopenia, as well as soft tissue swelling.

Psoriatic arthritis is manifested by erosions at the articular surface, which can result in a pencil-in-cup deformity. They may also occur at the joint capsule laterally. There is associated proliferative bone change including periosteal reaction.

Calcium pyrophosphate deposition disease can appear similar to gout with soft tissue swelling and periarticular calcification especially at the medial aspect of the first metatarsophalangeal joint. In advanced arthritis, hallux valgus deformity and metatarsosesamoid subluxation may be seen.

Ultrasound: Ultrasound may be more sensitive than radiography in detecting osteophytes and joint space narrowing in osteoarthritis. Furthermore, ultrasound detects synovitis on gray-scale imaging as well as increased power Doppler signal in the setting of inflammation. It is also useful to evaluate pathology at the metacarpophalangeal and interphalangeal joints for detection of tenosynovitis. It is more sensitive than radiography and the clinical exam in rheumatoid arthritis for erosions and inflammation (Szkudlarek et al. 2004).

In gouty arthritis, deposition of monosodium urate crystal on the cartilaginous surface as well as tophaceous material within the first metatarsophalangeal joint, may be seen (Thiele and Schlesinger 2007). In addition, erosions, effusions, and synovial hypertrophy with hypervascularity on power Doppler imaging may be seen. The findings are specific for gout and provide a noninvasive means of diagnosis. Ultrasound is more sensitive than plain films to diagnose gouty arthritis.

CT: CT is slightly more sensitive than plain films for erosions. It is less sensitive for synovitis compared to ultrasound or MRI. Paraarticular nodules or calcification may be seen in gout. CT can define erosions and tophus size in gout (Dalbeth and McQueen 2009).

MRI: MRI is the most sensitive modality in rheumatoid arthritis for visualizing early inflammatory and destructive changes, which include erosions, synovitis, bone marrow edema, tenosynovitis, and ethesitis (Szkudlarek et al. 2004).

In gout, standard characteristics of arthritis may be seen including joint effusion, bone marrow and soft tissue edema, as well as enhancement of the paraarticular surface. In addition, tophi are seen on MRI, which have a variable appearance on MRI depending on the degree of calcification and water content. MRI is useful to monitor tophus size during treatment (Fig. 8.60).

MRI is usually used to demonstrate Freiberg's infraction especially if plain films are normal.

Scintigraphy: Bone scan demonstrates increased activity at the joint. It is sensitive, but not specific for the type of arthritis.

Indications

The three main indications for first metatarsophalangeal joint injection are: (1) Arthritis (gout, osteo, CPPD, rheumatoid)**; (2) turf toe (traumatic arthrosis seen in football lineman)**; (3) synovitis**.

8.3 Lower Extremity Nerve Blocks

8.3.1 Obturator Nerve Block (Fig. 8.61)

8.3.1.1 Anatomy

The obturator nerve is derived from the ventral rami L2 to L4. It combines within the psoas and arises as a single nerve from the medial margin of the psoas continuing inferiorly and anteriorly with respect to the sacral ala. It continues posterior to the common iliac vasculature and courses adjacent to the lateral wall of

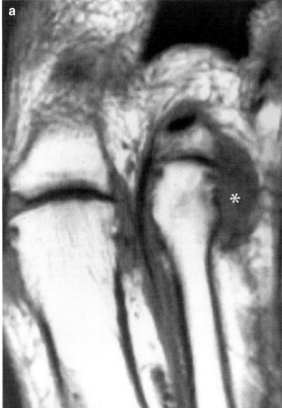

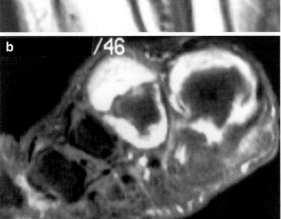

Fig. 8.60 Gout. First and second metatarsophalangeal joints. Long-axis T1-weighted (**a**), and contrast-enhanced fat-saturated T1-weighted (**b**) MR images demonstrate a tophus adjacent to the second metatarsophalangeal joint (*asterisk*) with low signal intensity on (**a**) and high signal intensity on (**b**). Note the presence of a second enhancing tophus in the first metatarsophalangeal joint in (**b**) (Rosenberg et al. 2000)

the lesser pelvis. The nerve is localized lateral to the ureter and internal iliac vasculature. It then splits into anterior and posterior branches after entry into the superior portion of the obturator foramen.

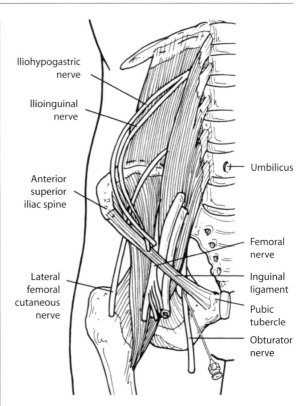

Fig. 8.61 Obturator nerve injection (Weiss 2007q, Fig. 6-23)

8.3.1.2 Function

The obturator nerve provides sensation to the skin over the medial portion of the thigh that may continue inferiorly to the knee. It also supplies motor innervation to the abductor muscles (obturator externus, adductor longus, adductor brevis, adductor magnus, and adductor gracilis).

8.3.1.3 Clinical Presentation

Obturator nerve entrapment/injury presents as exercise-related groin pain and pain in the adductor origin in the pubic bone. The pain may radiate to the medial thigh all the way to the knee. There may also be decreased sensation in the medial thigh. The patient may present with difficulty in walking or instability in the lower extremity. There may also be pain in the adductor origin in the pubic bone, which may radiate from the medial thigh to the knee. There may be weakness of the muscles innervated by the obturator nerve if neuropathy is severe.

8.3.1.4 Etiology

Etiologies can include fractures/tumor**, pelvic trauma**, delivery (compression by the fetal head or fetal lower limb during delivery), surgery** (total hip arthroplasty**), prolonged lower limb malposition.

8.3.1.5 Differential Diagnosis

Differential diagnoses include upper lumbar radiculopathy**, femoral neuropathy**, ilioinguinal neuropathy, iliohypogastric neuropathy, and genitofemoral neuropathy.

8.3.1.6 Injection Site

Injection is made using a medial proximal thigh approach 4 cm lateral to the pubic tubercle with the direction of the needle slightly inferior into the superomedial aspect of the obturator foramen.

8.3.1.7 Imaging/Radiology

Plain film radiographs: Plain films have limited usefulness but may exclude acetabular fracture or subchondral cysts. Flouroscopy can guide injection.

Ultrasound: Sonography can demonstrate cysts. It is also capable of directly visualizing the nerve. In addition, it may be useful in guiding cyst aspiration and obturator nerve block (Akkaya et al. 2009).

MRI: The external obturator, gracilis, and adductor muscles may demonstrate increased signal intensity (denervation edema) on T2-weighted and STIR sequences and fatty atrophy on T1-weighted sequences (Fig. 8.62). The nerve may be seen (though not reliably) as a hypointense dark cord-like structure on T1-weighted sagittal images in the pelvic fatty tissue lateral to the urinary bladder (Marhofer et al. 2000). Acetabular labral cysts may be identified as being responsible for compression of the nerve.

8.3.1.8 Indications

The main indication for obturator nerve injection is obturator neuralgia/neuropathy.

8.3.1.9 Complications

Hematoma due to puncture of the obturator artery can be a complication of obturator nerve injection.

8.3.2 Femoral Nerve Injection (Fig. 8.63)

8.3.2.1 Anatomy

The femoral nerve is the largest branch of the lumbar plexus, which originates from the L2 through L4 nerve

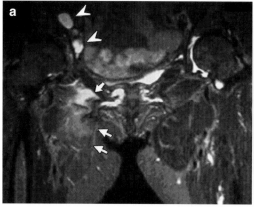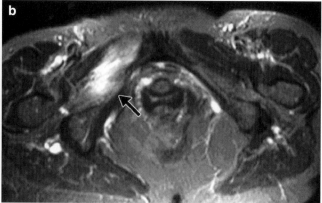

Fig. 8.62 (**a, b**) Obturator neuropathy in a 75-year-old-woman with pain in the right groin and anteromedial thigh. (**a**) Coronal STIR image (TR/TE, 6,000/60; inversion time, 130 ms) shows cystic lesion (*arrowheads*) on lateral wall of the lesser pelvis and increased signal intensity in the external obturator and adductor muscles (*arrows*). (**b**) Axial STIR image (TR/TE, 6,000/60; inversion time, 130 ms) shows increased signal intensity in the external obturator and adductor muscles (*arrow*) (Yukata et al. 2005)

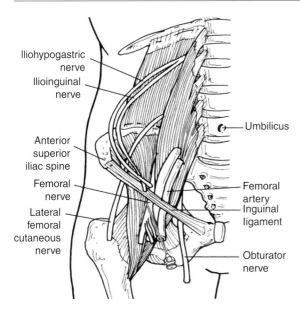

Iliohypogastric nerve

Ilioinguinal nerve

Anterior superior iliac spine

Femoral nerve

Lateral femoral cutaneous nerve

Umbilicus

Femoral artery

Inguinal ligament

Obturator nerve

Fig. 8.63 Femoral nerve injection (Weiss 2007r, Fig. 6-25)

roots. It is formed at the lateral margin of the psoas and dives inferiorly between this muscle and the iliacus. It continues below the inguinal ligament lateral to the common femoral artery (Fig. 8.64).

8.3.2.2 Function

The femoral nerve provides sensory branches in the superior thigh to supply the anterosuperior thigh. It supplies muscular branches to the quadriceps. Its major branch is the lateral femoral cutaneous nerve. There is also a medial femoral cutaneous branch, which supplies sensation to the medial distal thigh and knee. It also supplies the suprapatellar and patellar region in addition to the saphenous nerve.

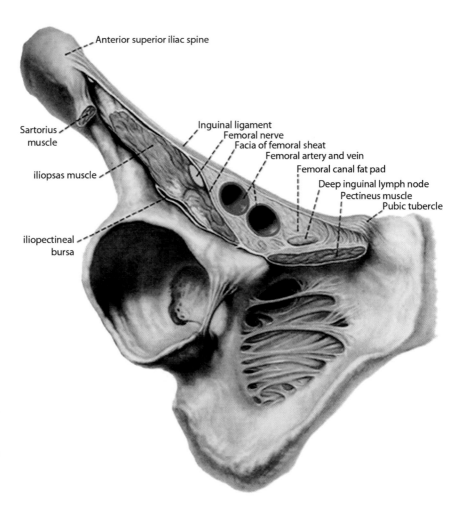

Anterior superior iliac spine

Sartorius muscle

iliopsas muscle

iliopectineal bursa

Inguinal ligament
Femoral nerve
Facia of femoral sheat
Femoral artery and vein
Femoral canal fat pad
Deep inguinal lymph node
Pectineus muscle
Pubic tubercle

Fig. 8.64 Illustration of the femoral canal and femoral sheath. The long adductor muscle, which is not shown, lies medial and anterior to the pectineal muscle (Shadbolt et al. 2001)

8.3.2.3 Clinical Presentation

Femoral neuropathy results in inguinal pain as well as anterior thigh and anteromedial leg pain/numbness. There can be associated sensory loss/pain in the saphenous nerve distribution as well as quadriceps weakness. Entrapment neuropathy usually occurs at or below the inguinal ligament.

8.3.2.4 Etiology

Femoral nerve pathology may originate from injury, pelvic or inguinal. This may be iatrogenic such as needle punctures or due to surgical retractors. The most common etiology, however, is diabetic amyotrophy. Injury can also occur in the setting of total hip arthroplasty** (heat injury from methylmethacrylate), pelvic surgery**, difficult childbirth, pelvic fractures**, acute hyperextension of the thigh, pelvic radiation**, and appendiceal** or renal abscesses**/tumors**, as well as retroperitoneal hemorrhage** or inguinal hemorrhage** as in post-catheterization or PTCA**.

8.3.2.5 Differential Diagnosis

Differential diagnose include lumbar plexopathy**, lumbar radiculopathy**, obturator neuropathy**, lateral femoral cutaneous neuropathy**, and genitofemoral neuropathy**.

8.3.2.6 Injection Site

Lateral aspect of the femoral canal at the inguinal ligament.

8.3.2.7 Imaging/Radiology

Ultrasound: Ultrasound may be useful for mass lesions along the course of the femoral nerve. It may also be useful for guidance in performing femoral nerve block; in addition, it can be useful in guidance for decompression of causative cystic structures such as the iliopsoas bursa (Gruber et al. 2003).

CT: In emergencies, CT is useful in the evaluation of hemorrhage (causing femoral nerve injury) related to surgery/arterial catheterization or trauma, as well as other forms of abdominal pathology (acute or chronic) including tumor, abscess, or aneurysm (Fig. 8.65).

MRI: MRI is similarly useful for the evaluation of mass lesions if CT is negative. (Weiss and Tolo 2008) Denervation edema in the quadriceps muscle may be suggestive of femoral neuropathy.

8.3.2.8 Indication

The chief indication for femoral nerve injection is femoral neuropathy.

8.3.3 Saphenous Nerve Injection
(*Figs. 8.66 and 8.67*)

8.3.3.1 Anatomy

The saphenous nerve originates from the femoral nerve as its longest branch in the groin and follows the course of a superficial femoral artery under the sartorius to the adductor canal at the inferior aspect of the adductor magnus. The nerve then deviates from the course of the superficial femoral artery at this site to the medial aspect of the knee. It becomes subcutaneous by traversing the connective tissue at the superficial aspect of the adductor canal 10 cm proximal to the medial femoral epicondyle. A branch forms the infrapatellar plexus whereas the main nerve extends into the medial leg and foot.

8.3.3.2 Function

The saphenous nerve innervates the skin at the medial and anterior aspect of the knee as well as the medial and dorsal aspect of the foot. It provides no motor supply.

8.3.3.3 Clinical Presentation

Entrapment neuropathy of the saphenous nerve is manifested by aching in the thigh and medial knee with paresthesias in the distribution of the nerve in the

Fig. 8.65 CT scans of a 77-year-old-woman with right groin and thigh hematoma after PTCA. Hematoma primarily involves the medial muscles, including the pectineus, adductor magnus, and adductor longus (Trerotola et al. 1991). A hematoma of this kind can result in femoral nerve injury

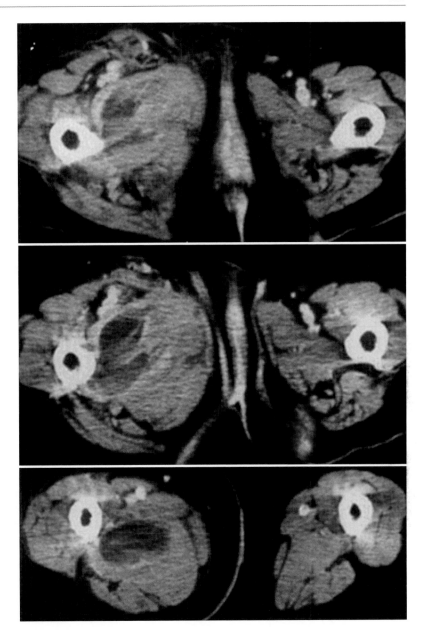

leg and foot. There may be associated numbness/paresthesia below the knee exacerbated by bending the knee or by any form of external compression. It may be associated with direct trauma.

8.3.3.4 Etiology

Etiologies include improperly protected knee or head support during surgery; entrapment of the saphenous nerve in Hunter's canal; compressive syndromes (femoral vessels, pes anserine bursitis**, tumor**); femoral popliteal bypass or saphenous vein stripping**; trauma**; tumor (exostoses**, leiomyosarcoma**); and meniscal cyst**.

8.3.3.5 Differential Diagnosis

Different diagnoses include lumbar radiculopathy**, lower extremity vascular insufficiency**, other etiologies of medial knee pain.

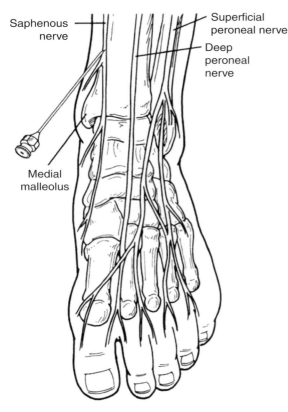

Fig. 8.66 Saphenous nerve injection at the ankle (Weiss 2007s, Fig. 6-27)

8.3.3.6 Injection Site

There are two main injection sites. (1) Distal medial thigh: The injection is usually performed along the course of the nerve proximal to the site of entrapment. This can be performed where it pierces the superficial connective tissue in Hunter's canal at the site of its sharp angulation (10 cm proximal to the medial femoral condyle). This is usually where there is point tenderness. (2) Medial ankle: Another site of injection is at the medial ankle adjacent to the medial malleolus volar aspect medial to the tibialis anterior.

8.3.3.7 Imaging/Radiology

Ultrasound: Sonography may be useful for guidance. It may also be able to delineate mass lesions including cysts along the course of the nerve (Tsui and Ozelsel 2009).

   MRI: This modality can directly visualize the saphenous nerve throughout its course. It is also able to evaluate mass lesions throughout the course of the saphenous nerve and exclude other pathology (Fig. 8.68).

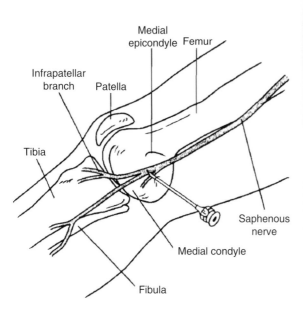

Fig. 8.67 The course of the saphenous nerve is shown as it passes over the medial condyle of the femur, splitting into terminal sensory branches. Note the site of injection at the medial aspect of the knee joint (Raj and Lou, Fig. 26-9)

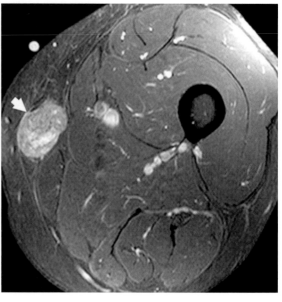

Fig. 8.68 Leiomyosarcoma arising from the saphenous vein in a 53-year-old-man. Axial gadolinium-enhanced T1-weighted (675/17) fat-suppressed SE MR image shows homogeneous moderate enhancement of the mass (*arrow*) (Murphey et al. 1999). Such an invasive tumor can result in pain mediated by the saphenous nerve

8.3.3.8 Indications

Saphenous neuropathy is the main indication for saphenous nerve injection.

8.3.4 Sciatic Nerve Injection in the Popliteal Fossa (Fig. 8.69)

8.3.4.1 Anatomy

The sciatic nerve courses into the thigh under the lower margin of the gluteus maximus. It continues inferiorly adjacent to the adductor magnus and is covered by the long head of the biceps femoris. The nerve then divides in the popliteal fossa into the tibial nerve and common peroneal nerve. The tibial nerve arises from the sciatic nerve. The tibial nerve then courses through the popliteal fossa deep to the arch of the soleus.

The tibial nerve provides innervation through branches within the popliteal fossa to the gastrocnemius, popliteus, soleus, and plantaris muscles, a branch to the knee joint, as well as a sensory branch that turns into the sural nerve. The sural nerve is supplemented by branches of the common peroneal nerve and travels through the posterior leg to supply the outer portion of the foot. The tibial nerve lies adjacent to the tibia, inferior to the soleus, and supplies the tibialis posterior, flexor hallucis longus, and the flexor digitorum longus. The tibial nerve continues into the foot running behind to the medial malleolus. Here the nerve travels adjacent to the posterior tibial artery (posterior tibial nerve) surrounded by the flexor retinaculum.

The common, superficial, and deep peroneal nerve anatomy is discussed in their respective sections.

8.3.4.2 Function

Below the knee, the sciatic nerve also provides motor supply to flex and extend the ankle. Furthermore, it provides sensory supply to the posterolateral aspect of the knee, as well as the entire lower leg, toes, foot, and knee.

8.3.4.3 Injection Site

A transverse view with ultrasound is obtained with the patient in a prone position of the popliteal fossa crease. Proximal and distal scanning is used to identify the branching point of the sciatic nerve into its tibial and peroneal divisions. The sciatic nerve is blocked prior to its division. It is seen as a hyperechoic structure lateral to the popliteal artery.

8.3.4.4 Imaging/Radiology

Ultrasound: Sonography provides a useful technique to localize the sciatic nerve as it passes through the popliteal fossa prior to its bifurcation (Fig. 8.70).

8.3.4.5 Indications

Analgesia for surgical procedures of the foot and ankle, palliation of pain due to malignancy, and acute pain due to injuries of the lower extremity are the main indications for this injection.

8.3.5 Common Peroneal Nerve Block (Fig. 8.71)

8.3.5.1 Anatomy

The common peroneal nerve enters the peroneal or fibular tunnel formed by the origin of the peroneus

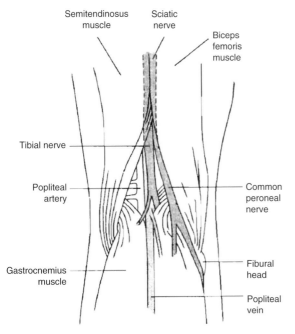

Fig. 8.69 Sciatic nerve at the popliteal fossa (Raj and Lou, Fig. 26-22)

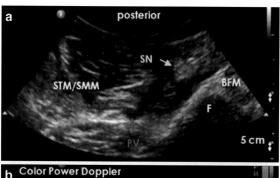

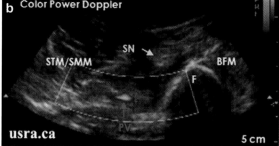

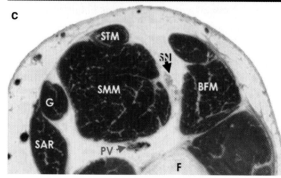

Fig. 8.70 (**a–c**) *BFM* biceps femoris muscle; *F* femur; *G* gracilis muscle; *PV* popliteal vessels; *SAR* sartorius muscle; *SN* sciatic nerve (*arrow*); *SMM* semimembranosus muscle; *STM* semitendinosus muscle (http://www.usra.ca/sb_sciaticpopliteal). (Reproduced with permission from Vincent Chan, MD, FRCPC)

longus tendon. The nerve can be compressed, as it lies adjacent to the neck of the fibula within the peroneal tunnel. This occurs during plantar flexion or foot inversion. It is the most common nerve entrapment syndrome of the lower extremity (Fig. 8.72).

8.3.5.2 Function

The common peroneal nerve (L4-S2) provides sensory supply to the anterolateral leg and dorsum of the foot. It also provides motor supply to the short head of the biceps femoris (flexor of the leg), tibialis anterior, fibularis, and extensor muscles that dorsiflex and invert the foot as well as adduct the toes.

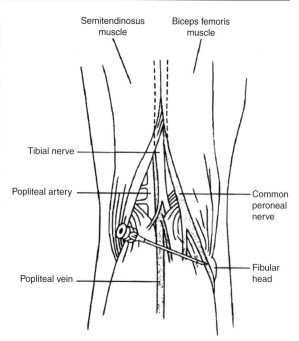

Fig. 8.71 Common peroneal nerve block (Raj and Lou, Fig. 26-21)

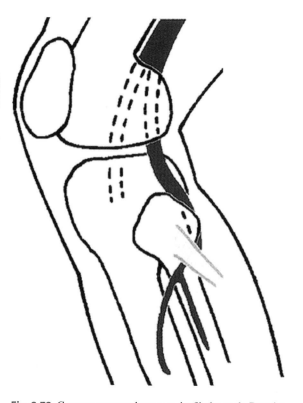

Fig. 8.72 Common peroneal nerve at the fibular neck. Drawing of the anterolateral aspect of the leg shows the course of the common peroneal nerve (*dark gray region*) and its superficial and deep branches. The *light gray region* represents the origin of the peroneus longus muscle (Martinoli et al. 2000)

8.3.5.3 Clinical Presentation

Common peroneal nerve entrapment is manifested by pain and tenderness overlying the peroneal tunnel. There is pain overlying the sensory distribution of the nerves worsened by foot inversion. There is numbness over the dermatome supplied by the nerve with foot-drop and flattening of the foot, during walking, in more advanced stages.

8.3.5.4 Etiology

In addition to repetitive use injury (running, paddling, and squatting), it is seen in the setting of trauma (fibular head fracture**, knee dislocation**, etc.), surgery (post total knee arthroplasty**, tibial osteotomy**, etc.), as well as cystic lesions such as synovial cyst** or ganglion cyst**. It may also be seen in the setting of tumors, which could be soft tissue** or osseous** (exostosis**), as well as popliteal artery aneurysm**. It may also be seen in anatomic variations as well as in the setting of rapid weight loss.

8.3.5.5 Differential Diagnosis

Differential diagnoses include tibial stress fracture**, lumbar radiculopathy **/sciatica, and shin splints.

8.3.5.6 Injection Site

A lateral approach is used with the leg slightly flexed. The needle is placed toward the neck of the fibula using palpation.

8.3.5.7 Imaging/Radiology

Plain film radiographs: Plain films may demonstrate calcified lesions or bony abnormalities (osteochondroma), as well as fracture in the trauma setting. However, they are usually negative.

Ultrasound: High-resolution ultrasound may delineate the common peroneal nerve from its origin in the popliteal fossa to the superior fibula. It may identify mass lesions (ganglion cyst, etc.) and nerve pathology due to inflammation along the course of the nerve. Duplex and color ultrasonography can detect a popliteal aneurysm within the popliteal fossa (Fig. 8.73).

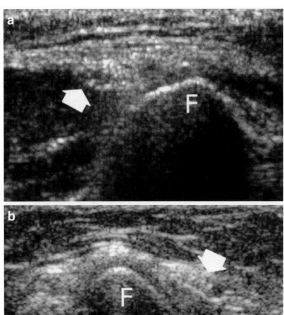
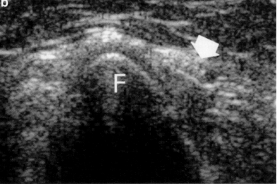

Fig. 8.73 Common peroneal nerve at the fibular neck. (**a, b**) Transverse 5- to 12-MHz US scans show the common peroneal nerve (*arrow*) before (**a**) and after (**b**) winding around the fibular neck. Note the close relationship of the nerve to the osseous surface of the fibula (*F*) (Martinoli et al. 2000)

CT: CT is sensitive for bony abnormality along the course of the peroneal nerve. The nerve is not directly seen as in ultrasound or MRI.

MRI: MRI can identify the common peroneal nerve and its divisions. MRI can also evaluate the distal thigh and leg including the popliteal fossa for mass lesions (ganglion cyst, etc.) and nerve pathology including inflammation (Fig. 8.74). MRI can detect a biceps femoris variation involving the posterior and distal extension of this muscle. This creates a tunnel through which the common peroneal nerve traverses, resulting in peroneal nerve compression. Denervation atrophy and edema in the musculature can also be detected (Hochman et al. 2004).

8.3.5.8 Indications

The main indications for common peroneal nerve injection include common peroneal neuropathy (this may be helpful in some patients as opposed to a surgical approach) and sciatic radicular pain (questionable evidence).

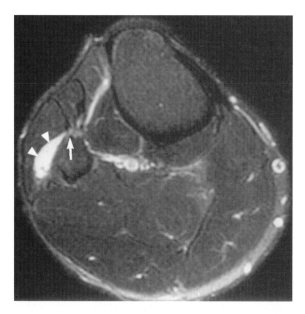

Fig. 8.74 Nerve sheath ganglion in a 25-year-old-man with peroneal nerve distribution symptoms. MR image shows a fluid-appearing mass (*arrowheads*) adjacent to the anterolateral proximal fibula and peroneal nerve (*arrow*) (Murphey et al. 1999)

8.3.6 Injection of the Superficial Peroneal Nerve (for Superficial Peroneal Tunnel Syndrome) (*Fig. 8.75*)

8.3.6.1 Anatomy

The superficial peroneal nerve branches off the common peroneal nerve at the neck of the fibula. It then continues anteriorly in the leg between the peroneus longus and brevis muscles to innervate these muscles. It then penetrates the deep fascia in the lower leg to divide into medial and dorsal cutaneous nerves and continues further distally. The superficial branch then continues into the dorsum of the foot external to the extensor retinaculum (the extensor retinaculum is an extension of the anterior leg fascia that prevents the extensor tendon at the anterior ankle from bowstringing). The superficial branch of the superficial peroneal nerve continues along the anterolateral aspect of the ankle. It is anterior to the fibula and lateral to the extensor hallucis longus. Tethering usually occurs where the superficial peroneal nerve penetrates the deep fascia. This is the peroneal tunnel where the superficial peroneal nerve may become entrapped.

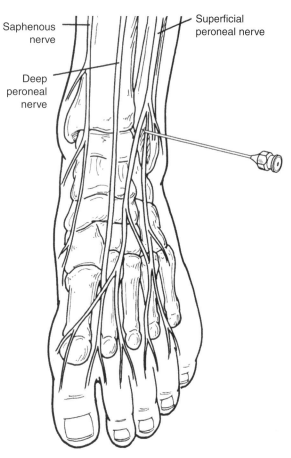

Fig. 8.75 Superficial peroneal nerve injection (Weiss 2007t, Fig. 6-33)

8.3.6.2 Function

The distal portion of the nerve at the ankle provides sensation to most of the dorsum of foot except for the first webspace between the first and second toes. The proximal portion of the nerve provides sensation to the lateral leg.

The nerve provides motor supply to the peroneus longus and brevis, which evert the foot. Foot eversion may therefore be affected if the proximal portion of the superficial peroneal nerve is affected. There is however no motor innervation at the ankle and below.

8.3.6.3 Clinical Presentation

Superficial peroneal neuropathy results in forefoot pain as well as numbness and paraesthesias in the dorsum of the foot. There is sparing of the first webspace. Weakness may indicate proximal compression of the superficial peroneal nerve or deep peroneal nerve involvement.

8.3.6.4 Etiology

Etiologies include prolonged compression (tight shoes); overstretching injury due to prolonged inversion or plantarflexion (tension neuropathy), which can occur in dancers; distal tibial fracture**; trauma**; and repetitive ankle injury**.

8.3.6.5 Differential Diagnosis

Differential diagnoses include lumbar radiculopathy**, sciatic neuropathy, peripheral neuropathy, common peroneal neuropathy**, more proximal deep peroneal neuropathy**, lumbar plexopathy**, and hypertrophy of the extensor hallucis brevis** resulting in compression and anterior compartment syndrome.

8.3.6.6 Injection Site

The needle is placed at the anterolateral ankle along the level of the malleoli at the outer aspect of the extensor hallucis longus tendon and volar aspect of the fibula.

8.3.6.7 Imaging/Radiology

Plain film radiographs: Plain films exclude fracture in the setting of trauma.

Ultrasound: Ultrasound can detect the nerve throughout its course and may demonstrate nerve enlargement indicating pathology (Canella et al. 2009).

CT: CT can exclude bony abnormality or soft tissue mass.

MRI: MRI can directly visualize the superficial peroneal nerve. It excludes mass lesions and nerve pathology (Delfaut et al. 2003) (Fig. 8.76).

8.3.6.8 Indications

The main indication for nerve block is superficial peroneal neuropathy at the anterior or anterolateral ankle.

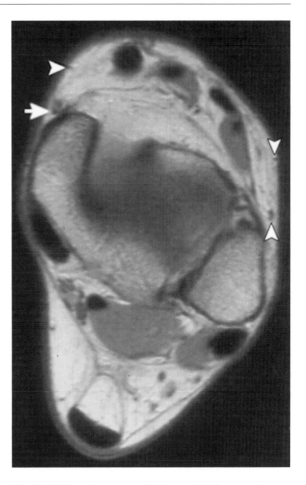

Fig. 8.76 Normal anatomy of the superficial peroneal nerve (SPN) at the ankle. Coronal oblique spin-echo T1-weighted MR image shows the subcutaneous SPN branches (*arrowheads*) and the great saphenous vein (*arrow*) (Delfaut et al. 2003)

8.3.7 Injection of the Deep Peroneal Nerve (Anterior Tarsal Tunnel Syndrome) (Fig. 8.77)

8.3.7.1 Anatomy

Anterior tarsal tunnel syndrome involves the portion of the deep peroneal nerve underneath the inferior extensor retinaculum at the ankle. The nerve may be compressed at the dorsum of the foot. The common peroneal nerve divides into the superficial and deep branches inferior to the head of the fibula. The deep peroneal nerve continues within the anterior compartment of the leg and then proceeds below the extensor retinaculum at the ankle adjacent to the extensor

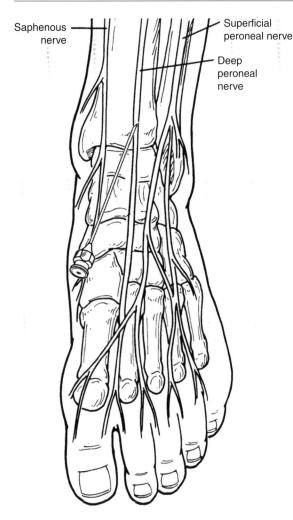

Saphenous nerve

Superficial peroneal nerve

Deep peroneal nerve

Fig. 8.77 Deep peroneal nerve injection (Weiss 2007u, Fig. 6-31)

hallucis longus at its medial aspect and the extensor digitorum longus at its lateral aspect. It bifurcates just at or in the close vicinity of the ankle joint into the sensory branch for the first interspace and the motor branch of the extensor digitorum brevis.

8.3.7.2 Function

The deep peroneal nerve provides motor innervation to the muscles of the anterior compartment of the leg except the peroneus longus and the peroneus brevis. The extensor digitorum brevis is also innervated. Distal to the extensor retinaculum at the ankle, the nerve provides sensory supply to the extensor aspect of the first webspace (involving the first two toes).

8.3.7.3 Clinical Presentation

Anterior tarsal tunnel syndrome presents as pain in the dorsomedial aspect of the foot distally worse at rest. There is numbness and tingling in the first webspace. Weakness is usually not demonstrated. In advanced cases, weakness of the extensor digitorum brevis may occur. Superior compression of the nerve outside of the anterior tarsal tunnel should be suspected when there is weakness of the muscles other than the extensor digitorum brevis (such as anterior compartment muscles of the leg).

8.3.7.4 Etiology

Etiologies include trauma** (soccer players), tight shoes (skiers), osteophytes** of the talonavicular joint, chronic prolonged compression (Muslim prayer), space occupying lesions such as ganglia**, repetitive motion, and inversion injury**.

8.3.7.5 Differential Diagnosis

Differential diagnoses include lumbar radiculopathy**, sciatic neuropathy, peripheral neuropathy, common peroneal neuropathy**, more proximal deep peroneal neuropathy**, superficial peroneal neuropathy**, lumbar plexopathy**, and hypertrophy of the extensor hallucis brevis** resulting in compression.

8.3.7.6 Injection Site

The needle is placed adjacent to the inner edge of the extensor hallucis tendon along the anterior aspect of the ankle at the level of the malleoli. The extensor retinaculum is traversed since the nerve is deep to it.

8.3.7.7 Imaging/Radiology

Plain film radiographs: Plain films can demonstrate osteophyte at the talonavicular, naviculocuneiform, and cuneometatarsal joint.

Ultrasound: Ultrasound demonstrates soft tissue anatomy including nerve thickening indicating nerve injury or damage. It is also useful for guidance.

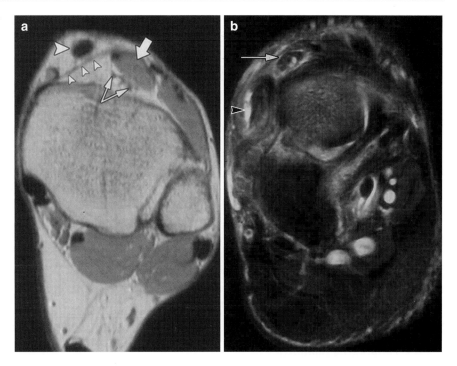

Fig. 8.78 (**a**) Normal anatomy of the anterior tarsal tunnel. Proton-density-weighted MR image (3,500/19) shows the anterior tibial tendon (*large arrowhead*), extensor hallucis longus muscle and tendon (*thick arrow*), inferior extensor retinaculum (*small arrowheads*), dorsal pedis artery, and lateral and medial terminal branches of the DPN (*thin arrows*). (**b**) Inflammatory arthritis and multiple tenosynovitis in a patient with vague foot pain and swelling. Contrast-enhanced fat-saturated T1-weighted MR image (700/12) shows tenosynovitis of the extensor digitorum longus tendon (*arrowhead*) and contrast material uptake surrounding the deep peroneal neurovascular bundle (*arrow*) (Delfaut et al. 2003)

CT: This modality may demonstrate bony anatomy, especially osteophyte and fractures in the setting of trauma. It may also demonstrate soft tissue masses.

MRI: MRI is superior for demonstrating soft tissue anatomy. The neurovascular bundle can be directly visualized within the anterior tarsal tunnel. Soft tissue swelling, hematoma, tenosynovitis of the extensor digitorum longus, arthritis, ganglion cyst, and varicosities may be seen (Delfaut et al. 2003) (Fig. 8.78).

8.3.7.8 Indications

Entrapment of the deep peroneal nerve (anterior tarsal tunnel syndrome)** is the main indication for deep peroneal nerve injection.

8.3.8 *Injection of the Sural Nerve*
(Fig. 8.79)

8.3.8.1 Anatomy

The sural nerve (L5-S1) is formed by branches of the common peroneal nerve and tibial nerve. The nerve starts inferior to the knee and courses subcutaneously

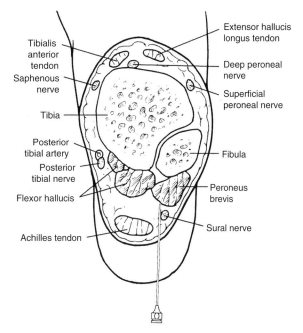

Fig. 8.79 Sural nerve injection (Weiss 2007v, Fig. 6-35)

in the back of the leg. It is in the posterior midline in the lower leg with the Achilles tendon medial to it and then courses behind the lateral malleolus continuing below the peroneal tendon sheath.

8.3.8.2 Function

The sural nerve provides sensory supply to the posterolateral leg and lateral foot including the fifth toe.

8.3.8.3 Clinical Presentation

Sural nerve injury results in numbness of the lateral foot and fifth toe as well as associated pain.

8.3.8.4 Etiology

Etiologies include soft tissue or osseous trauma to the lateral foot, as well as peroneal tendon or Achilles tendon injury. Damage may also occur after small saphenous vein ablation or posterolateral ankle surgery.

8.3.8.5 Differential Diagnosis

Differential diagnoses include S1 radiculopathy** (affects the posterior thigh as well as the sural nerve distribution), peripheral, sciatic, tibial**, peroneal**, and lumbar plexopathy**.

8.3.8.6 Injection Site

Injection is performed in the posterior distal leg at the level of the lateral malleolus just lateral to the Achilles tendon margin.

8.3.8.7 Imaging/Radiology

Plain film radiographs: These may demonstrate fracture of the posterior malleolus.

Ultrasound: The nerve may demonstrate increased cross-sectional area (Cartwright et al. 2008). Cyst and other mass lesions may be identified. It may also provide guidance for sural nerve block (Redborg et al. 2009).

CT: CT can exclude adjacent bony abnormality or soft tissue mass.

MRI: MRI can correctly visualize the nerve and is superior in evaluating for mass lesions including ganglion cyst. It may also identify soft tissue injury or

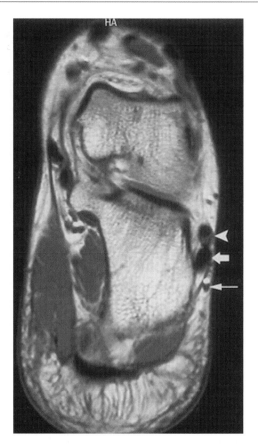

Fig. 8.80 Normal anatomy of the sural nerve. Proximal coronal oblique spin-echo T1-weighted MR image (400/12) shows the sural nerve and vessels (*thin arrow*) near the peroneus brevis (*arrowhead*) and peroneus longus (*thick arrow*) tendons (Delfaut et al. 2003)

compression due to Achilles tendon or peroneal tendon pathology (Delfaut et al. 2003) (Fig. 8.80).

8.3.9 Posterior Tibial Nerve Injection (Tarsal Tunnel) (Fig. 8.81)

8.3.9.1 Anatomy

The posterior tibial nerve (L4-S3) is the most frequently entrapped nerve in the foot and ankle. There may be entrapment of the posterior tibial nerve itself or one of its branches. In proximal tarsal tunnel syndrome, the site of entrapment is in the fibroosseous tunnel behind the medial malleolus. In distal tarsal tunnel syndrome, the site of entrapment is at the distal

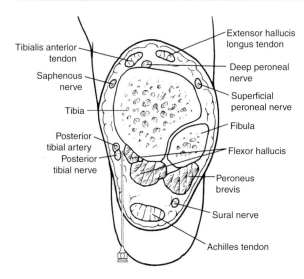

Tibialis anterior tendon

Saphenous nerve

Tibia

Posterior tibial artery

Posterior tibial nerve

Extensor hallucis longus tendon

Deep peroneal nerve

Superficial peroneal nerve

Fibula

Flexor hallucis

Peroneus brevis

Sural nerve

Achilles tendon

Fig. 8.81 Posterior tibial nerve (tarsal tunnel) injection (Weiss 2007w, Fig. 6-29)

branches involving either the medial or lateral plantar nerves. The tarsal tunnel is bounded by the inner aspect of the talus, lower and inner margin of the navicular, the sustentaculum tali, and the medial aspect of the calcaneus. The flexor retinaculum forms the fibrous component of the canal. The posterior tibial nerve itself originates from the sciatic nerve. The nerve travels in the leg below the knee between the two gastrocnemius muscle heads. It then courses in the deep posterior compartment under the soleus muscle. In the proximal leg, it traverses between the posterior tibial and flexor digitorum longus muscles. In the distal leg, it is surrounded by the flexor digitorum longus and flexor hallucis longus. It then courses posterior to the medial malleolus in the tarsal tunnel where it bifurcates into the medial and lateral plantar nerves.

8.3.9.2 Function

At the level of the tarsal tunnel the nerve, prior to its bifurcation, incorporates the innervation of both the medial and lateral plantar nerves. The lateral plantar nerve provides motor function to the quadratus plantae, flexor digiti minimi, adductor hallucis, interossei, three lumbricals, and abductor digiti minimi. The sensory innervation is to the lateral plantar region of the foot and the fifth and lateral half of the fourth digit of the foot. The medial plantar nerve provides motor function to the

first lumbrical, abductor hallucis, flexor digitorum brevis, and flexor hallucis brevis. The sensory innervation is to the medial plantar aspect of the foot and the first three toes as well as the medial half of the fourth toe.

8.3.9.3 Clinical Presentation

Proximal tarsal tunnel syndrome results in widespread pain in the foot. There is burning pain in the plantar foot with paresthesia/numbness. The pain is worse with weightbearing and relieved by rest. It can radiate to the medial leg. The pain is also worsened with dorsiflexion. In distal tarsal tunnel syndrome, there is chronic burning heel pain associated with weightbearing when the lateral plantar nerve is involved. When the medial plantar nerve is involved, there is pain involving the medial aspect of the arch, which radiates to the medial toes. The pain is also associated with weightbearing.

8.3.9.4 Etiology

Tarsal tunnel syndrome can be associated with any form of external compression including ganglion cyst**, traumatic soft tissue or osseous injury**, varicosities**, benign and malignant tumors**, as well as a congenitally narrow tarsal canal**. The nerve can also be compressed by arterial** or muscular variation**. In addition, it can be compressed by nearby tendon pathology**, tarsal coalition**, or arthritis**.

8.3.9.5 Differential Diagnosis

Differential diagnoses include S1 radiculopathy**, peripheral neuropathy complex regional pain syndrome (reflex sympathetic dystrophy)**, plantar fasciitis**, calcaneal bursitis**, tendinopathy**, tenosynovitis**, and peripheral arterial disease**.

8.3.9.6 Injection Site

The injection is performed just posterior to the medial malleolus overlying the posterior tibial nerve 2 cm proximal to the site of pain. Injection is made into the subcutaneous tissue, relatively superficially.

8.3.9.7 Imaging/Radiology

Plain film radiographs: Axial radiographs of the hind-foot can reveal osteophytes, tarsal coalition, and other bone pathology.

CT: This modality is the most accurate at revealing bony pathology.

Ultrasound: Sonography can be useful for depicting the tarsal tunnel structures and evaluating mass lesions.

MRI: MRI can superbly demonstrate the tarsal tunnel on T1- and T2-weighted sequences in the anatomical axial, sagittal, and coronal planes. MRI is excellent at depicting mass lesions and excluding other etiologies in the differential diagnosis (Hochman and Zilberfarb 2004) (Fig. 8.82).

8.3.9.8 Indications

The main indication for injection is tarsal tunnel syndrome** which could be caused by any condition compressing the space of the tarsal tunnel containing the posterior tibial nerve.

8.3.10 Injection of the Interdigital Nerves for Morton's Neuroma (*Fig. 8.83*)

8.3.10.1 Anatomy

Morton's neuroma represents an interdigital enlargement of the interdigital nerve, which travels below and in between the metatarsal heads or toes. The interdigital nerves originate from the medial and lateral plantar nerves. Morton's neuroma usually occurs between the third and fourth metatarsal space, but can also occur at other interspaces. The pathology is due to chronic compression of the interdigital nerve between the transverse intermetatarsal ligament and the plantar aspect of the foot.

8.3.10.2 Function

The interdigital nerve provides sensory innervation of the toes.

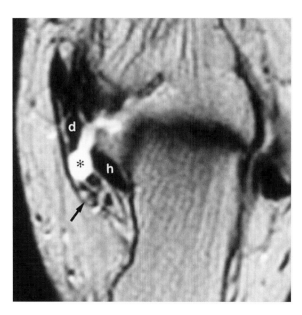

Fig. 8.82 Tarsal tunnel syndrome secondary to ganglion cyst. Axial T2-weighted MR image reveals a ganglion cyst (*asterisk*) interposed between the flexor digitorum longus (*d*) and flexor hallucis longus (*h*) tendons and abutting the adjacent neurovascular bundle (*arrow*) (Rosenberg et al. 2000)

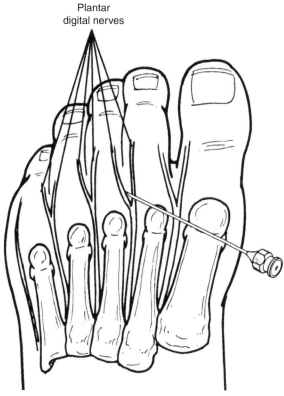

Fig. 8.83 Lower extremity digital nerve injection (Weiss 2007x, Fig. 6-38)

8.3.10.3 Clinical Presentation

Morton's neuroma presents as intermittent, gradually progressive neuropathic pain (burning pain associated with tingling or numbness). There may also be a sensation of a foreign body within the shoe. The Mulder click test is performed by feeling a sudden mass at the plantar foot between the distal metatarsals when they are compressed.

8.3.10.4 Etiology

This pathology is caused by wearing shoes with a narrowed toe box or chronic repetitive trauma from running or racket sports.

8.3.10.5 Differential Diagnosis

Differential diagnoses include stress fracture**, tendon sheath ganglion**, bursitis** involving the metatarsophalangeal joint junction, fibromas**, and tumors**.

8.3.10.6 Injection Site

The needle is placed into the extensor aspect of the foot between adjacent distal metatarsals.

8.3.10.7 Imaging/Radiology

Plain film radiographs: These can help specify the diagnosis by ruling out bone pathology (including fracture) or radiopaque foreign body. The presence of a mass may be indirectly demonstrated through the visualization of a larger than normal gap between the metatarsals.

Ultrasound: Ultrasonography is useful when the diagnosis is not straightforward or unclear. Morton's neuroma is seen on ultrasound as an ovoid hypoechoic structure aligned with a long axis of the metatarsal. This can be seen if it is greater than 5 mm in diameter (Lee et al. 2007). The equivalent of the Mulder click test can assist in the diagnosis during realtime or dynamic imaging. Ultrasound is also useful in excluding bursitis and synovitis; however, it is operator dependent.

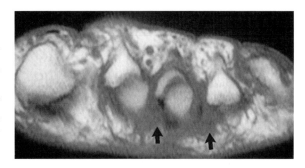

Fig. 8.84 Multiple Morton neuromas. Oblique coronal T1-weighted MR image of the foot demonstrates low-signal-intensity masses in the second and third intermetatarsal spaces (*arrows*) (Rosenberg et al. 2000)

MRI: MRI is usually reserved for atypical clinical presentations as well in the setting of suspected Morton's neuroma. It is the preferred modality by most radiologists in the US. Morton's neuroma presents as an ovoid structure with low signal intensity on T1- and T2-weighted images with variable enhancement on T1-weighted fat-saturated images (Fig. 8.84). It is clinically relevant when larger than 5 mm in diameter. MRI has been shown to affect clinical decision-making and alter treatment plan in a large percentage of patients with suspected Morton's neuroma (Zanetti et al. 1999). Its accuracy has be shown to be greater than 90%.

8.3.10.8 Indications

The chief indication for intervention is Morton neuroma**.

References

Chatha DS, Cunningham PM, Schweitzer ME. MR imaging of the diabetic foot: diagnostic challenges. Radiol Clin North Am. 2005;43(4):747-59

Weiss LD. Easy injections. Philadelphia: Elsevier, 2007a, p. 41

Weiss LD. Easy injections. Philadelphia: Elsevier, 2007b, p. 42

Peterson JJ, Fenton DS, Czervionke LF. Mayo Foundation for Medical Education and Research. Image-guided musculoskeletal intervention. Philadelphia: Saunders/Elsevier, 2008

Manaster BJ. From the RSNA Refresher Courses. Radiological Society of North America. Adult chronic hip pain: radiographic evaluation. Radiographics. 2000;20 Spec No:S3-25

Pourbagher MA, Ozalay M, Pourbagher A. Accuracy and outcome of sonographically guided intra-articular sodium hyaluronate injections in patients with osteoarthritis of the hip. J Ultrasound Med. 2005;24(10):1391-5

Shadbolt CL, Heinze SB, Dietrich RB. Imaging of groin masses: inguinal anatomy and pathologic conditions revisited. Radiographics. 2001;21 Spec No:S261-71

Petersilge CA. From the RSNA Refresher Courses. Radiological Society of North America. Chronic adult hip pain: MR arthrography of the hip. Radiographics. 2000;20 Spec No:S43-52

Schmid MR, Nötzli HP, Zanetti M, Wyss TF, Hodler J. Cartilage lesions in the hip: diagnostic effectiveness of MR arthrography. Radiology. 2003;226(2):382-6

Mauffrey C, Pobbathy. Hip Joint Injection Technique Using Anatomic Landmarks: Are We Accurate? A Prospective Study. Int J Orthop Surg. 2006;3(1). http://www.ispub.com/ostia/index.php?xmlFilePath=journals/ijos/vol3n1/hip.xml

Fluoroscopically guided steroid injection effective in hip osteoarthritis. http://www.medicexchange.com/mall/departmentpage.cfm/MedicExchangeUSA/_81696/2365/departments-contentview

Wisniewski SJ, Grogg B. Femoroacetabular impingement: an overlooked cause of hip pain. Am J Phys Med Rehabil. 2006;85(6):546-9

Crawford JR, Villar RN. Current concepts in the management of femoroacetabular impingement. J Bone Joint Surg Br. 2005; 87(11):1459-62

Liang C, Ma R. Ultrasound-guided intra-articular hylan G-F 20 injection for hip pain due to avascular necrosis: a case report. Arch Phys Med Rehabil. 2008, 89(11):e74-e74

Weiss LD. Easy injections. Philadelphia: Elsevier, 2007c, p. 91

Kong A, Van der Vliet A, Zadow S. MRI and US of gluteal tendinopathy in greater trochanteric pain syndrome. Eur Radiol. 2007;17(7):1772-83. Epub 2006 Dec 6

Pfirrmann CW, Chung CB, Theumann NH, Trudell DJ, Resnick D. Greater trochanter of the hip: attachment of the abductor mechanism and a complex of three bursae–MR imaging and MR bursography in cadavers and MR imaging in asymptomatic volunteers. Radiology. 2001;221(2):469-77

Fang C, Teh J. Imaging of the hip. Imaging. 2003;15:205-16

Cvitanic O, Henzie G, Skezas N, Lyons J, Minter J. MRI diagnosis of tears of the hip abductor tendons (gluteus medius and gluteus minimus). AJR Am J Roentgenol. 2004;182(1): 137-43

Feldman F, Staron RB. MRI of seemingly isolated greater trochanteric fractures. AJR Am J Roentgenol. 2004;183(2):323-9

Jones DL, Erhard RE. Diagnosis of trochanteric bursitis versus femoral neck stress fracture. Phys Ther. 1997;77(1):58-67

Morelli V, Smith V. Groin injuries in athletes. Am Fam Physician. 2001;64(8):1405-14

Adler RS, Buly R, Ambrose R, Sculco T. Diagnostic and therapeutic use of sonography-guided iliopsoas peritendinous injections. AJR Am J Roentgenol. 2005;185(4):940-3

Weiss LD. Easy injections. Philadelphia: Elsevier, 2007d, p. 94

Cho KH, Lee SM, Lee YH, Suh KJ, Kim SM, Shin MJ, Jang HW. Non-infectious ischiogluteal bursitis: MRI findings. Korean J Radiol. 2004;5(4):280-6

Robinson P, Salehi F, Grainger A, Clemence M, Schilders E, O'Connor P, Agur A. Cadaveric and MRI study of the musculotendinous contributions to the capsule of the symphysis pubis. AJR Am J Roentgenol. 2007;188(5):W440-5

O'Connell MJ, Powell T, McCaffrey NM, O'Connell D, Eustace SJ. Symphyseal cleft injection in the diagnosis and treatment of osteitis pubis in athletes. AJR Am J Roentgenol. 2002; 179(4):955-9

Omar IM, Zoga AC, Kavanagh EC, Koulouris G, Bergin D, Gopez AG, Morrison WB, Meyers WC. Athletic pubalgia and "sports hernia": optimal MR imaging technique and findings. Radiographics. 2008;28(5):1415-38

Ross JJ, Hu LT. Septic arthritis of the pubic symphysis: review of 100 cases. Medicine (Baltimore). 2003;82(5):340-5

Weiss LD. Easy injections. Philadelphia: Elsevier, 2007e, p. 45

Weiss LD. Easy injections. Philadelphia: Elsevier, 2007f, p. 46

Mesgarzadeh M, Schneck CD, Bonakdarpour A. Magnetic resonance imaging of the knee and correlation with normal anatomy. Radiographics. 1988;8(4):707-33

Jacobson JA, Girish G, Jiang Y, Sabb BJ. Radiographic evaluation of arthritis: degenerative joint disease and variations. Radiology. 2008;248(3):737-47

Calmbach WL, Hutchens M. Evaluation of patients presenting with knee pain: part II. Differential diagnosis. Am Fam Physician. 2003a;68(5):917-22

Zuber TJ. Knee joint aspiration and injection. Am Fam Physician. 2002;66(8):1497-500; 1503-4; 1507

Calmbach WL, Hutchens M. Evaluation of patients presenting with knee pain: part I. History, physical examination, radiographs, and laboratory tests. Am Fam Physician. 2003b; 68(5):907-12

Weiss LD. Easy injections. Philadelphia: Elsevier, 2007g, p. 81

Haims AH, Medvecky MJ, Pavlovich R Jr, Katz LD. MR imaging of the anatomy of and injuries to the lateral and posterolateral aspects of the knee. AJR Am J Roentgenol. 2003; 180(3):647-53

Khaund R, Flynn SH. Iliotibial band syndrome: a common source of knee pain. Am Fam Physician. 2005;71(8):1545-50. Review

Weiss LD. Easy injections. Philadelphia: Elsevier, 2007h, p. 98

Lee P, Hunter TB, Taljanovic M. Musculoskeletal colloquialisms: how did we come up with these names? Radiographics. 2004;24(4):1009-27

Weiss LD. Easy injections. Philadelphia: Elsevier, 2007i, p. 83

Stacy GS, Dixon LB. Pitfalls in MR image interpretation prompting referrals to an orthopedic oncology clinic. Radiographics. 2007;27(3):805-26; discussion 827-8

Ward EE, Jacobson JA, Fessell DP, Hayes CW, van Holsbeeck M. Sonographic detection of Baker's cysts: comparison with MR imaging. AJR Am J Roentgenol. 2001;176(2):373-80

Weiss LD. Easy injections. Philadelphia: Elsevier, 2007j, p. 96

Unlu Z, Ozmen B, Tarhan S, Boyvoda S, Goktan C. Ultrasonographic evaluation ofpes anserinus tendino-bursitis in patients with type 2 diabetes mellitus. J Rheumatol. 2003; 30(2):352-4

Beaman FD, Peterson JJ. MR imaging of cysts, ganglia, and bursae about the knee. Radiol Clin North Am. 2007;45(6):969-82; vi

Janzen DL, Peterfy CG, Forbes JR, Tirman PF, Genant HK. Cystic lesions around the knee joint: MR imaging findings. AJR Am J Roentgenol. 1994;163(1):155-61

Weiss LD. Easy injections. Philadelphia: Elsevier, 2007k, p. 48

Robinson P, White LM. Soft-tissue and osseous impingement syndromes of the ankle: role of imaging in diagnosis and management. Radiographics. 2002;22(6):1457-69; discussion 1470-1

Weiss LD. Easy injections. Philadelphia: Elsevier, 2007l, p. 78

Schweitzer ME, Karasick D. MR imaging of disorders of the Achilles tendon. AJR Am J Roentgenol. 2000;175(3):613-25

Cheung Y, Rosenberg ZS, Magee T, Chinitz L. Normal anatomy and pathologic conditions of ankle tendons: current imaging techniques. Radiographics. 1992;12(3):429-44

Ryan M, Wong A, Taunton J. Favorable outcomes after sonographically guided intratendinous injection of hyperosmolar dextrose for chronic insertional and midportion achilles tendinosis. AJR Am J Roentgenol. 2010;194(4):1047-53

Weiss LD. Easy injections. Philadelphia: Elsevier, 2007m, p. 53

Weiss LD. Easy injections. Philadelphia: Elsevier, 2007n, p. 51

Frey C, Feder KS, DiGiovanni C. Arthroscopic evaluation of the subtalar joint: does sinus tarsi syndrome exist? Foot Ankle Int. 1999;20(3):185-91

Lee KB, Bai LB, Park JG, Song EK, Lee JJ. Efficacy of MRI versus arthroscopy for evaluation of sinus tarsi syndrome. Foot Ankle Int. 2008;29(11):1111-6

Lektrakul N, Chung CB, Lai Ym, Theodorou DJ, Yu J, Haghighi P, Trudell D, Resnick D. Tarsal sinus: arthrographic, MR imaging, MR arthrographic, and pathologic findings in cadavers and retrospective study data in patients with sinus tarsi syndrome. Radiology. 2001;219(3):802-10

Rosenberg ZS, Beltran J, Bencardino JT. From the RSNA Refresher Courses. Radiological Society of North America. MR imaging of the ankle and foot. Radiographics. 2000;20 Spec No:S153-79

Weiss LD. Easy injections. Philadelphia: Elsevier, 2007o, p. 75

Zhu F, Johnson JE, Hirose CB, Bae KT. Chronic plantar fasciitis: acute changes in the heel after extracorporeal high-energy shock wave therapy–observations at MR imaging. Radiology. 2005;234(1):206-10. Epub 2004 Nov 24

Weiss LD. Easy injections. Philadelphia: Elsevier, 2007p, p. 56

Szkudlarek M, Narvestad E, Klarlund M, Court-Payen M, Thomsen HS, Østergaard M. Ultrasonography of the metatarsophalangeal joints in rheumatoid arthritis: comparison with magnetic resonance imaging, conventional radiography, and clinical examination. Arthritis Rheum. 2004;50(7):2103-12

Thiele RG, Schlesinger N. Diagnosis of gout by ultrasound. Rheumatology (Oxford). 2007;46(7):1116-21. Epub 2007 Apr 27

Dalbeth N, McQueen FM. Use of imaging to evaluate gout and other crystal deposition disorders. Curr Opin Rheumatol. 2009;21(2):124-31

Weiss LD. Easy injections. Philadelphia: Elsevier, 2007q, p. 136

Akkaya T, Ozturk E, Comert A, Ates Y, Gumus H, Ozturk H, Tekdemir I, Elhan A. Ultrasound-guided obturator nerve block: a sonoanatomic study of a new methodologic approach. Anesth Analg. 2009;108(3):1037-41

Marhofer P, Nasel C, Sitzwohl C, Kapral S. Magnetic resonance imaging of the distribution of local anesthetic during the three-in-one block. Anesth Analg. 2000;90(1):119-24

Yukata K, Arai K, Yoshizumi Y, Tamano K, Imada K, Nakaima N. Obturator neuropathy caused by an acetabular labral cyst: MRI findings. AJR Am J Roentgenol. 2005;184(3 Suppl):S112-4

Weiss LD. Easy injections. Philadelphia: Elsevier, 2007r, p. 138

Gruber H, Peer S, Kovacs P, Marth R, Bodner G. The ultrasonographic appearance of the femoral nerve and cases of iatrogenic impairment. J Ultrasound Med. 2003;22(2):163-72

Trerotola SO, Kuhlman JE, Fishman EK. CT and anatomic study of postcatheterization hematomas. Radiographics. 1991;11(2):247-58

Weiss JM, Tolo V. Femoral nerve palsy following iliacus hematoma. Orthopedics. 2008;31(2):178

Weiss LD. Easy injections. Philadelphia: Elsevier, 2007s, p. 141

Raj PP, Lou L, Erdine S et al. Radiographic Imaging for Regional Anesthesia and Pain Management ISBN 0-443-06596-9

Tsui BC, Ozelsel T. Ultrasound-guided transsartorial perifemoral artery approach for saphenous nerve block. Reg Anesth Pain Med. 2009;34(2):177-8; author reply 178

Murphey MD, Smith WS, Smith SE, Kransdorf MJ, Temple HT. From the archives of the AFIP. Imaging of musculoskeletal neurogenic tumors: radiologic-pathologic correlation. Radiographics. 1999;19(5):1253-80

Martinoli C, Bianchi S, Gandolfo N, Valle M, Simonetti S, Derchi LE. US of nerve entrapments in osteofibrous tunnels of the upper and lower limbs. Radiographics. 2000;20 Spec No:S199-213; discussion S213-7. Erratum in: Radiographics 2000;20(6):1818

Hochman MG et al. Nerves in a pinch: imaging of nerve compression syndromes. Radiol Clin N Am. 2004;42:221-45

Weiss LD. Easy injections. Philadelphia: Elsevier, 2007t, p. 149

Canella C, Demondion X, Guillin R, Boutry N, Peltier J, Cotten A. Anatomicstudy of the superficial peroneal nerve using sonography. AJR Am J Roentgenol. 2009;193(1):174-9

Delfaut EM, Demondion X, Bieganski A, Thiron MC, Mestdagh H, Cotten A. Imaging of foot and ankle nerve entrapment syndromes: from well-demonstrated to unfamiliar sites. Radiographics. 2003;23(3):613-23

Weiss LD. Easy injections. Philadelphia: Elsevier, 2007u, p. 147

Weiss LD. Easy injections. Philadelphia: Elsevier, 2007v, p. 152

Cartwright MS, Passmore LV, Yoon JS, Brown ME, Caress JB, Walker FO. Cross-sectional area reference values for nerve ultrasonography. Muscle Nerve. 2008;37(5):566-71

Redborg KE, Sites BD, Chinn CD, Gallagher JD, Ball PA, Antonakakis JG, Beach ML. Ultrasound improves the success rate of a sural nerve block at the ankle. Reg Anesth Pain Med. 2009;34(1):24-8

Weiss LD. Easy injections. Philadelphia: Elsevier, 2007w, p. 144

Hochman MG, Zilberfarb JL. Nerves in a pinch: imaging of nerve compression syndromes. Radiol Clin North Am. 2004;42(1):221-45

Weiss LD. Easy injections. Philadelphia: Elsevier, 2007x, p. 154

Lee MJ, Kim S, Huh YM, Song HT, Lee SA, Lee JW, Suh JS. Morton neuroma: evaluated with ultrasonography and MR imaging. Korean J Radiol. 2007;8(2):148-55

Zanetti M, Strehle JK, Kundert HP, Zollinger H, Hodler J. Morton neuroma: effect of MR imaging findings on diagnostic thinking and therapeutic decisions. Radiology. 1999;213(2):583-8

Index

Printing and Binding: Stürtz GmbH, Würzburg